Genetic Disorders Sourcebook,
1st Edition

Genetic Disorders Sourcebook,
2nd Edition

Head Trauma Sourcebook

Headache Sourcebook

Health Insurance Sourcebook

Health Reference Series Cumulative
Index 1999

Healthy Aging Sourcebook

Healthy Heart Sourcebook for Women

Heart Diseases & Disorders
Sourcebook, 2nd Edition

Household Safety Sourcebook

Immune System Disorders Sourcebook

Infant & Toddler Health Sourcebook

Injury & Trauma Sourcebook

Kidney & Urinary Tract Diseases &
Disorders Sourcebook

Learning Disabilities Sourcebook

Liver Disorders Sourcebook

Lung Disorders Sourcebook

Medical Tests Sourcebook

Men's Health Concerns Sourcebook

Mental Health Disorders Sourcebook,
1st Edition

Mental Health Disorders Sourcebook,
2nd Edition

Mental Retardation Sourcebook

Obesity Sourcebook

Ophthalmic Disorders Sourcebook

Oral Health Sourcebook

Osteoporosis Sourcebook

Pain Sourcebook, 1st Edition

Pain Sourcebook, 2nd Edition

Pediatric Cancer Sourcebook

Physical & Mental Issues in Aging
Sourcebook

Podiatry Sourcebook

Pregnancy & Birth Sourcebook

Prostate Cancer

Public Health Sourcebook

Reconstructive & Cosmetic Surgery
Sourcebook

Rehabilitation Sourcebook

Respiratory Diseases & Disorders
Sourcebook

Sexually Transmitted Diseases
Sourcebook, 1st Edition

Sexually Transmitted Diseases
Sourcebook, 2nd Edition

Skin Disorders Sourcebook

Sleep Disorders Sourcebook

Sports Injuries Sourcebook

Stress-Related Disorders Sourcebook

Substance Abuse Sourcebook

Surgery Sourcebook

Transplantation Sourcebook

Traveler's Health Sourcebook

Women's Health Concerns Sourcebook

Workplace Health & Safety Sourcebook

Worldwide Health Sourcebook

Teen Health Series

Diet Information for Teens

Drug Information for Teens

Mental Health Information
for Teens

Sexual Health Information
for Teens

Lung
Disorders
SOURCEBOOK

Health Reference Series

First Edition

Lung Disorders SOURCEBOOK

Basic Consumer Health Information about Emphysema, Pneumonia, Tuberculosis, Asthma, Cystic Fibrosis, and Other Lung Disorders, Including Facts about Diagnostic Procedures, Treatment Strategies, Disease Prevention Efforts, and Such Risk Factors as Smoking, Air Pollution, and Exposure to Asbestos, Radon, and Other Agents

Along with a Glossary and Resources for Additional Help and Information

Edited by
Dawn D. Matthews

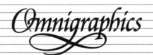

615 Griswold Street • Detroit, MI 48226

Bibliographic Note

Because this page cannot legibly accommodate all the copyright notices, the Bibliographic Note portion of the Preface constitutes an extension of the copyright notice.

Edited by Dawn D. Matthews

Health Reference Series

Karen Bellenir, *Managing Editor*
David A. Cooke, MD, *Medical Consultant*
Elizabeth Barbour, *Permissions Associate*
Dawn Matthews, *Verification Assistant*
Carol Munson, *Permissions Assistant*
Laura Pleva, *Index Editor*
EdIndex, Services for Publishers, *Indexers*

* * *

Omnigraphics, Inc.

Matthew P. Barbour, *Senior Vice President*
Kay Gill, *Vice President—Directories*
Kevin Hayes, *Operations Manager*
David P. Bianco, *Marketing Consultant*

* * *

Peter E. Ruffner, *President and Publisher*

Frederick G. Ruffner, Jr., *Chairman*

Copyright © 2002 Omnigraphics, Inc.

ISBN 0-7808-0339-6

Library of Congress Cataloging-in-Publication Data

Lung disorders sourcebook : basic consumer health information about emphysema, pneumonia, tuberculosis, asthma, cystic fibrosis, and other lung disorders, including facts about diagnostic procedures, treatment strategies, disease prevention efforts, and such risk factors as smoking, air pollution, and exposure to asbestos, radon, and other agents; along with a glossary and resources for additional help and information / edited by Dawn D. Matthews.-- 1st ed.
    p. cm. -- (Health reference series)
  ISBN 0-7808-0339-6
    1. Lungs--Diseases--Popular works. I. Matthews, Dawn D. II. Health reference series
  (Unnumbered)

RC736 .L864 2002
616.2'4--dc21

                                                                          2002016976

Printed in the United States

Table of Contents

Part III: Diagnosis

Part IV: Treatment

Part V: Risks and Prevention

Part VI: Additional Help and Information

Preface

About This Book

Lung disease is responsible for one in seven deaths in the United States. Additionally, an estimated 25 million Americans live with chronic lung conditions. Medical problems at birth or during infancy and childhood can affect lung development. Later in life, the lungs may be damaged by smoking, allergies, contact with hazardous substances, or accidents. These problems, along with the effects of bacteria and viruses, can result in a wide variety of respiratory diseases and disorders, including asthma, bronchitis, chronic obstructive pulmonary disease (COPD), emphysema, influenza, lung cancer, pneumonia, and tuberculosis (TB).

The *Lung Disorders Sourcebook* offers information about the various types of lung disorders and diagnosis, treatment, and prevention issues. It provides information about risks in the home and workplace and offers advice for preventing lung disorders that are acquired by asbestos, radon, and other environmental exposures. Explanations of the medical tests used to diagnose lung disorders are included, as well as information on the proper use of nebulizers, inhalers, and medicines commonly used to treat lung disorders. A glossary and directories of resources for further help and information are also provided.

How to Use This Book

This book is divided into parts and chapters. Parts focus on broad areas of interest. Chapters are devoted to single topics within a part.

Part I: Introduction provides facts about lung structure and function. It discusses environmental effects on lung disease, the origins of lung disease, and who is most at risk.

Part II: Types of Lung Disorders gives helpful information about many types of lung disorders, including asthma, cystic fibrosis, primary pulmonary hypertension (PPH), tuberculosis, and numerous other lung disorders and conditions.

Part III: Diagnosis describes the various tests used to diagnose lung disorders. These include x-rays, lung scans, pulmonary function tests, arterial blood gas testing, and others.

Part IV: Treatment provides facts about the different methods of treating lung disorders, including information on medications, inhalers, oxygen therapy, and surgical procedures.

Part V: Risks and Prevention offers information about the risks of cigarette smoking, indoor air pollution, and occupational hazards. It also provides information about preventing lung disorders.

Part VI: Additional Help and Information includes a glossary of related terms and directories of resources for additional information on some of the most common types of lung disorders.

Bibliographic Note

This volume contains documents and excerpts from publications issued by the following government agencies: Centers for Disease Control and Prevention (CDC), Department of Health and Human Services (DHHS); Environmental Protection Agency (EPA); Food and Drug Administration (FDA); National Cancer Institute (NCI); National Institute for Occupational Safety and Health (NIOSH); National Institute of Child Health and Human Development (NICHD); National Institute of Environmental Health Sciences (NIEHS); National Institute on Aging (NIA); National Institutes of Health (NIH); National Heart, Lung, and Blood Institute (NHLBI); and Occupational Safety and Health Association (OSHA).

In addition, this volume contains copyrighted articles from the American Academy of Family Physicians; the American Lung Association; DrKoop.Com, Inc.; the Endocrine Society; Jefferson Health System; Loyola University Health System; the Mayo Foundation; the Methodist Health Care System; Micromedex Thomson Healthcare; the

National Jewish Medical and Research Center; Medscape Inc.; Patricia Wrean and Marie Goldenberg; Sir Charles Gairdner Hospital; and the Yale University School of Medicine.

Full citation information is provided on the first page of each chapter. Every effort has been made to secure all necessary rights to reprint the copyrighted material. If any omissions have been made, please contact Omnigraphics to make corrections for future editions.

Acknowledgements

Thanks go to Karen Bellenir, Liz Barbour, and Carol Munson for their help with the many details involved in the production of this book.

Note from the Editor

This book is part of Omnigraphics' *Health Reference Series*. The series provides basic information about a broad range of medical concerns. It is not intended to serve as a tool for diagnosing illness, in prescribing treatments, or as a substitute for the physician/patient relationship. All persons concerned about medical symptoms or the possibility of disease are encouraged to seek professional care from an appropriate health care provider.

Our Advisory Board

The *Health Reference Series* is reviewed by an Advisory Board comprised of librarians from public, academic, and medical libraries. We would like to thank the following board members for providing guidance to the development of this series:

Dr. Lynda Baker, Associate Professor of Library and Information Science, Wayne State University, Detroit, MI

Nancy Bulgarelli, William Beaumont Hospital Library, Royal Oak, MI

Karen Imarisio, Bloomfield Township Public Library, Bloomfield Township, MI

Karen Morgan, Mardigian Library, University of Michigan-Dearborn, Dearborn, MI

Rosemary Orlando, St. Clair Shores Public Library, St. Clair Shores, MI

Medical Consultant

Medical consultation services are provided to the *Health Reference Series* editors by David A. Cooke, MD. Dr. Cooke is a graduate of Brandeis University, and he received his M.D. degree from the University of Michigan. He completed residency training at the University of Wisconsin Hospital and Clinics. He is board-certified in Internal Medicine. Dr. Cooke currently works as part of the University of Michigan Health System and practices in Brighton, MI. In his free time, he enjoys writing, science fiction, and spending time with his family.

Health Reference Series *Update Policy*

The inaugural book in the *Health Reference Series* was the first edition of *Cancer Sourcebook* published in 1992. Since then, the Series has been enthusiastically received by librarians and in the medical community. In order to maintain the standard of providing high-quality health information for the layperson, the editorial staff at Omnigraphics felt it was necessary to implement a policy of updating volumes when warranted.

Medical researchers have been making tremendous strides, and it is the purpose of the *Health Reference Series* to stay current with the most recent advances. Each decision to update a volume will be made on an individual basis. Some of the considerations will include how much new information is available and the feedback we receive from people who use the books. If there is a topic you would like to see added to the update list, or an area of medical concern you feel has not been adequately addressed, please write to:

Editor
Health Reference Series
Omnigraphics, Inc.
615 Griswold
Detroit, MI 48226

The commitment to providing on-going coverage of important medical developments has also led to some format changes in the *Health Reference Series*. Each new volume on a topic is individually titled and called a "First Edition." Subsequent updates will carry sequential edition numbers. To help avoid confusion and to provide maximum flexibility in our ability to respond to informational needs, the practice of consecutively numbering each volume has been discontinued.

Part One

Introduction

Chapter 1

The Lungs: A Historical View

Introduction

Breathing for most of us is something we do without being aware
of it. We pay no attention to this continuous activity as we work, play,
or sleep. Our lungs are responsible for this essential natural function
that gets oxygen into the bloodstream so that it can be delivered to
the cells of our body.

During a normal day, we breathe nearly 25,000 times. The more than
10,000 liters of air we inhale is mostly oxygen and nitrogen. In addition,
there are small amounts of other gases, floating bacteria, and viruses.
It also contains the products of tobacco smoke, automobile exhaust, and
other pollutants from the atmosphere in varying amounts.

Air pollutants can affect our lungs in many ways. They may simply cause irritation and discomfort. But sometimes inhaled materials can cause illness or death. The lungs have a series of built-in
mechanical and biological barriers that keep harmful materials from
entering the body. In addition, specific defense mechanisms can inactivate some disease-causing materials.

However, sometimes the normal lung defenses and barriers in the
lungs do not work as well as they should. Medical problems at birth or
during infancy and growth can affect lung development. Later in life the
lungs may be damaged by smoking, occupational exposures, or accidents.
These abnormalities allow air pollutants to break through the lung's
defenses. The result can be respiratory problems or diseases.

Excerpted from "The Lungs in Health and Disease," National Heart, Lung,
and Blood Institute (NHLBI), NIH Publication Number 97-3279, 1997.

A Historical View

Nearly 2,000 years ago, Claudius Galen, a Greek physician, wrote that the lung was an instrument of voice and respiration. He thought that the purpose of respiration was to cool the heart by "the substance of the air." His concept was that breathing in (inspiration) supplied a cooling substance to the heart while breathing out (expiration) removed hot material from it.

At the end of the 16th century, a Dutch scientist, Fabricius, expressed the view that the function of the lungs was to prepare air for the heart.

Until the middle of the 17th century, the lungs were thought to be a solid, compact, fleshy mass. At that time Marcello Malpighi, an Italian anatomist, and Thomas Willis, an English clinician, noted independently that the lungs were a system of canals made up of membranes, air passages, and blood vessels.

Many of the currently used terms for the components of the lung such as lobules, alveoli, arteries, and veins come from these authors. In 1628, William Harvey, a British physician and physiologist, described his theory of circulation and proposed that the blood was pumped through the lungs by the expansion and contraction of the lungs during breathing.

Our knowledge about the lungs has come a long way during the more than 300 years since Malpighi, Willis, and Harvey. Today we know that the lungs are a pair of cone-shaped, soft, spongy, pinkish, organs. They get oxygen into the blood and remove carbon dioxide, a waste-product of the body. We have also learned that a major function of the lungs is to protect the body from potentially harmful airborne agents and toxic chemicals that our body may produce.

We now know that the lungs have both "respiratory" and "nonrespiratory" functions. The respiratory function of the lungs is "gas exchange." This is the term for the transfer of oxygen from the air into the blood and the removal of carbon dioxide from the blood.

The nonrespiratory functions of the lungs are mechanical, biochemical, and physiological. The lungs provide the first line of defense against airborne irritants and bacterial, viral, and other infectious agents. They also remove volatile substances and particles of matter generated within the body. The lungs control the flow of water, ions, and large proteins across its various cellular structures. Together with the liver, they remove various products of the body's metabolic reactions. The lungs also manufacture a variety of essential hormones and other chemicals that have precise biological roles.

4

Chapter 2

Lung Structure and Function

The lungs are shaped like cones and textured like a fine grained sponge that can be inflated with air. They sit within the thoracic cage where they stretch from the trachea (windpipe) to below the heart. About 10 percent of the lung is solid tissue, the remainder is filled with air and blood.

This unique structure of the lung is delicate enough for gas exchange and yet strong enough to maintain its shape and enable it to perform the many functions vital for keeping us healthy. Two "plumbing" systems, the airways for ventilation (exchange of air between the lungs and the atmosphere) and the circulatory system for perfusion (blood flow), are coordinated by special muscles and nerves. This arrangement enables the lung to perform its primary function of rapidly exchanging oxygen from inhaled air with the carbon dioxide from the blood.

Air enters the body through the nose or the mouth, and travels down the throat and trachea into the chest through a pair of air tubes called bronchi (plural for bronchus). The bronchi divide and subdivide into successive generations of narrower and shorter branching tubes of unequal length and diameter. The final destination for inhaled air is the network of about 3 million air sacs, called alveoli, located at the ends of the lungs' air passages. Between the trachea and alveoli, the lungs look like an inverted tree.

The first (main) branching of the trachea leads to the left and right lungs. The two lungs fill most of the chest cavity. Between the lungs

Excerpted from "The Lungs in Health and Disease," National Heart, Lung, and Blood Institute (NHLBI), NIH Publication Number 97-3279, 1997.

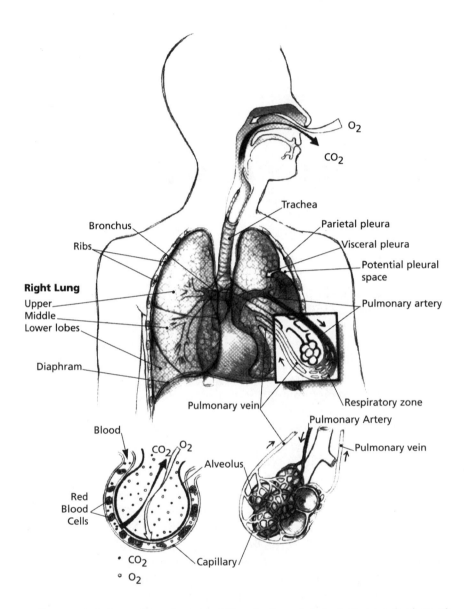

Figure 2.1. Lung Structure and Respiration. Inhaled air travels through the airways to the alveoli. Blood is pumped out of the heart through the pulmonary arteries to a network of capillaries that surround the alveoli. The oxygen of the inhaled air diffuses out of the alveoli into the bood while carbon dioxide in the blood moves into the alveoli to be exhaled. The oxygen-rich blood is returned to the heart through the pulmonary veins.

are located the heart, the major blood vessels, the trachea, the esophagus (tube leading from the throat to the stomach), and lymph nodes. The thorax (chest wall) surrounds and supports the lungs.

Movement of the air into the lungs is controlled by the respiratory muscles of the thorax. These muscles, collectively called the ventilatory apparatus, include the diaphragm (the muscle that separates the chest and abdominal contents) and the muscles that move the ribs. When the respiratory muscles contract, the chest enlarges like a bellows sucking in air (inhalation). As air fills the lungs they expand automatically. The lungs return to their original (resting) size when we exhale. The performance of the ventilatory apparatus is coordinated by specific nerve sites, called respiratory centers, located in the brain and the neck.

The respiratory centers respond to changes in oxygen, carbon dioxide, and acid levels in the blood. Normal concentrations of these chemicals in arterial blood are maintained by changing the breathing rate.

The right lung is slightly larger than the left lung and is divided into three sections or lobes; the left lung has only two lobes. Each lobe is subdivided into two to five bronchopulmonary segments. The segments are further subdivided into lobules served by smaller branches of the bronchi.

The outside of the lung and the inside of the chest cavity are lined by a single continuous membrane called the pleura. The portion of the pleura surrounding the lungs is called the visceral pleura, while the portion lining the chest cavity is called the parietal pleura. The potential space between the lungs and the inside of the chest cavity is called the pleural space or pleural cavity. The pleural space is moistened with a fluid that lubricates the pleurae as they slide back and forth on each other during ventilation. Normally the pleural space contains only a small amount of fluid and is free of any gas, blood, or other matter.

Blood vessels, bronchi, and nerves come together at the entrance of the lung called the hilum. Bronchopulmonary lymph nodes, important for the drainage of the lungs, are located here. The extensive nervous system of the lungs extends from the hilum to almost all of the lungs' structural units.

The Conducting Airways

The first 16 subdivisions of the bronchi ending in terminal bronchioles are called the conducting airways. Terminal bronchioles are the smallest airways without alveoli. They further divide into respiratory bronchioles, ending in alveolar ducts. Respiratory bronchioles have occasional alveoli budding from their walls, while alveolar ducts are completely lined with alveoli. The last seven branchings of the bronchioles where gas exchange occurs are called the respiratory zone. The terminal respiratory unit of the lung from the respiratory bronchiole to the alveolus is called the acinus.

Gas Exchange

Gas exchange between inhaled air and blood takes place in the alveoli. Blood is brought to the alveoli through a fine network of pulmonary capillaries where it is spread in a thin film. The barrier separating the air and blood is extremely thin, 50 times thinner than a sheet of tissue paper. A large surface area (80 square meters, as large as a tennis court) is available for gas exchange. In the resting state, it takes just about a minute for the total blood volume of the body (about 5 liters) to pass through the lungs. It takes a red cell a fraction of a second to pass through the capillary network. Gas exchange occurs almost instantaneously during this short period.

The Lung of the Unborn Baby (Fetus)

Most of the respiratory needs of the fetus are provided by the mother. The fetal lung is filled with amniotic fluid and has none of the gas exchange function that it will have after birth. It is thus different from the fetal heart, kidneys, and liver, all of which begin their lifelong functions early in fetal life and increase their capabilities as the baby grows in its mother's womb.

The main functions of the fetal lung are to produce amniotic fluid and a material called surfactant that reduces the surface tension of the fluids that line the bronchioles and alveoli. Surfactant is necessary to clear liquid from the fetal lungs so that they can fill with air when the baby begins to breathe immediately after birth. Along with the first breath, a variety of circulatory and respiratory changes begin. These changes are necessary for the baby to live outside its mother's womb.

Surfactant production must continue after birth, since it maintains the mechanical stability of alveoli and prevents their collapse. Lack or deficiency of surfactant in infants causes Respiratory Distress Syndrome (RDS), a disease in which it becomes harder and harder for the baby to breathe. Lack of surfactant is also a factor in adult lung disease.

Cellular and Molecular Aspects

At the cellular and molecular level, the components of the lung are maintained by a unique arrangement of diverse structural proteins and cellular elements. This includes some 40 different types of cells, glands, muscles, and molecules, strategically arranged in intricate but orderly patterns in various parts of the lung. The controlled complexity of the various parts of the lungs facilitates their many functions.

Oxygen-poor blood is pumped from the right ventricle of the heart through a system of pulmonary arteries, arterioles, and capillaries to the alveoli, and the oxygen-rich blood is returned to the left heart through a collecting system of venules and veins. This extensive system, called the pulmonary circulation, filters clots, fat particles, and cellular debris from the bloodstream. It also moves liquid and large and small molecules across the pulmonary blood vessels, providing oxygen and nutrients, and facilitating various metabolic functions of the lung including the synthesis of substances such as surfactant.

The lungs also have a second blood supply from the bronchial circulation. The purpose of this blood supply is to provide nutrients especially for the large airways. Bronchial circulation represents only a small portion (1-2 percent) of the cardiac output. In this system, bronchial arteries bring oxygenated blood from the left side of the heart to the airways (bronchi, bronchioles) and the supporting structures (connective tissue) of the lung. Bronchial venous blood is returned, just like the venous blood from the rest of the body, to the right atrium.

Bronchial circulation is believed to be more important in the fetal lung than in the adult lung. Conducting airways receive their blood supply from branches of bronchial arteries, while the terminal respiratory units receive blood from branches of the pulmonary arteries.

Gas exchange occurs by diffusion of gases across the alveolar membranes into and out of the blood as it flows through the capillaries. Oxygen-poor blood discards its carbon dioxide into the alveoli, and hemoglobin, an oxygen-carrying protein in the red blood cells, binds with oxygen from inhaled air (becomes "arterialized"). Although the red blood cells are exposed to alveolar air only for a fraction of a second, gas exchange between alveoli and capillaries takes place very efficiently because there is an extremely large surface area between the blood and the air.

The bronchi contain specialized connective tissue (cartilage), while bronchioles are noncartilaginous. The bronchi mostly serve nonrespiratory roles such as ridding the airways of irritating particles;

their only respiratory function is to carry air from the external environment to the distal sites of gas exchange.

The arteries and capillaries that bring blood to the alveoli are lined with a layer of delicate specialized cells called endothelial cells. The air-blood barrier is composed of three tissue layers—an endothelium lining the capillaries; an epithelium lining the airspaces; and, between them, an interstitial layer composed of connective tissue, interstitial extracellular matrix, and mesenchymal cells. The interstitial layer also contains special cells—alveolar macrophages, lymphocytes, and inflammatory cells—that can defend or injure the lungs, depending on the situation. Dispersed throughout the interstitium are proteins, lipids, carbohydrates, and other substances derived from plasma and cells.

The endothelium acts as a barrier retarding the passage of fluid, proteins, and other blood components from the vessel lumen into the interstitium and air spaces of the lung. In addition, the endothelial cells perform many of the nonrespiratory functions of the lung, particularly the transformation of a variety of bioactive substances.

The walls of the conducting airways are mostly composed of epithelial lining, connective tissue elements, and a smooth muscle sleeve. The exact proportion of these constituents varies depending on whether the walls are in the large bronchi, the bronchioles, or the alveoli. The epithelium also contains unique mixtures of cells with distinct functions. These functions vary depending on the level of the airway at which the cells are located.

The lungs' first line of defense against injury from inhaled agents is a mix of anatomic barriers, nonspecific mechanical and cellular defenses, antimicrobial secretions, and circulating and resident scavenger (phagocytic) cells that engulf or digest particulates. Removal of particles from the conducting airways (nose to respiratory bronchioles) is carried out by "mucociliary clearance," helped by airway secretions. A film of mucus produced in the lungs envelops the particles which are then continuously moved by the rhythmic beating motions of cilia (hair-like structures that extend from the surface of the cells) to the oropharynx where they are swallowed or coughed out. These defenses are present at birth.

Operating beyond the nonspecific defenses, are specific acquired immune mechanisms that are latent until activated by natural (maternal transfer or infections) or artificial exposures (vaccinations) to foreign materials. These highly specific defenses of the lung are initiated by complex interactions between foreign substances (antigens) and specialized cells. These interactions result in antibody-mediated or cell-mediated immunities that provide uniquely specific defenses against certain organisms or agents.

Research supported by the National Heart, Lung, and Blood Institute is generating new knowledge on previously unrecognized physiological and metabolic processes and mediators operating in the lung. Scientists now realize that the lung, an organ once thought to be merely an inert balloon serving as a receptacle for air, is in reality a powerhouse of concerted and interrelated mechanical, physiological, neurological, immunological, pharmacological, and metabolic functions necessary to sustain life.

Chapter 3

The Environment and Lung Disease

How well or how poorly our lungs perform, and whether or not we are able to maintain our overall health, depends, in great part, on the quality of the air we breathe. Exposure to any one of a number of forms of indoor or outdoor air pollution adds up to a wide range of health risks for many populations.

Environmental Justice: A Critical Issue for Minority Communities

While air pollution is a health risk faced by all Americans, health advocates and experts are aware that poor and ethnic communities carry the burden of the greatest risk. A 1990 report of the U. S. Environmental Protection Agency (EPA) Environmental Equity Workgroup stated that, "Racial minority and low-income populations experience higher than average exposures to selected air pollutants, hazardous waste facilities, contaminated fish, and agricultural pesticides in the workplace."

Industrial and electricity generating facilities, for example, are major sources of harmful air pollution. Studies show that these facilities are disproportionately concentrated in counties with high percentages of minorities. Of all the U.S. counties considered urban, only 12 percent had minority populations of greater than 31 percent. However, these areas contain 21 percent of the 3,000 major air-polluting facilities in the nation.

13

Data also indicate that people of color are disproportionately represented in nonattainment areas (districts failing to meet national standards for clean air).* While information is unavailable for all communities, Table 3.1 gives some idea of levels of exposure to particularly dangerous pollutants.

Table 3.1. Percent Minorities Living in Highly Polluted Areas

Pollutant	Whites	Blacks	Hispanics
Particulates	14.7	16.5	34.0
Carbon Monoxide	33.6	46.0	57.1
Ozone	52.5	62.2	71.2
Lead	6.0	9.2	18.5

Source: EPA, Environmental Equity: Reducing the Risks for All Communities, June 1993, Vol. 1.

In addition, while 33 percent of Whites were found to live in areas that exceeded federal health standards for two or more pollutants, 50 percent of Blacks and 60 percent of Hispanics lived in these areas. Even greater differences were found for areas that violate air quality standards for three and four pollutants. Environmental risks for Hispanic children also include labor-related factors. In interviews conducted with Mexican American farm-worker youths in New York State, for example, 48% reported having worked in fields with pesticides and 36% reported being sprayed with pesticides either directly or by drift while working in fields or orchards.

Indoor Air Pollution

Elements within our homes and workplace have been recognized as a threat to respiratory health. The major culprits are:

- **Environmental tobacco smoke ("secondhand smoke").** All the perils posed by smoking apply not only to the smoker but to those in the smoker's environment, as well.

- **Radon** is a naturally occurring gas resulting from the radioactive decay of radium, which is itself a decay product of uranium.

Radon, in turn, breaks down into components known as radon progeny, sometimes called "radon daughters," which emit high-energy alpha particles. These emissions, which are odorless and colorless, are often present in the home and increase the risk of lung cancer. (An important note: radon is believed to be the second leading cause of lung cancer—however, its effects on minority populations has not been quantified.) Smokers exposed to radon substantially increase their risk of lung cancer in comparison to exposed nonsmokers.

- **Combustion products** (aside from tobacco smoke), include carbon monoxide (CO), nitrogen dioxide (NO2), and sulfur dioxide (SO2); they stem from such sources as stoves, furnaces, fireplaces, heaters, and dryers. Carbon monoxide, which is both colorless and odorless—can be a particularly insidious and rapid killer; fatal and near-fatal carbon monoxide poisonings have occurred most often in winter, as a result of misuse or malfunction of heating devices.

- **Biologicals.** Excreta and dander, from living organisms such as insects, other animals (both pets and pests), pollen, molds, and dust mites that are likely to be the cause of allergic reactions. In office buildings, heating, cooling, and ventilation systems are frequent sources.

- **Volatile organic compounds** are emitted as gases from solids or liquids. Sources include formaldehyde-containing building materials, as well as an array of home and office products ranging from cosmetics, paints, and cleaners to pesticides, copiers and printers, glues and adhesives, and craft supplies.

- **Lead dust** is a particular danger to children and fetuses. It can cause impaired physical and mental development, as well as acute illness in both children and adults. Within older buildings (the type most likely to be found in poverty-ridden urban areas) lead dust comes from old, lead-based paint that is still on the walls. While the primary impact is not on the lungs, the respiratory system is the major route of entry into the body for lead particles. Lead poisoning via ingestion by small children (nibbling on old chips or putting lead-dust-covered objects in the mouth) has been most widely publicized—but it is the absorption of lead via the lung in children that is most devastating. Lead absorption rates in children, via the lung, are 95 percent, versus 30 to 40 percent for ingested lead.

- **Asbestos**, in homes and other buildings. As noted in the occupational lung disease section of this report., asbestos has been shown to be a major threat to worker's health. If present and disturbed, it can pose the same risk in the home. It was once widely used in shingles, fireproofing, heating systems, floor and ceiling tiles of older buildings. When asbestos-containing material is damaged or disintegrates, microscopic fibers are dispersed into the air.

* The EPA sets air quality standards under the Clean Air Act. The EPA also identifies communities failing to meet national standards (nonattainment areas). The criteria for acceptable and unacceptable levels of airborne pollutants are generally based on measurement of a 24-hour average for any given point in time.

Chapter 4

Lung Diseases: How They Begin

The most common clinical signs of lung diseases are cough, chest pain, chest tightness, shortness of breath (dyspnea), and abnormal breathing patterns. When any of these symptoms appear, it may signal that some vital functions of the lung have been disturbed. Because most individuals have enormous reserves of lung tissue, the disturbances in lung defenses or function may have begun some time before the clinical symptoms begin to appear.

Respiratory problems can have a number of causes. They usually arise from acute or chronic inhalation of toxic agents in the workplace or other settings, accidents, or harmful lifestyles such as smoking. Infections, genetic factors, or anything else that directly or indirectly affects lung development and function can also cause respiratory symptoms. In some lung diseases, the lung itself has been damaged. Others result from diseases of the nervous system or the muscles. These disorders interfere with the normal function of the respiratory muscles so that, although the lung itself is normal, breathing is difficult.

Facts about Some Lung Diseases

Estimates of the number of known lung diseases vary from a few dozen to several hundred. Lung diseases are classified and counted either as individual, specific diseases, or as groups of diseases that share common features. These features may be their sites, etiologies

Excerpted from "The Lungs in Health and Disease," National Heart, Lung, and Blood Institute (NHLBI), NIH Publication Number 97-3279, 1997.

(initiating events), pathophysiology (abnormalities of function), or clinical features (signs and symptoms).

Most doctors find it convenient to deal with lung diseases in groups, based on the particular pulmonary (lung) component that is diseased. Examples are diseases of the airways, diseases of the interstitium (the space between tissues), or disorders of the pulmonary circulation, the ventilatory apparatus, or gas exchange.

Often, many of these diseases occur together, particularly if they are caused by infection, inflammation, or cancer. In such cases they present an overlapping, progressive series of a mixture of clinical symptoms.

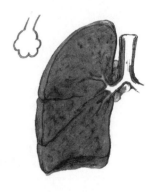

Figure 4.1. *Normal Lung*

Diseases of the Airways

Airways diseases are lung disorders that are primarily due to a continuing obstruction of airflow. Acute or chronic airflow obstruction or limitation can be caused by a variety of structural changes in the airways. Asthma, chronic bronchitis, emphysema, bronchiolitis, cystic fibrosis, and bronchiectasis are some common airways diseases.

The term chronic obstructive pulmonary disease (COPD) is commonly used for chronic bronchitis and emphysema that exist together in many patients and in which the airway obstruction is mostly irreversible. COPD is the fourth most common and the most rapidly increasing cause of death in the United States.

- In *asthma*, reversible airway obstruction is caused by inflammation, contraction of the airway smooth muscle, increased mucus secretion, and plugging of the bronchioles.

- In *chronic bronchitis*, airway obstruction results from chronic and excessive secretion of abnormal airway mucus, inflammation, bronchospasm, and infections.

- In *emphysema*, a structural element (elastin) in the terminal bronchioles is destroyed leading to collapse of the airway walls and inability to exhale "stale" air.

- *Bronchiolitis* in children is due to viral infections that cause obstructive inflammatory changes in the bronchioles.

- In *bronchiolitis* obliterans (obliteration of bronchioles, occurring in transplanted lung or after bone marrow transplantation), inflammatory changes that occur in transplanted lungs eventually cause blocking of the lumen (air channel) of the bronchioles; this is a sign that the new lung is being rejected.

- *Cystic fibrosis* is a genetic disease in which thickened airway mucus, pulmonary infections, and inflammation lead to bronchiectasis and airway obstruction.

- In *bronchiectasis*, airway obstruction is due to chronic abnormal dilation (stretching) of the bronchi and the destruction of the elastic and muscular components of the bronchial walls; it is usually caused by repeated lung infections.

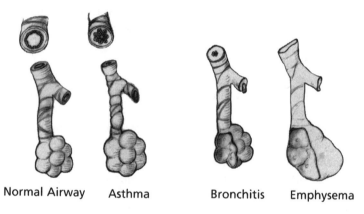

Normal Airway   Asthma   Bronchitis   Emphysema

Figure 4.2. *Normal airway and airway obstructed by disease.*

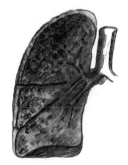

Figure 4.3. *Emphysema*

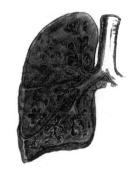

Figure 4.4. *Bronchiectasis*

Diseases of the Interstitium

The interstitium (the space between tissues) of the lungs includes portions of the connective tissue of the blood vessels and air sacs. Major chronic diseases of the lower respiratory tract in which fibrosis (scarring of the lung tissue) occurs affect the interstitial tissue. Sarcoidosis and pulmonary fibrosis are examples of the more than 150 interstitial lung diseases. Another term for these diseases is "stiff lung" disease. The most common symptoms are shortness of breath after exercise and a nonproductive cough. Some patients with interstitial lung diseases have fever, fatigue, muscle and joint pain, and abnormal chest sounds. As these diseases advance, heart function is affected.

Some interstitial lung diseases are caused by occupational or environmental exposure to inorganic dusts. Workers who inhale particles of silica are at risk for silicosis; similarly, workers in beryllium mines may develop berylliosis. Interstitial lung diseases may also be caused by inhaling organic dusts such as bacteria.

Lung disease that results from breathing in animal proteins is called hypersensitivity pneumonitis. Drugs, poisons, infections, and radiation have also been known to cause these diseases. However, approximately two-thirds of the cases of interstitial lung diseases have no known cause and are therefore termed "idiopathic."

Interstitial lung diseases begin with inflammation of the lung cells. This may be caused by an immune response or injury. The lungs stiffen as a result of inflammation of the air sacs (alveolitis) and scarring (fibrosis).

Disorders of Gas Exchange and Blood Circulation

Pulmonary edema occurs when excess fluid collects in the tissues and air spaces of the lungs. The fluid interferes with gas exchange, thus causing the patient to be short of breath and to possibly have wheezing and a persistent cough. Pulmonary edema may result from diseases of the heart or may occur as complications of other illnesses such as widespread viral or other infections, drug toxicity, exposure to high altitudes, kidney failure, or hemorrhagic shock.

Pulmonary embolism is the sudden blocking of the blood flow in one of the arteries in the lung. The highly branched network of blood vessels in the lung filters the blood as it flows through it. Sometimes the blood carries a blood clot, a fat globule, an air bubble, or a piece of tissue that is large enough to block a blood vessel leading to the lung's network of capillaries. Gas exchange then can no longer occur in this section of the lung. The result is shortness of breath or even heart failure. The most common form of pulmonary embolism is a thromboembolism. It occurs when a blood clot travels from the legs or pelvis to the pulmonary blood vessels.

Respiratory failure is the inability of the lungs to perform gas exchange. It occurs either when the muscles of the ventilatory system fail or when the structures that perform gas exchange are unable to function. Patients with neuromuscular diseases such as muscular dystrophy and polio may have normal lungs, but they can develop respiratory failure because their disease-weakened muscles are unable to pump air into their lungs. When gas exchange is impaired, not enough oxygen gets into the blood to fuel the body's metabolic activity. This condition is called hypoxemia. Chronic hypoxemia causes the blood vessels in the lung to contract; the result is pulmonary hypertension. Hypoxemia may also weaken the heart and the circulatory system. Any lung disease, if not adequately treated, can lead to respiratory failure.

Adult or acute respiratory distress syndrome (ARDS) was once called "shock lung." It is a type of pulmonary edema that is not related to heart problems. It has many causes such as severe infections, exposure to toxic fumes, circulatory collapse, sepsis (presence of disease-causing organisms or their toxic products in blood or other tissues), shock following severe blood loss, and bone fractures. During ARDS, there is severe damage to the alveolar surfaces, the blood-air barrier becomes leaky, and protein-containing fluid fills the alveoli so that they can no longer conduct gas exchange.

Respiratory distress syndrome of the newborn (RDS) is a type of respiratory failure that develops most commonly in premature or low birth weight babies whose lungs have not yet made enough surfactant. The surfactant is critical for opening the baby's alveoli with its first breath and keeping them open. As the lungs collapse, respiratory distress occurs.

Pulmonary hypertension is a disorder in which the blood pressure in the pulmonary arteries is abnormally high. In severe pulmonary hypertension, the right side of the heart must work harder than usual to pump blood against the high pressure.

When this continues for long periods, the right heart enlarges and functions poorly, and fluid collects in the ankles (edema) and the belly. Eventually the left side of the heart begins to fail. Heart failure caused by pulmonary disease is called cor pulmonale. The most common causes of cor pulmonale are various combinations of emphysema, chronic bronchitis, and/or fibrosis.

When pulmonary hypertension occurs in the absence of any other disease, it is called primary pulmonary hypertension. It affects more women than men; its cause is not known.

Pulmonary hypertension that results from another disease of the heart or lungs (for example, congenital heart disease, pulmonary thromboembolism, COPD, or interstitial fibrosis) is called secondary pulmonary hypertension.

Lung Disorders from Unusual Atmospheric Pressure

At high altitudes, the air pressure is less than at sea level, and the air contains less oxygen. Some individuals traveling to high altitudes experience a variety of symptoms while they adapt to changes in the atmosphere. The symptoms are probably due to excess fluid accumulation in the tissues.

- *Acute mountain sickness* causes dizziness, headache, and drowsiness; lethargy, shortness of breath, and nausea and vomiting may also occur.

- *High altitude cerebral edema* (fluid in brain tissue) is diagnosed when a person has symptoms of severe headache, confusion, nausea, and vomiting. Seizures may occur that can lead to coma and even death.

- *High altitude pulmonary edema* (fluid in the lung tissue) may cause cough and shortness of breath on exercise or, when severe, progressive shortness of breath even at rest, suffocation, and death.

When people dive into deep water below sea level, they become exposed to increased atmospheric pressures. This causes greater than normal amounts of nitrogen to become dissolved in their blood. If the diver returns too quickly to the surface, the excess nitrogen leaves the blood in the form of bubbles that lodge in the blood vessels of vital organs, causing necrosis (cell death) in surrounding tissue. Although this condition (decompression sickness) typically involves the limbs near a joint and is known as the bends, it can also occur in the chest, lung, or brain.

Disorders of the Pleura

Pleural effusion means an accumulation of fluid in the pleural space. It may result from heart failure, cancer, pulmonary embolism, or inflammation. If the pleurae themselves are inflamed, the condition is called pleurisy. Pleurisy causes severe chest pain with every breath and may occur with pleural effusion. If blood is the accumulating fluid, the condition is referred to as hemothorax. If the accumulating liquid is pus, it is called empyema.

When air accumulates in the pleural spaces, the condition is called pneumothorax. Mechanical injuries or diffuse diseases of the lung that distort lung architecture can lead to pneumothorax. Such diseases include emphysema, asthma, and cystic fibrosis. The most common symptom of pneumothorax is sudden pain on one side of the lung accompanied by shortness of breath.

Infections

Infections are a major cause of respiratory illness. They can be caused by bacteria or viruses and can affect not only the lung but also the nose, sinuses, ears, teeth, and gums. Infections may also complicate other lung diseases.

Pneumonia, or inflammation of the lungs, is the most common type of infectious disease of the lung. Infectious pneumonias are usually identified by naming the cause of the infection or the pattern of the infection in the respiratory tract. More than half the cases of pneumonia are caused by the bacterium, *Streptococcal pneumoniae* (pneumococcus) and are called pneumococcal pneumonia.

Influenza A is the cause of a significant number of cases of pneumonia in the elderly during the winter months. Another well known form of pneumonia is Legionnaires' disease, which is caused by the organism, *Legionella pneumophila*.

The inflammatory response of the lung in pneumonia varies depending on the type of infection, and might include:

- lobar consolidation: solidification of the lung as air spaces are filled with fluid and cellular material, and

- interstitial inflammation.

Pneumonia is sometimes accompanied by:

- necrosis: tissue changes accompanying cell death,

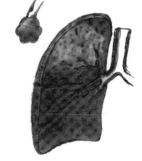

Figure 4.5. *Lobar Pneumonia.*

- cavitation: hollow spaces walled off by scar tissue,

- abscess: pus formation, and

- granuloma formation: production of tumor-like masses of different kinds of cells due to a chronic inflammatory response.

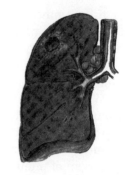

Tuberculosis is a granulomatous infectious disease caused by an organism called *Mycobacterium tuberculosis*.

Figure 4.6. Abscess (Bacterial or Tubercular)

Lung Cancer

Deaths from lung cancer were virtually unknown in the United States until 1900, but have steadily increased since then.

Currently, lung cancer is responsible for almost one-third of all cancer deaths in this country. The incidence of lung cancer may have reached its peak in men, but it is continuing to rise in women. More than 90 percent of patients with lung cancer are, or have been, cigarette smokers. Smoking marijuana increases the risk of cancer for cigarette smokers. Quitting cigarette smoking reduces the incidence of lung cancer, but the level of risk reaches that of a nonsmoker only after the person has remained a nonsmoker for 10 to 15 years.

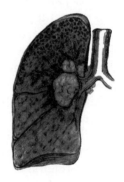

Figure 4.7. Cancer

Types of Lung Cancer

Cancers of the cells that line the major bronchi or their primary branches are called squamous cell carcinomas. This type of cancer metastasizes (spreads) mostly to other sites within the thorax.

Adenocarcinomas are cancers of the glandular cells that line the respiratory tract. They most often start at the outer edges of the lungs and spread to the brain, the other lung, liver, and bones.

Large cell carcinomas usually begin in the outermost parts of the lung. By the time they are diagnosed, they are often seen as large, bulky tumors.

Small cell carcinomas, also called "oat cell" cancers, usually begin in the bronchi. Small cell carcinomas metastasize widely to the mediastinum, liver, bones, bone marrow, central nervous system, and pancreas.

Diagnosing Lung Diseases

When a person's symptoms suggest lung disease, a chest x-ray is usually the first examination the doctor orders. Then various tests are performed to identify the disease and to determine how severe it is. These tests include:

- pulmonary function tests;
- microscopic examination of lung tissue, cells, and fluids using a light microscope and an electron microscope; and
- biochemical and cellular studies of respiratory fluids removed from the lung by lavage (washing).

To determine how well the lungs are working, doctors can measure respiratory or gas exchange functions, airway or bronchial activity, particle clearance rates, and permeability of the blood-air barrier.

Spirometry

Spirometry, like the measurement of blood pressure, is useful for assessing lung function as well as general health. It is the simplest and most common of the lung function tests.

Spirometry measures how much and how quickly air can be expelled following a deep breath. It is performed by having the patient breathe out forcefully into a device called a spirometer. At the same time a machine makes a tracing of the rate at which the air leaves the lung. Diseases of airflow obstruction and of lung stiffening give characteristic tracings with spirometry.

Measures of the amount of air that can be expelled following a deep breath, forced vital capacity (FVC), and the amount of air that can be forcibly exhaled in 1 second, forced expiratory volume in 1 second (FEV1), are the most useful numbers derived from spirometry. The ratio of FEV1 to FVC is often used to assess patients for airflow obstruction. It is normally 75 to 85 percent, depending on the patient's age. The ratio is reduced in obstructive diseases, while it is preserved or even increased in restrictive disorders. A lower than normal FEV1 is a sign that a lung disease is present. A falling FEV1 is a sign that a person's lung disease is getting worse.

The "normal" values for FVC and FEV1 for a patient depend on the individual's age, gender, height, and race. They are higher for younger than for older people, higher for tall than for short individuals, higher for men than for women, and higher for whites than blacks or Asians. Therefore, the numbers are presented as percentages of the average expected in someone of the same age, height, sex, and race. This is called percent predicted. Any number smaller than 85 percent of predicted is considered abnormal.

If these numbers are abnormal, the patient is referred for additional pulmonary function tests to find out why. These may include checking the patient's response to bronchodilators, absolute lung volumes, and blood levels of oxygen and carbon dioxide which tell how well gas exchange is occurring. Other important measures of lung function are arterial blood gas tensions ($PaO2$ and $PaCO2$) and the diffusing capacity of the lung for carbon monoxide (DLCO).

Some doctors recommend having spirometry before age 25 to get baseline numbers. However, if you are a smoker, are occupationally exposed to irritants, or have symptoms of cough, wheeze, or shortness of breath, you should be checked with a spirometer at intervals of 3 to 5 years or more frequently if your doctor recommends it.

Abnormal spirometry numbers at any age means that you are at risk for early lung disease and even potentially fatal lung cancer, heart disease, or stroke. You should immediately stop smoking if you still smoke, and talk to your doctor about other measures you may need to take depending on the reasons for your abnormal numbers.

Preventing Lung Diseases

Because respiratory problems are so often caused by environmental exposure to irritants and infectious agents, smoking tobacco, and occupations that involve inhaling dangerous substances, many lung diseases can be prevented by following some simple guidelines:

- Do not smoke tobacco or other products.

- Avoid exposure to dusts and irritants that can harm your lungs.

- Wear proper protective devices if you must work in environments that contain respiratory irritants.

- Have spirometry done as often as recommended by your doctor to get to know your numbers.

Chapter 5

Who Can Get Respiratory Failure?

Almost everyone who has a critically ill friend or relative may expect to hear the term, respiratory failure. Although failure to breathe normally was recognized even in ancient times as an ominous sign, the term, "respiratory failure," did not appear in the medical literature until the 1960s.

Doctors now understand that respiratory failure is a serious disorder caused by a variety of different medical problems that may or may not start in the lung. Healthy people as well as patients with either pulmonary (lung) or nonpulmonary diseases can develop respiratory failure.

The recognition of respiratory failure as a life-threatening problem led to the development of the concept of the intensive care unit (ICU) in modern hospitals. ICU personnel and equipment support vital functions to give patients their best chance for recovery. Today's sophisticated ICU facilities with their novel mechanical life support devices evolved as doctors and scientists learned more and more about the causes of respiratory failure and how to treat it.

This chapter is a brief overview of the unique changes in lung function that are typical of respiratory failure and the widely different medical conditions that can cause those changes. It also discusses the methods that are used to restore normal respiration and prolong life,

Excerpted from "Respiratory Failure," National Heart, Lung, and Blood Institute (NHLBI), NIH Publication Number 95-3531, 1995. Despite the age of this document, it still provides important information about the risk factors for respiratory failure.

and the related dilemma of deciding if and when to withdraw or withhold life support from a hopelessly sick patient.

Who Can Get Respiratory Failure

Many different medical conditions can lead to respiratory failure. Following are a few examples of people who may develop respiratory failure.

- A patient with a long history of asthma, emphysema, or chronic obstructive lung disease

- A patient who is undergoing major surgery in the abdomen, heart, or lung

- A person who has taken an overdose of sleeping pills or certain depressant drugs

- A premature baby who weighs less than 3 pounds

- A baby with bronchopulmonary dysplasia

- A patient suffering from AIDS

- A person who has received multiple physical injuries

- A person who has suffered extensive burns

- A person who has bled extensively from a gunshot wound

- A person who has almost drowned

- A patient with severe heart failure

- A patient with severe infections

- A person who is extremely obese

Breathing and Respiratory Failure

The term, "respiratory failure," is used when the lungs are unable to perform their basic task—gas exchange. This process involves transfer of oxygen from inhaled air into the blood and of carbon dioxide from the blood into the lungs, with the result that the arterial blood, blood circulating through the body from the heart, has enough oxygen to nourish the tissues.

Gas exchange occurs in tiny air sacs in the lung, called alveoli. When a person breathes in (inspiration), air is brought into the alveoli by the action of the respiratory muscles—the diaphragm, the muscles between the ribs, and the accessory muscles (those between the neck and the chest wall). These are collectively called "the ventilatory apparatus." The activity of the respiratory muscles is controlled by respiratory centers in the brain. The brain's respiratory centers in turn are controlled by chemoreceptors, special cells that are sensitive to the amounts of carbon dioxide or oxygen in the blood. The chemoreceptors that are sensitive to oxygen concentration are located in the large arteries in the neck in the carotid bodies. When they sense a fall in the level of oxygen in the blood, they send messages that stimulate the respiratory center in the brain so that there will be an increase in the rate or depth of breathing.

Whenever any part of the ventilatory apparatus and/or the respiratory centers fails to work properly, the result can be respiratory failure. Both adults and babies can develop respiratory failure. In infants, however, respiratory failure occurs mostly in premature babies whose lungs have not yet fully developed.

What Happens during Respiratory Failure

When the process of gas exchange is faulty, there is not enough oxygen in the blood (hypoxemia) to fuel the body's metabolic activity. In addition, sometimes there is also an accumulation of carbon dioxide, a waste product of metabolism, in the blood and tissues (hypercapnia).

Hypercapnia makes blood more acidic; this condition is called acidemia. Eventually the body tissues become acidic. This condition, called acidosis, injures the body's cells and interferes with the functions of the heart and central nervous system. Ultimately, lack of oxygen in the blood causes death of the cells in the brain and other tissues. If not adequately treated, respiratory failure is fatal.

Hypoxemic Respiratory Failure

When a lung disease causes respiratory failure, gas exchange is reduced because of changes in ventilation (the exchange of air between the lungs and the atmosphere), perfusion (blood flow), or both. Activity of the respiratory muscles is normal. This type of respiratory failure which results from a mismatch between ventilation and perfusion is called hypoxemic respiratory failure. Some of the alveoli get less fresh air than they need for the amount of blood flow, with the net result of a fall in oxygen in the blood. These patients tend to have more difficulty with the transport of oxygen than with removing carbon dioxide. They often overbreathe (hyperventilate) to make up for the low oxygen, and this results in a low CO2 level in the blood (hypocapnia). Hypocapnia makes the blood more basic or alkaline which is also injurious to the cells.

Hypercapnic Respiratory Failure

Respiratory failure due to a disease of the muscles used for breathing ("pump or ventilatory apparatus failure") is called hypercapnic respiratory failure. The lungs of these patients are normal. This type of respiratory failure occurs in patients with neuromuscular diseases such as myasthenia gravis, stroke, cerebral palsy, poliomyelitis, amyotrophic lateral sclerosis, muscular dystrophy, postoperative situations limiting ability to take deep breaths, and in depressant drug overdoses. Each of these disorders involves a loss or decrease in neuromuscular function, inefficient breathing and limitation to the flow of air into the lungs.

Blood oxygen falls and the carbon dioxide increases because fresh air is not brought into the alveoli in needed amounts. In general, mechanical devices that help move the chest wall help these patients.

Conditions That May Progress to Respiratory Failure

Almost all lung diseases including asthma, chronic obstructive pulmonary disease (COPD), AIDS-related pneumonia, other pneumonias and lung infections, and cystic fibrosis may eventually lead to respiratory failure particularly if the diseases are inadequately treated. These patients find it very hard to breathe and the result is low oxygen and high carbon dioxide blood levels.

People whose normal lungs have been injured, such as from exposure to noxious gases, steam, or heat during a fire, can subsequently go into respiratory failure. Adult respiratory distress syndrome (ARDS), also referred to as acute respiratory distress syndrome, is a form of acute respiratory failure caused by extensive lung injury following a variety of catastrophic events such as shock, severe infection, and burns. ARDS can occur in individuals with or without previous lung disease.

Hyaline membrane disease or respiratory distress syndrome of the newborn (RDS), the most common respiratory illness affecting premature babies, is another kind of respiratory failure. In this condition, the baby's lungs do not have enough surfactant, a substance that makes it possible for air to pass into the alveoli by lowering surface tension and preventing their collapse.

Symptoms of Respiratory Failure

The clinical features of respiratory failure vary widely in individual patients because so many different conditions can lead to this disorder. There are no physical signs unique to respiratory failure. At extremely low arterial oxygen ($PaO2$) levels, patients have rapid heart rates, rapid breathing rates, and they are confused, sweaty, and cyanotic (blue). Chronically low arterial oxygen makes patients irritable, and elevated carbon dioxide produces headaches and sleepiness. Difficult, rapid, or labored breathing (dyspnea) is a consistent symptom in the awake patient.

The functions of the heart and blood vessels are often severely impaired in patients with respiratory failure. In some cases, chronic hypoxemia produces narrowing of the blood vessels in the lung which, along with the lung damage or the associated treatments, may weaken the heart and the circulatory system. Some of the signs of inadequate circulation are constriction of blood vessels in the skin, cold extremities, and low urine output.

Diagnosis of Respiratory Failure

It is impossible to estimate the extent of hypoxemia and hypercapnia by observing a patient's signs and symptoms, and mild hypoxemia and hypercapnia may go entirely unnoticed. Blood oxygen must fall markedly before changes in breathing and heart rate occur.

The way to diagnose respiratory failure, therefore, is to measure oxygen ($PaO2$) and carbon dioxide ($PaCO2$) in the arterial blood. However the levels that indicate respiratory failure are somewhat arbitrary. Depending on age, a $PaO2$ less than 60 mm Hg or $PaCO2$ greater than 45 mm Hg generally mean that the patient is in respiratory failure.

Part Two

Types of Lung Disorders

Chapter 6

Alpha-1 Antitrypsin Deficiency

What Is Alpha-1 Antitrypsin Deficiency?

Alpha-1 antitrypsin is a protein that is made in the liver. The liver releases this protein into the bloodstream.

Alpha-1 antitrypsin protects the lungs so they can work normally. Without enough alpha-1 antitrypsin, the lungs can be damaged, and this damage may make breathing difficult. Alpha-1 antitrypsin deficiency is an inherited (passed down from parents) disorder that causes low levels of, or no alpha-1 antitrypsin in the blood.

How Do Normal Lungs Work?

Air usually enters the nose and mouth and goes down the air tube (trachea) to two main air passages (bronchi). These passages allow air to go into the right and left lung. Each bronchus branches out into grape-like air sacs called alveoli. Through the alveoli, oxygen enters the bloodstream during breathing in (inspiration), and carbon dioxide, a waste product, leaves the body during breathing out (expiration).

White blood cells normally found in our bodies help protect us from infection. But white blood cells also release an enzyme, called neutrophil elastase, that can damage the lungs. In normal lungs, alpha-1

Text in this chapter is from an undated fact sheet produced by the National Heart, Lung, and Blood Institute (NHLBI), available on the internet at http://www.nhlbi.nih.gov/health/public/lung/other/antitryp.htm; cited October 2001.

antitrypsin protects the lungs from the harmful effects of neutrophil elastase.

What Happens If There Isn't Enough Alpha-1 Antitrypsin?

When the lungs do not have enough alpha-1 antitrypsin, neutrophil elastase is free to destroy lung tissue. As a result, the lungs lose some of their ability to expand and contract (elasticity). This leads to emphysema and sometimes makes breathing difficult. Shortness of breath may occur.

The speed at which lung tissue is destroyed varies with each person. What is known is that tobacco smoking worsens the lung damage.

How Does Smoking Worsen Lung Damage Caused by the Disorder?

Tobacco smoke irritates and damages the lungs, prompting the body to send more white blood cells to protect them. The more white blood cells there are, the more neutrophil elastase is made, causing even more lung damage.

Also, the smoke itself changes alpha-1 antitrypsin so that it cannot do as good a job protecting the lungs from harm. Smokers with alpha-1 antitrypsin deficiency have a faster rate of lung damage. So if you smoke, stop.

What Are the Risk Factors for the Disorder?

Alpha-1 antitrypsin deficiency is not contagious, and you cannot "catch it" from someone. The disorder is inherited, which means that it is passed on genetically from a relative. All persons who have relatives with this disorder should consider being tested to find out whether they carry the gene for it.

How Is the Disorder Inherited?

Everyone receives one gene for alpha-1 antitrypsin from each parent. The M gene is the most common type of gene, and it is normal. The person who inherits an M gene from each parent has normal levels of alpha-1 antitrypsin.

The Z gene is the most common defect that causes the disorder. If a person inherits one M gene and one Z gene, that person is a carrier of the disorder. While such a person may not have normal levels of alpha-1 antitrypsin, there should be enough to protect the lungs.

The person who inherits the Z gene from each parent is called "type ZZ." This person has very low alpha-1 antitrypsin levels, allowing elastase to damage the lungs.

In rare cases, a person's body may not produce any alpha-1 antitrypsin. This condition is also inherited, and it is called "null-null type." Another type is called "dysfunctional." In this case, the alpha-1 antitrypsin levels are normal but it does not work the way it should. This type of the disorder is very uncommon.

What Are the Signs and Symptoms of the Alpha-1 Antitrypsin Deficiency?

A person with this disorder can be short of breath during daily activities. This is because the air sacs have been destroyed, and the lungs trap air as they expand and contract during breathing.

Can This Disorder Be Treated?

There are several ways you can protect your lungs from the effects of the disorder:

- receive immunizations for flu and pneumonia

- receive early treatment for lung infections by seeing your doctor at the first sign of a cold or other lung problem

- avoid tobacco smoke, noxious fumes, dust, and pollution

- stay fit by doing regular exercise

- increase your alpha-1 antitrypsin level. Speak with your doctor about alpha-1 antitrypsin replacement therapy

You can also reduce symptoms of shortness of breath by doing the following:

- using medications (for example, bronchodilators, or inhaled steroids) prescribed by your doctor to help open your airways

- using oxygen if your doctor prescribes it

- doing pulmonary rehabilitation (including breathing techniques). Call your local lung association to find out more.

Research is being conducted at National Institutes of Health (NIH) to learn more about alpha-1 antitrypsin deficiency. Scientists are studying how the disorder affects the body as well as new and future treatments. Someday, gene therapy may be able to correct the inherited problem.

If you have questions about alpha-1 antitrypsin deficiency, feel free to ask your nurse or doctor.

Chapter 7

Anthrax

What Is Anthrax?

Bacillus anthracis, the etiologic agent of anthrax, is a large, gram-positive, non-motile, spore-forming bacterial rod. The three virulence factors of *B. anthracis* are edema toxin, lethal toxin and a capsular antigen. Human anthrax has three major clinical forms: cutaneous, inhalation, and gastrointestinal. If left untreated, anthrax in all forms can lead to septicemia and death.

What Is the Case Definition for Anthrax?

A confirmed case of anthrax is defined as:

1. A clinically compatible case of cutaneous, inhalational, or gastrointestinal illness that is laboratory-confirmed by isolation of *B. anthracis* from an affected tissue or site, or

2. A clinically compatible case of cutaneous, inhalational, or gastrointestinal disease with other laboratory evidence of *B. anthracis* infection based on at least two supportive laboratory tests.

Information in this chapter is compiled from documents produced by the Centers for Disease Control and Prevention (CDC) after the identification of several anthrax cases in October 2001. Further information and additional updates can be found on the CDC website at http://www.cdc.gov.

History

How many anthrax cases have we had in the United States in the last 50 years?

From January 1955 to December 1999, there were 236 reported cases of anthrax, most of them cutaneous, in 30 states and the District of Columbia.

When was the last case of inhalational anthrax in the United States?

The last case of inhalational anthrax in the United States, before 2001, was in 1976 in California. A home craftsman, who worked with yarn, died. *Bacillus anthracis* was isolated from some of the imported yarns used by the patient.

When was the last case of cutaneous anthrax?

The last case of cutaneous anthrax, before 2001, occurred in North Dakota, in 2000. It was the only case since 1992. To find out more about this case, read the following article: "Human Anthrax Associated With an Epizootic Among Livestock-North Dakota, 2000" (*MMWR* 2000; 5[32]:677; Available at http://www.cdc.gov/mmwr/preview/mmwrhtml/mm5032a1.htm.

Can you list the most recent cases of anthrax in the Southeast of the United States?

Before October 2001, the last cases of anthrax, all cutaneous, were:

- Florida, 1973
- South Carolina, 1974
- North Carolina, 1987

Signs and Symptoms

What are the signs and symptoms of anthrax?

Symptoms of disease vary depending on how the disease was contracted, but symptoms usually occur within 7 days.

Cutaneous anthrax is the most common naturally occurring type of infection (>95%) and usually occurs after skin contact with contaminated meat, wool, hides, or leather from infected animals. The incubation period ranges from 1-12 days. The skin infection begins as a small papule, progresses to a vesicle in 1-2 days followed by a necrotic ulcer. The lesion is usually painless, but patients also may have fever, malaise, headache, and regional lymphadenopathy. Most (about 95%) anthrax infections occur when the bacterium enters a cut of abrasion on the skin. Skin infection begins as a raised bump that resembles a spider bite, but (within 1-2 days) it develops into a vesicle and then a painless ulcer, usually 1-3 cm in diameter, with a characteristic black necrotic (dying) area in the center. Lymph glands in the adjacent area may swell. About 20% of untreated cases of cutaneous anthrax will result in death. Deaths are rare if patients are given appropriate antimicrobial therapy.

Inhalational anthrax is the most lethal form of anthrax. Anthrax spores must be aerosolized in order to cause inhalational anthrax. Studies show that 4,000-5,000 spores must be present to cause an infection. The incubation period of inhalational anthrax among humans is unclear, but it is reported to range from 1 to 7 days, possibly ranging up to 60 days. It resembles a viral respiratory illness and initial symptoms include sore throat, mild fever, muscle aches and malaise. These symptoms may progress to respiratory failure and shock with meningitis frequently developing.

Gastrointestinal anthrax usually follows the consumption of raw or undercooked contaminated meat and has an incubation period of 1-7 days. It is associated with severe abdominal distress followed by fever and signs of septicemia. The disease can take an oropharyngeal or abdominal form. Involvement of the pharynx is usually characterized by lesions at the base of the tongue, sore throat, dysphagia, fever, and regional lymphadenopathy. Lower bowel inflammation usually causes nausea, loss of appetite, vomiting and fever, followed by abdominal pain, vomiting blood, and bloody diarrhea.

What specific symptoms should I watch for?

People should watch for the following symptoms:

- Fever (temperature greater than 100 degrees F) The fever may be accompanied by chills or night sweats.

- Flu-like symptoms.

- Cough, usually a non-productive cough, chest discomfort, shortness of breath, fatigue, muscle aches.

- Sore throat, followed by difficulty swallowing, enlarged lymph nodes, headache, nausea, loss of appetite, abdominal distress, vomiting, or diarrhea.

- A sore, especially on your face, arms or hands, that starts as a raised bump and develops into a painless ulcer with a black area in the center.

Is anthrax contagious?

No. Anthrax is not contagious; the illness cannot be transmitted from person to person.

What are the case fatality rates for the various forms of anthrax?

Early treatment of cutaneous anthrax is usually curative, and early treatment of all forms is important for recovery. Patients with cutaneous anthrax have reported case fatality rates of 20% without antibiotic treatment and less than 1% with it. Although case-fatality estimates for inhalational anthrax are based on incomplete information, the rate is extremely high, approximately 75%, even with all possible supportive care including appropriate antibiotics. Estimates of the impact of the delay in post-exposure prophylaxis or treatment on survival are not known. For gastrointestinal anthrax, the case-fatality rate is estimated to be 25%-60% and the effect of early antibiotic treatment on that case-fatality rate is not defined.

Exposure

What is the difference between exposure to anthrax and disease caused by anthrax?

A person can be said to be exposed to anthrax when that person comes in contact with the anthrax bacteria and a culture taken from that person is positive for anthrax. A person can be exposed without having disease. A person who might have come in contact with anthrax, but without a positive culture would be said to be potentially exposed. Disease caused by anthrax occurs when there is some sign of illness, such as the skin lesion that occurs with cutaneous anthrax.

A person who is exposed to anthrax but is given appropriate antibiotics can avoid developing disease.

Can I be exposed to anthrax via mail?

Letters containing *Bacillus anthracis* (anthrax) have been received by mail in several areas in the United States. In some instances, anthrax exposures have occurred, with several persons becoming infected. To prevent such exposures and subsequent infection, all persons should learn how to recognize a suspicious package or envelope and take appropriate steps to protect themselves and others.

What kind of mail should be considered suspicious?

Identifying Suspicious Packages and Envelopes

Some characteristics of suspicious packages and envelopes include the following:

- Inappropriate or unusual labeling
    Excessive postage
    Handwritten or poorly typed addresses
    Misspellings of common words
    Strange return address or no return address
    Incorrect titles or title without a name
    Not addressed to a specific person
    Marked with restrictions, such as "Personal," "Confidential," or "Do not x-ray"
    Marked with any threatening language
    Postmarked from a city or state that does not match the return address

- Appearance
    Powdery substance felt through or appearing on the package or envelope
    Oily stains, discolorations, or odor
    Lopsided or uneven envelope
    Excessive packaging material such as masking tape, string, etc.

- Other suspicious signs
    Excessive weight
    Ticking sound
    Protruding wires or aluminum foil

If a package or envelope appears suspicious, DO NOT OPEN IT.

What should people do who get a letter or package with powder?

Handling of Suspicious Packages or Envelopes

- Do not shake or empty the contents of any suspicious package or envelope.

- Do not carry the package or envelope, show it to others or allow others to examine it.

- Put the package or envelope down on a stable surface; do not sniff, touch, taste, or look closely at it or at any contents which may have spilled.

- Alert others in the area about the suspicious package or envelope. Leave the area, close any doors, and take actions to prevent others from entering the area. If possible, shut off the ventilation system.

- WASH hands with soap and water to prevent spreading potentially infectious material to face or skin. Seek additional instructions for exposed or potentially exposed persons.

- If at work, notify a supervisor, a security officer, or a law enforcement official. If at home, contact the local law enforcement agency.

- If possible, create a list of persons who were in the room or area when this suspicious letter or package was recognized and a list of persons who also may have handled this package or letter.

- Give this list to both the local public health authorities and law enforcement officials.

Can anthrax spores be killed on letters in the mail by microwave, UV light, or ironing?

While some of these methods may kill some spores, it is not known what procedures to use (e.g., length of time, temperature, etc.). Furthermore, because of insufficient data on the efficacy of these methods in inactivating anthrax spores, CDC does not recommend these techniques for reliable decontamination.

Testing

Can I get screened or tested to find out whether I have been exposed to anthrax?

There is no screening test for anthrax; there is no test that a doctor can do for you that says you've been exposed to or carry it. The only way exposure can be determined is through a public health investigation. The tests that you hear or read about, such as nasal swabs and environmental tests, are not tests to determine whether an individual should be treated. These kinds of tests are used only to determine the extent of exposure in a given building or workplace.

If the patient is suspected of being exposed to anthrax, should he/she be quarantined or should other family members be tested?

Direct person-to-person spread of anthrax is extremely unlikely and anthrax is not contagious.

Therefore, there is no need to quarantine individuals suspected of being exposed to anthrax or to immunize or treat contacts of persons ill with anthrax, such as household contacts, friends, or coworkers, unless they also were also exposed to the same source of infection.

Does CDC collect samples to test the bacteria?

CDC is engaging its partners in the Laboratory Response Network (LRN) in states all across the United States. The LRN is a collaborative partnership and multilevel system linking state and local public health laboratories with advanced capacity laboratories—including clinical, military, veterinary, agricultural, water, and food-testing laboratories—to rapidly identify threat agents, including anthrax. Local clinical laboratory testing is confirmed at state and large metropolitan public health laboratories. CDC conducts the definitive or highly specialized testing for major threat agents. There are 100 laboratories in the network; none of them are commercials labs.

What's the turnaround time for an anthrax test in an environmental sample—for example, the time it takes to confirm that a substance in an envelope was indeed anthrax?

Before testing can begin, samples must be collected and arrive in the laboratory in a form suitable for testing. Testing itself is a two-step process. The initial screening tests may be positive within two hours if the sample is large and the concentration of bacteria is high. The confirmation tests take much longer, depending in part on how fast the bacteria grow, but are usually available 24-36 hours after the sample is received in the laboratory.

Does CDC recommend the use of home test kits for anthrax?

Hand-held assays (sometimes referred to as "Smart Tickets") are sold commercially for the rapid detection of *Bacillus anthracis*. These assays are intended only for the screening of environmental samples. First responder and law enforcement communities are using these as instant screening devices and should forward any positive samples to authorities for more sensitive and specialized confirmatory testing. The results of these assays should not be used to make decisions about patient management or prophylaxis. The utility and validity of these assays are unknown.

At this time, CDC does not have enough scientific data to recommend the use of these assays. The analytical sensitivity of these assays is limited by the technology, and data provided by manufacturers indicate that a minimum of 10,000 spores is required to generate a positive signal. This number of spores would suggest a heavy contamination of the area (sample). Therefore a negative result does not rule out a lower level of contamination. Data collected from field use also indicate specificity problems with some of these assays. Some positive results have been obtained with spores of the non-anthrax Bacillus bacteria that may be found in the environment.

For these reasons, CDC has been asked to evaluate the sensitivity and specificity of the commercially available rapid, hand-held assays for *B. anthracis*. When this study is completed, results will be made available. Conclusions from this study are not expected in the near future.

Diagnosis

How is anthrax diagnosed?

Anthrax is diagnosed by isolating *B. anthracis* from the blood, skin lesions, or respiratory secretions or by measuring specific antibodies in the blood of persons with suspected cases. In patients with symptoms compatible with anthrax, providers should confirm the diagnosis by obtaining the appropriate laboratory specimens based on the clinical form of anthrax that is suspected (i.e., cutaneous, inhalational, or gastrointestinal).

- Cutaneous—vesicular fluid and blood

- Inhalational— blood, cerebrospinal fluid (if meningeal signs are present) or chest X-ray

- Gastrointestinal—blood

What are the standard diagnostic tests used by the laboratories?

- Presumptive identification to identify to Genus level (*Bacillus* family of organisms) requires Gram stain and colony identification.

- Presumptive identification to identify to species level (*B. anthracis*) requires tests for motility, lysis by gamma phage, capsule production and visualization, hemolysis, wet mount and malachite green staining for spores.

- Confirmatory identification of *B. anthracis* carried out by CDC may include phage lysis, capsular staining, and direct fluorescent antibody (DFA) testing on capsule antigen and cell wall polysaccharide.

When is a nasal swab indicated?

Nasal swabs and screening may assist in epidemiologic investigations, but should not be relied upon as a guide for prophylaxis or treatment. Epidemiologic investigation in response to threats of exposure to *B. anthracis* may employ nasal swabs of potentially exposed persons as an adjunct to environmental sampling to determine the extent of exposure.

Preventive Therapy

What is the therapy for preventing inhalational anthrax?

Interim recommendations for postexposure prophylaxis for prevention of inhalational anthrax after intentional exposure to *B. anthracis* may be found in the MMWR issue at http://www.cdc.gov/mmwr/preview/mmwrhtml/mm5041a1.htm

What is Cipro (ciprofloxacin)?

Ciprofloxacin, or Cipro as it is commonly known, is a broad-spectrum, synthetic antimicrobial agent active against several microorganisms. The use of ciprofloxacin is warranted only under the strict supervision of a physician.

Does ciprofloxacin have an expiration date?

Yes. Antibiotics, just like all medicines, have expiration dates. If you received your ciprofloxacin through a pharmacist, the expiration date should be listed on the bottle. If you can't find it or have questions about the expiration date, contact your pharmacist directly.

What are the side effects of Cipro?

Adverse health effects include vomiting, diarrhea, headaches, dizziness, sun sensitivity, and rash. Hypertension, blurred vision, and other central nervous system effects occur in <1% of patients and may be accentuated by caffeine or medications containing theophylline.

What are the guidelines for changing from ciprofloxacin to another antibiotic?

Considerations for choosing an antimicrobial agent include effectiveness, resistance, side effects, and cost. As a measure to preserve the effectiveness of ciprofloxacin against anthrax and other infections, use of doxycycline for preventive therapy may be preferable. As always, the selection of the antimicrobial agent for an individual patient should be based on side-effect profiles, history of reactions, and the clinical setting.

Should people buy and store antibiotics?

There is no need to buy or store antibiotics, and indeed, it can be detrimental to both the individual and to the community. First, only people who are exposed to anthrax should take antibiotics, and health authorities must make that determination. Second, individuals may not stockpile or store the correct antibiotics. Third, under emergency plans, the Federal government can ship appropriate antibiotics from its stockpile to wherever they are needed.

Treatment

What is the treatment for patients with inhalational and cutaneous anthrax?

Treatment protocols for cases of inhalational and cutaneous anthrax associated with this bioterrorist attack are found in the *MMWR*, 10/26/2001; 50(42), 909-919.

What if I develop side effects from the antibiotic?

If you develop side effects from the antibiotic, call your health care provider immediately. Depending on the type of side effects, you may be able to continue taking the medicine, or may be switched to an alternative antibiotic. If necessary, your physician may contact your State Department of Health for consultation on possible alternate antibiotics.

Has CDC tested the anthrax isolates for sensitivity to different antibiotics?

Yes. Antibiotic sensitivity testing performed at CDC has determined that the strain of anthrax was sensitive to a wide range of antibiotics, including penicillin and ciprofloxacin, giving public health officials important treatment information.

What are the risks of using tetracyclines and fluoroquinolones in children; are alternatives available?

Risks of using tetracyclines and fluoroquinolones in children must be weighed carefully against the risk for developing a life-threatening disease due to *B. anthracis*. Both agents can have adverse health reactions in children. If adverse reactions are suspected, therapy may be changed to amoxicillin or penicillin.

Vaccine

Is the anthrax vaccine available to the public?

A vaccine has been developed for anthrax that is protective against invasive disease, but it is currently only recommended for high-risk populations. CDC and academic partners are continuing to support the development of the next generation of anthrax vaccines.

Who should be vaccinated against anthrax?

The Advisory Committee on Immunization Practices (ACIP) has recommend anthrax vaccination for the following groups:

- Persons who work directly with the organism in the laboratory.

- Persons who work with imported animal hides or furs in areas where standards are insufficient to prevent exposure to anthrax spores.

- Persons who handle potentially infected animal products in high-incidence areas; while incidence is low in the United States, veterinarians who travel to work in other countries where incidence is higher should consider being vaccinated.

- Military personnel deployed to areas with high risk for exposure to the organism.

What is the protocol for anthrax vaccination?

The immunization consists of three subcutaneous injections given 2 weeks apart, followed by three additional subcutaneous injections given at 6, 12, and 18 months. Annual booster injections of the vaccine are recommended thereafter.

Are there adverse reactions to the anthrax vaccine?

Mild local reactions occur in 30% of recipients and consist of slight tenderness and redness at the injection site. Severe local reactions are infrequent and consist of extensive swelling of the forearm in addition to the local reaction. Systemic reactions occur in fewer than 0.2% of recipients.

Reporting

What is the protocol for investigating and reporting possible anthrax exposures?

Physicians should report any suspected cases of *B. anthracis* to their local or state public health officials IMMEDIATELY. Subsequent notification procedures for these officials may be found at the Web Site: http://www.bt.cdc.gov/EmContact/Protocols.asp.

Response

How is CDC responding to the anthrax reports?

The Federal government is coordinating the overall response to the anthrax reports. CDC continues to work with state and local health departments and other federal agencies to protect the public's health and facilitate the epidemiologic investigations.

CDC has deployed a large number of epidemiologists, laboratorians, and other program staff to areas with possible anthrax exposures to assist local health professionals conducting these investigations. CDC also has professional staff in Atlanta working around the clock to track the exposures, process specimens, answer questions, and provide technical assistance and support. As CDC learns of an emerging situation involving a possible exposure to anthrax, the agency works with state and local health departments and other federal agencies to determine an appropriate response.

What is CDC's role on "rapid response teams"?

CDC teams are on stand-by and available to assist with investigations into outbreaks, confirmation of cases and exposures, and cleanup of *B. anthracis* and other biologic and chemical agents. These teams work closely with local health officials in the areas of laboratory capacity, epidemiologic response, disease surveillance, and communication.

What is the approach to cleanup of buildings?

The Environmental Protection Agency (EPA) has lead responsibility for issues related to environmental cleanup of hazardous materials and weapons of mass destruction with the assistance of 16 different federal agencies and departments including HHS/CDC working with the State and local agencies. The decision for a most efficient approach to cleanup will be defined based upon the sampling results, review of cleanup options, environmental media, etc.

Does CDC cooperate with international health organizations like the World Health Organization (WHO) to help in other countries with anthrax cases?

CDC has assisted authorities in other countries investigating cases of bioterrorism-related anthrax. During October 12-November 13, 2001, CDC received 111 requests from 66 countries. Of these, 47 requests were laboratory related; 43 were general requests for bioterrorism information; 13 were for environmental or occupational health guidelines; and eight were about developing bioterrorism preparedness plans. The largest proportion of requests were from Central and South America (26%). Of the 66 countries, 15 received laboratory assistance, including testing or arrangements for testing of suspected isolates at a CDC-supported laboratory or a reference laboratory in another country. Forty-two countries received telephone or email consultation regarding specific tests for suspected *B. anthracis* isolates. Requests for information regarding bioterrorism-related issues outside the United States should be directed to the International Team of CDC's Emergency Operations Center (e-mail, eocinternational@cdc.gov).

Worker Safety

What are CDC's recommendations for protecting mail handlers?

CDC and the US Postal Service are collaborating to ensure that all mail handlers and postal workers are protected against exposure to anthrax.

Sources

What is the importance of knowing the genetic information about anthrax?

Genetic information about *B. anthracis*, particularly to determine genetic similarity among strains, is an important part of a disease investigation, but it is not immediately required for taking action to prevent or treat anthrax in those who may have been exposed to or infected by *B. anthracis*. Genetic information is often used to determine the similarity of strains if a common source is suspected.

Does the similarity in strains from Florida, New York, and Washington, D.C. mean that they came from the same source or are these just the most common strains?

The strains of anthrax identified in Florida, New York, and Washington, D.C., are similar and consistent with a naturally occurring strain that shows no evidence of genetic alteration or bioengineering. All are sensitive and susceptible to the antibiotics recommended by CDC for those who have been exposed to or infected with *B. anthracis*.

Children and Anthrax

Recent news reports of anthrax cases in several U.S. cities may have created fear among both children and adults. CDC has prepared this fact sheet to provide parents with information and resources to 1) help their children cope with their fears about anthrax and 2) make decisions related to anthrax and their children.

How to Reduce Children's Fears

- Help your children feel safe. Let them talk about their fears and worries. Stick to family routines that help children feel comfortable and secure. Reassure them that parents, teachers, doctors, and government officials are doing everything possible to keep them safe and healthy.

- Limit children's viewing of television news. Children may be frightened, overwhelmed, or traumatized by news reports about bioterrorism. Supervise what they watch on television, and when they do watch, be sure to allow for family discussion time during and after viewing to let them air their fears and concerns.

- Arm yourself with the facts. Education is your best protection against unnecessary fear. Your children will be less fearful if they see that you are not afraid and if you spend time with them answering all of their questions.

What Every Parent Should Know

Anthrax is an illness caused by bacteria called *Bacillus anthracis.* These bacteria are found naturally in the soil. They can form a protective coat around themselves called spores, and they can release poisonous substances into the bodies of infected people.

You and your children cannot catch anthrax from each other or from any other person. Even if you were to become sick with anthrax, you could not pass on the illness to your children. Also, even if someone were to put the bacteria that causes anthrax in your workplace on purpose, it is highly unlikely that you would carry the bacteria home to your children on your clothes or hair.

People come into contact with (are "exposed" to) bacteria or become infected with bacteria that cause anthrax in three ways. They can be exposed and infected by breathing in (inhaling) the bacteria, by coming into contact with the bacteria through cuts or abrasions in the skin, or by eating something that contains the bacteria (usually undercooked meat from an infected animal). The chance of coming into contact with the bacteria in any of these ways is very low. Also, our bodies have defenses against bacteria, so not everyone who comes into contact with the bacteria will become ill with anthrax.

The signs and symptoms of anthrax infection in children older than 2 months of age are similar to those in adults. The illness affects children and adults in much the same way, though children may be more likely to suffer side effects from some of the antibiotics used to prevent or treat the disease.

Although you may be tempted to ask your doctor for a supply of antibiotics to keep on hand, neither the Centers for Disease Control and Prevention (CDC) nor the American Academy of Pediatrics recommends doing this. You should not obtain antibiotics for your children unless public health authorities have confirmed that it is likely that your children have come into contact with the bacteria that cause anthrax. Giving your children antibiotics when the antibiotics are not needed can do more harm than good. Many antibiotics have serious side effects in children, and using antibiotics when they are not needed can lead to the development of drug-resistant forms of bacteria in your children. If this happens, the antibiotics will not be able to kill the resistant bacteria the next time your child needs the same antibiotic to treat ear, sinus, or other infections that children frequently develop.

Currently, there is no anthrax vaccine for children. The anthrax vaccine used for adults has never been studied in children, and it is not recommended for people younger than 18 years old. It is currently available only for people in the military service, although public health officials are now considering its use for people in other high-risk professions.

The chances of your children coming into contact with bacteria that cause anthrax are extremely low. However, if public health officials confirm or suspect that you or your children have come into contact with the bacteria, your doctor or other health official will prescribe antibiotics to keep you and your children from developing anthrax. Early identification and treatment of anthrax in children is critical, so call your health care provider immediately with any questions or concerns. Remember: never give your child an antibiotic unless a doctor has examined your child and prescribed an antibiotic. Also, be sure to use any antibiotic exactly as directed by the doctor or pharmacy.

Where to Get More Information

The American Academy of Pediatrics Web site addresses numerous issues related to anthrax, bioterrorism, and children. You can access these topics at http://www.aap.org/advocacy/releases. Suggestions for helping children after a disaster are available at the Web site of the American Academy of Child and Adolescent Psychiatry at http://www.aacap.org/publications/factsfam/disaster.htm. CDC also offers information on a wide range of bioterrorism topics at http://www.bt.cdc.gov.

Chapter 8

Asthma

Controlling Your Asthma

If you have asthma, you are not alone. More than 14 million people in the United States have this lung disease. Of these, almost 5 million are children. Asthma is a problem among all races. But the asthma death rate and hospitalization rate for blacks are three times the rate of whites. Proper asthma care could prevent these problems for all.

This chapter can help you learn how to control your asthma or help a friend or family member with asthma.

Asthma Is a Serious Lung Disease

Asthma makes the sides of the airways in your lungs inflamed or swollen all the time. See the drawing below. Your airways react to things like smoke, dust, pollen, or other things. Your airways narrow or become smaller and you get common symptoms like those described below.

Asthma that is not well controlled can cause many problems. People miss work or school, go to the hospital, or even die because of their asthma. But you do not have to put up with the problems asthma can cause.

"Facts about Asthma," National Heart, Lung, and Blood Institute, NIH Publication No. 97-2339, 1997.

Your Asthma Can Be Controlled With Proper Care

With your doctor's help, you can control your asthma and become free of symptoms most of the time. But your asthma does NOT go away when your symptoms go away. You need to keep taking care of your asthma.

Your asthma cannot be cured—having asthma is a part of your life. So you need to make taking care of your asthma a part of your life. This is true even if your asthma is mild.

Common Symptoms of Asthma

You may have all of these symptoms, some of them, or just one. Symptoms can be mild or severe.

- Coughing
- Wheezing (a whistling noise when you breathe)
- Chest tightness (the feeling that someone is squeezing or sitting on your chest)
- Shortness of breath

How to Take Care of Your Asthma

1. Work with your doctor and see him or her at least every 6 months.
2. Take your asthma medicines exactly as your doctor tells you.
3. Watch for signs that your asthma is getting worse and act quickly.
4. Stay away from or control things that make your asthma worse.

How to Work with Your Doctor

- Agree on clear treatment goals with your doctor.
- Agree on what things you need to do. Then do them.
- Ask questions until you feel you know what your doctor wants you to do, when you should do it, and why. Tell your doctor if you think you will have trouble doing what is asked. You can work together to find a treatment plan that is right for you.

- Write down the things you are supposed to do before you leave the doctor's office, or soon after.

- Put up reminders to yourself to take your medicine on time. Put these notes in places where you will see them.

- See your doctor at least every 6 months to check your asthma and review your treatment. Call for an appointment if you need one.

Prepare a day or two before each doctor's visit:

- Talk about any changes in your home or work that may have made your asthma worse.

- Write down questions and concerns to discuss with your doctor. Include ALL of your concerns, even those you think are not a big deal.

- Bring your medicines and written action plan to each visit. If you use a peak flow meter, bring it to each visit.

Is Your Asthma Under Control?

Answer the following question with a yes or no. Do this just before each doctor's visit.

In the past 2 weeks:

1. Have you coughed, wheezed, felt short of breath, or had chest tightness:

   During the day? yes no

   At night, causing you to wake up? yes no

   During or soon after exercise? yes no

2. Have you needed more "quick-relief " medicine than usual? yes no

3. Has your asthma kept you from doing anything you wanted to do? yes no

   If yes, what was it?

4. Have your asthma medicines caused you any problems, like shakiness, sore throat, or upset stomach? yes no

Table 8.1. Asthma Long-Term-Control Medications

Generic Name	Brand Name
Steroids: Inhaled	
beclomethasone	Beclovent®, Vanceril®, Vanceril®—Double Strength
budesonide	Pulmicort Turbuhaler®
flunisolide	AeroBid®, AeroBid-M®
fluticasone	Flovent®
triamcinolone	Azmacort®
Cromolyn and Nedocromil: Inhaled	
cromolyn sodium	Intal®
nedocromil sodium	Tilade®
Leukotriene Modifiers: Tablets	
zafirlukast	Accolate®
zileuton	Zyflo®
Long-Acting Beta2-Agonists	
salmeterol (inhaled)	Serevent®
albuterol	Volmax®
(extended release tablet)	Proventil Repetabs®

Theophylline: Tablets or liquid

Aerolate® III	Aerolate® JR
Aerolate® SR	Choledyl® SA
Elixophyllin®	Quibron®-T
Quibron®-T/SR	Slo-bid®
Slo-Phyllin®	Theo-24®
Theochron®	Theo-Dur®
Theolair®	Theolair®-SR
T-Phyl®	Uni-Dur®
Uniphyl®	

In the past few months:

5. Have you missed school or work because of your asthma? yes no

6. Have you gone to the emergency room or hospital because of your asthma? yes no

What Your Answers Mean

All "no" answers—your asthma is under control.

One or more "yes" answers—something needs to be done.

Taking the Right Medicines at the Right Times

There are two main kinds of medicines for asthma: (1) those that help with the long-term control of asthma and (2) those that give short-term quick relief from asthma symptoms.

Long-term-control medicines will prevent symptoms and control asthma. But it often takes a few weeks before you feel the full effects of this medicine.

Ask your doctor about taking daily long-term-control medicine if you:

*   Have asthma symptoms three or more times a week, or

*   Have asthma symptoms at night three or more times a month.

If you need a long-term-control medicine, you will need to keep taking your medicine each day, even when you feel well. This is the only way you can keep your asthma under control.

Make taking your long-term-control medicine a part of your daily routine-just like eating, sleeping, and brushing your teeth.

The Long-Term-Control Medicines

The most effective long-term-control medicines are those that reduce swelling in your airways (inflammation). These medicines include inhaled steroids, cromolyn, and nedocromil.

Inhaled steroids and steroid tablets or liquids are the strongest long-term-control medicines. The steroids used for asthma are NOT the same as the unsafe steroids some athletes take to build muscles.

Inhaled steroids are used to prevent symptoms and control mild, moderate, and severe asthma. Inhaled steroids are safe when taken at recommended doses. This is because the medicine goes right to your lungs where you need it. This reduces the amount of medicine you need and the chance of any side effects.

Steroid tablets or liquids are used safely for short times to quickly bring asthma under control. They are also used longer term to control the most severe asthma.

Cromolyn and nedocromil are often the choice of medicine for children with mild asthma. Inhaled long-acting beta2-agonists are used to help control moderate-to-severe asthma and to prevent nighttime symptoms. Long-acting beta2-agonists do not reduce inflammation. Therefore, patients taking this medicine also need to take inhaled

Table 8.2. Asthma Quick-Relief Medications

Generic Name	Brand Name
Short-Acting Beta2-Agonists: Inhaled	
albuterol	Airet®
	Proventil®
	Proventil HFA®
	Ventolin®
	Ventolin® Rotacaps
bitolterol	Tornalate®
pirbuterol	Maxair®
terbutaline	Brethaire®
	Brethine® (tablet only)
	Bricanyl® (tablet only)
Anticholinergics: Inhaled	
ipratropium bromide	Atrovent®
Steroids: Tablets or Liquids	
methylprednisolone	Medrol®
prednisone	Prednisone
	Deltasone®
	Orasone®
	Liquid Pred®
	Prednisone Intensol®
prednisolone	Prelone
	Pediapred

steroids. Inhaled long acting beta2-agonists should not be used for quick relief of asthma attacks.

Sustained-release theophylline or sustained-release beta2-agonist tablets can help prevent nighttime symptoms. These medicines are used with inhaled steroids, nedocromil, or cromolyn. Theophylline is sometimes used by itself to treat mild asthma. The dose for theophylline must be checked over time to prevent side effects.

Zileuton and zafirlukast are a more recent type of long-term-control medicine. Studies so far show that it is used mainly for mild asthma in patients 12 years of age and older.

Inhaled quick-relief medicine quickly relaxes and opens your airways and relieves asthma symptoms. But it only helps for about 4 hours. Quick-relief medicine cannot keep symptoms from coming back—only long-term-control medicines can do that.

Take quick-relief medicine when you first begin to feel symptoms—like coughing, wheezing, chest tightness, or shortness of breath. Your doctor may tell you to use a peak flow meter to help you know when to take your inhaled quick relief medicines.

Do not delay taking your quick relief medicine when you have symptoms. This can keep you from having a really bad asthma attack. Tell your doctor if you notice you are using more of this medicine than usual. This is often a sign that your long-term-control medicine needs to be changed or increased.

How to Control Things That Make Your Asthma Worse

You can help prevent asthma attacks by staying away from things that make your asthma worse. This chapter suggests many ways to help you do this.

You need to find out what makes your asthma worse. Some things that make asthma worse for some people are not a problem for others. Ask your doctor to help you find out what else makes your asthma worse. Then, decide with your doctor what steps you will take. Start with the things in your bedroom that bother your asthma. Try something simple first.

Tobacco Smoke

If you smoke, ask your doctor for ways to help you quit. Ask family members to quit smoking, too.

- Do not allow smoking in your home or around you.
- Be sure no one smokes at a child's day care center.

Dust Mites

Many people with asthma are allergic to dust mites. Dust mites are like tiny "bugs" you cannot see that live in cloth or carpet. Things that will help the most:

- Encase your mattress in a special dust-proof cover.

- Encase your pillow in a special dust-proof cover or wash the pillow each week in hot water. Water must be hotter than 130°F to kill the mites.

- Wash the sheets and blankets on your bed each week in hot water.

Other things that can help:

- Reduce indoor humidity to less than 50 percent. Dehumidifiers or central air conditioners can do this.

- Try not to sleep or lie on cloth-covered cushions or furniture.

- Remove carpets from your bedroom and those laid on concrete, if you can.

- Keep stuffed toys out of the bed or wash the toys weekly in hot water.

Animal Dander

Some people are allergic to the flakes of skin or dried saliva from animals with fur or feathers. The best things to do:

- Keep furred or feathered pets out of your home. If you can't keep the pet outdoors, then keep the pet out of your bedroom and keep the bedroom door closed.

- Cover the air vents in your bedroom with heavy material to filter the air.

- Remove carpets and furniture covered with cloth from your home. If that is not possible, keep the pet out of the rooms where these are.

Cockroach

Many people with asthma are allergic to the dried droppings and remains of cockroaches.

- Keep all food out of your bedroom.

- Keep food and garbage in closed containers (never leave food out).

- Use poison baits, powders, gels, or paste (for example, boric acid). You can also use traps.

- If a spray is used to kill roaches, stay out of the room until the odor goes away.

Vacuum Cleaning

Try to get someone else to vacuum for you once or twice a week, if you can. Stay out of rooms while they are being vacuumed and for a short while afterward. If you vacuum, use a dust mask (from a hardware store), a double-layered or microfilter vacuum cleaner bag, or a vacuum cleaner with a HEPA filter.

Indoor Mold

- Fix leaky faucets, pipes, or other sources of water.

- Clean moldy surfaces with a cleaner that has bleach in it.

Pollen and Outdoor Mold

What to do during your allergy season (when pollen or mold spore counts are high):

- Try to keep your windows closed.

- Stay indoors with windows closed during the midday and afternoon, if you can. Pollen and some mold spore counts are highest at that time.

- Ask your doctor whether you need to take or increase anti-inflammatory medicine before your allergy season starts.

Smoke, Strong Odors, and Sprays

- If possible, do not use a wood-burning stove, kerosene heater, or fireplace.

- Try to stay away from strong odors and sprays, such as perfume, talcum powder, hair spray, and paints.

Exercise, Sports, Work, or Play

- You should be able to be active without symptoms. See your doctor if you have asthma symptoms when you are active-like when you exercise, do sports, play, or work hard.

- Ask your doctor about taking medicine before you exercise to prevent symptoms.

- Warm up for about 6 to 10 minutes before you exercise.

- Try not to work or play hard outside when the air pollution or pollen levels (if you are allergic to the pollen) are high.

Other Things That Can Make Asthma Worse

- *Flu:* Get a flu shot.

- *Sulfites in foods:* Do not drink beer or wine or eat shrimp, dried fruit, or processed potatoes if they cause asthma symptoms.

- *Cold air:* Cover your nose and mouth with a scarf on cold or windy days.

- *Other medicines:* Tell your doctor about all the medicines you may take. Include cold medicines, aspirin, and even eye drops.

For More Information about Asthma

National Asthma Education and Prevention Program
NHLBI Information Center, P.O. Box 30105
Bethesda, MD 20824-0105
Tel: 301-251-1222
Internet: http://www.nhlbi.nih.gov/nhlbi/nhlbi.htm

Allergy and Asthma Network/Mothers of Asthmatics, Inc.
Toll Free: 800-878-4403
Internet: http://www.podi.com/health/aanma

American Academy of Allergy, Asthma, and Immunology
Toll Free: 800-822-2762
Internet: http://www.aaaai.org

American College of Allergy, Asthma, and Immunology
Toll Free: 800-842-7777
Internet: http://allergy.mcg.edu

American Lung Association
Toll Free: 800-586-4872
Internet: http://www.lungusa.org

Asthma and Allergy Foundation of America
Toll Free: 800-727-8462
Internet: http://www.aafa.org

National Jewish Medical and Research Center (Lung Line)
Toll Free: 800-222-5864
Internet: http://www.njc.org

Chapter 9

Asthma and Older Adults

Asthma should not limit your enjoyment of life, no matter what your age. When you work with your doctor, your asthma can be controlled so that you can do the things you enjoy.

What Is Asthma?

Asthma is a disease of the lung airways. With asthma, the airways are inflamed (swollen) and react easily to certain things, like viruses, smoke, or pollen. When the inflamed airways react, they get narrow and make it hard to breathe. Common asthma symptoms are wheezing, coughing, shortness of breath, and chest tightness. When these symptoms get worse, it's an asthma attack.

Asthma symptoms may come and go, but the asthma is always there. To keep it under control, you need to work with your doctor and keep taking care of it.

Asthma and Aging

Many older adults have asthma. Some people develop it late in life. For others, it may be a continuing problem from younger years. The cause is not known.

"Living with Asthma: Special Concerns for Older Adults," developed by the National Asthma Education and Prevention Program of the National Heart, Lung, and Blood Institute (NHLBI), 1998.

Asthma in older adults presents some special concerns. For example, the normal effects of aging can make asthma harder to diagnose and treat. So can other health problems that many older adults have (like emphysema or heart disease). Also, older adults are more likely than younger people to have side effects from asthma medicines. (For example, recent studies show that older adults who take high doses of inhaled steroid medicines over a long time may increase their chance of getting glaucoma.) When some asthma and nonasthma medicines are taken by the same person, the drugs can combine to produce harmful side effects. Doctors and patients must take special care to watch out for and address these concerns through a complete diagnosis and regular checkups.

Diagnosing Asthma

If you have episodes of coughing, wheezing, shortness of breath, or chest tightness, have a complete checkup to find out what the problem is. It could be asthma or another medical problem.

Several tests may be needed to tell what is causing your symptoms. These tests include spirometry (to measure how open your airways are), a chest x-ray, an electrocardiogram (to show whether you have heart disease), and a blood test. Accurate diagnosis is important because asthma is treated differently from other diseases with similar symptoms.

Controlling Your Asthma

You can help get your asthma under control and keep it under control if you do a few simple things.

1. Talk openly with your doctor.

Say what you want to be able to do that you can't do now because of your asthma. Also, tell your doctor your concerns about your asthma, your medicines, and your health.

If you take medicine that you must inhale, be sure that you are doing it right. It must be timed with taking your breath in. And such common problems as arthritis or loss of strength may make it more difficult. Your doctor should check that you are doing it right and help you solve any problems.

It's also important to talk to your doctor about all the medicines you take—for asthma and for other problems—to be sure they will not cause harmful side effects. Be sure to mention eye drops, aspirin, and other medicines you take without a prescription. Also, tell your doctor about any symptoms you have, even if you don't think they are related to asthma. Being open with your doctor about your medicines and symptoms can help prevent problems.

Finally, be honest about any problems you may have hearing, understanding, or remembering things your doctor tells you. Ask your doctor to speak up or repeat something until you're sure of what you need to do.

2. Ask your doctor for a written treatment plan. Then be sure to follow it.

A written treatment plan will tell you when to take each of your asthma medicines and how much to take. If you have trouble reading small print, ask for your treatment plan (and other handouts) in larger type.

3. Watch for early symptoms and respond quickly.

Most asthma attacks start slowly. You can learn to tell when one is coming if you keep track of the symptoms you have, how bad they are, and when you have them. Your doctor also may want you to use a "peak flow meter," which is a small plastic tool that you blow into that measures how well you are breathing. If you respond quickly to the first signs that your asthma is getting worse, you can prevent serious asthma attacks.

4. Stay away from things that make your asthma worse.

Tobacco smoke and viruses can make asthma worse. So can other things you breathe in, such as pollen. Talk to your doctor about what makes your asthma worse and what to do about those things. Ask about getting a flu shot and a vaccine to prevent pneumonia.

5. See your doctor at least every 6 months.

You may need to go more often, especially if your asthma is not under control. Regular visits will let your doctor check your progress and, if needed, change your treatment plan. Your doctor also can check other medical problems you may have.

Bring your treatment plan and all your medicines to every checkup. Show your doctor how you take your inhaled medicines to make sure you're doing it right.

If You Need Help

If you ever feel depressed or under stress because of your asthma or other reasons, ask for help. Talking to close friends, family members, support groups, or counselors can help you feel better and help you keep your asthma under control.

Chapter 10

Beryllium Disease

What Is Beryllium?

Beryllium is a naturally occurring metal which is found in beryl and bertrandite rock. It is extremely lightweight and hard, is a good electrical and thermal conductor, and is non-magnetic. These properties make beryllium suitable for many industrial uses, which include:

- Metal working—(pure beryllium, copper and aluminum alloys, jet brake pads, aerospace components)
- Ceramic manufacturing—(semi-conductor chips, ignition modules, crucibles, jet engine blades, rocket covers)
- Electronic industry—(transistors, heat sinks, x-ray windows)
- Atomic energy industry—(heat shields, nuclear reactors, nuclear weapons)
- Laboratory work—(research and development, metallurgy, chemistry)
- Extraction—(ore and scrap metal)
- Dental alloys—(crowns, bridges, dental plates)

Prior to 1951, it was used in fluorescent lamp work.

What Is Beryllium Disease (Berylliosis)?

Beryllium disease primarily affects the lungs. The disease occurs when people inhale beryllium dust or fumes. Skin disease, with poor wound healing, rash or wart-like bumps can also occur. A person can develop beryllium disease even after being away from the beryllium industry for many years. There are two forms of beryllium disease:

- Acute Beryllium Disease usually has a quick onset, and resembles pneumonia or bronchitis. It is now rare due to improved industrial protective measures designed to reduce exposure levels.

- Chronic Beryllium Disease has a very slow onset. It still occurs in one to six percent of exposed people. It is caused by an allergic reaction to beryllium. Even brief or small exposures can lead to this disease.

Does Beryllium Cause Cancer?

Beryllium has been shown to cause cancer in several species of animals. Workers in some beryllium producing facilities have had an increased rate of lung cancer, as have beryllium cases in the U.S. Beryllium Case Registry. Beryllium has recently been classified as a human carcinogen by the International Agency for Research on Cancer (IARC).

What Are My Chances of Getting Beryllium Disease?

Only 1-6% of exposed people will develop beryllium disease. However, certain work tasks have been associated with disease rates as high as 16%. Recent genetic research has shown that approximately 40% of the population have a genetic marker that has been associated with susceptibility to disease in some individuals. Beryllium disease occurs among people exposed to dust or fumes from beryllium metal, metal oxides, alloys, ceramics or salts. Even very small amounts of exposure to beryllium can cause disease in some people. You are at risk of developing beryllium sensitization even after you leave beryllium exposure. The risk continues the rest of your life, even if you tested normal for beryllium sensitization at one time.

What Are the Signs and Symptoms of Beryllium Disease?

Beryllium disease is often accompanied by several abnormalities. Some symptoms that you may notice include:

- Cough
- Shortness of breath, especially with activity
- Fatigue
- Weight loss and/or loss of appetite
- Fevers
- Night sweats

Signs of beryllium disease that your doctor may notice include:

- Abnormal lung sounds heard with a stethoscope.
- Many small lung scars on a chest x-ray.
- Abnormal breathing tests (pulmonary function tests).
- Allergy (sensitization) to beryllium, which is measured in the blood or in lung washings with a test called the beryllium lymphocyte proliferation test (BeLPT).
- A particular type of scar called a granuloma found in lung or skin tissue when biopsied and examined under a microscope.

If you have been exposed to beryllium, and develop unexplained cough, shortness of breath, fatigue or skin rash, you should inform your doctor of your past beryllium exposure or seek information from a doctor who specializes in occupational lung diseases.

Beryllium disease is easily confused with another lung disease called sarcoidosis. Past exposure to beryllium and evidence of beryllium sensitization (on the BeLPT) differentiates beryllium disease from sarcoidosis.

How Do I Find Out If I Have Beryllium Disease?

Screening for beryllium disease usually begins with:

- A chest x-ray
- A blood test for beryllium sensitization (BeLPT)

The blood test detects abnormalities earlier than breathing tests or chest x-rays. This test is not routinely done in other medical laboratories. It is done only in a few centers that study and treat patients with beryllium disease. Doctors and patients may order the test from anywhere that overnight courier service to Denver, Colorado is available.

Contact the Clinical Immunology Laboratory at National Jewish Medical and Research Center at 303-398-1344 for information on ordering the beryllium lymphocyte proliferation test (BeLPT).

What Is the Treatment for Chronic Beryllium Disease?

Treatment is very effective in controlling the disease; however, a complete cure, with or without treatment, is rare.

Patients who are sensitized to beryllium, but who do not yet have disease do not need treatment. However, they do need to be checked by a doctor regularly for signs of disease.

Patients who have early beryllium disease, who do not yet have symptoms might not require treatment. However, they need to be checked by a doctor regularly.

Patients with beryllium disease who do have symptoms and abnormal breathing tests are usually treated with prednisone, a type of steroid that fights inflammation. Treatment with this medication usually stabilizes the disease and often improves symptoms.

Beryllium particles imbedded in the skin often must be removed before skin wounds will heal.

How Does Beryllium Disease Progress?

Beryllium sensitization often leads to disease, even in people who are no longer working with beryllium. Most people with beryllium sensitization have granuloma scars in their lungs, and sometimes in other organs also. In some individuals, the disease progresses very slowly, over many years; in others it may progress much more rapidly. The onset of symptoms after the first beryllium exposure can vary greatly. The time between first exposure to beryllium and the onset of symptoms can vary from a few months to forty years. Once a person has been exposed to beryllium, there is a lifelong risk of developing the disease.

What Can I Do to Avoid Beryllium Exposure?

It is not possible to determine your exact risk for developing beryllium disease, however here are some general guidelines that you can follow to minimize your exposure.

- Avoid breathing beryllium dust or fumes by working in well-ventilated, well-exhausted areas where beryllium air monitoring is done routinely. Use all ventilation and exhaust equipment available in order to reduce exposures to the lowest possible level.

- Whenever possible, work with non-beryllium metals, alloys, ceramics and salts.

- Do not eat, drink or smoke in areas where beryllium is in use.

- Before entering work areas where beryllium is used, change into work-clothes, including shirt, pants and shoes. At the end of the work shift take a shower and thoroughly clean your hands and hair before changing into street clothing.

- Use approved respirators for tasks that may result in high exposures.

- Avoid generating beryllium dust unless the process is well protected and has been sampled for exposure levels.

National Jewish Medical and Research Center offers a comprehensive beryllium screening and surveillance program to help patients, doctors and employers manage beryllium-related health issues. Physicians with expertise in identification and treatment of beryllium disease may be consulted through the Division of Environmental and Occupational Health Sciences at National Jewish Medical and Research Center in Denver, Colorado. To consult with a physician, or for more information on the beryllium program, please call 303-398-1722.

Chapter 11

Bronchiectasis

Bronchiectasis (pronounced brong-ke-ek'-tas-is) is a chronic disease that damages the muscle and elastic tissue of the airways within the lungs. Permanent dilation of the airways can be a result of the damaged bronchial wall. Dilation can be a uniform enlargement, or irregular and result in the formation of pouches. The pouches in the airways are susceptible to infection because bacteria thrive in these warm, dark and moist areas. When small infections accumulate, you may become very ill. Early diagnosis and treatment of bronchiectasis is very important.

You may be born with bronchiectasis, or you may acquire it as an adult or child through one or more of the following ways:

1. Accidental inhalation of an object into your lungs, causing inflammation.

2. Obstruction in your airways because of a growth or tumor.

3. Gastroesophageal reflux (heartburn) which occurs when the valve or sphincter connecting your esophagus and stomach is too relaxed; this allows a backward flow of stomach contents to enter your lungs and irritate the airways.

---

4. Having another chronic lung condition, such as cystic fibrosis, allergic aspergillosis, tuberculosis, whooping cough (pertussis), or an immune deficiency disease or repeated episodes of flu and pneumonia.

5. Kartagener's Syndrome, a rare inherited disease that combines bronchiectasis, loss of ability to clear mucus and chronic sinusitis.

Bronchiectasis Develops in Several Stages

First, injury to the walls of the airway occurs from any mechanism. Second, the immune defenses of the respiratory tract weaken and lose ability to clear mucus, making the airways susceptible to infections. Repeated lung infections cause permanent damage to the elastic tissue within the bronchial wall. And finally, chronic weakness and pouching of the airway walls develop.

What Are the Symptoms?

Symptoms of bronchiectasis include a recurring cough with mucus. The mucus may be discolored and foul smelling, sometimes containing blood. Fatigue, weight loss, shortness of breath and abnormal chest sounds can occur. Also, many persons with bronchiectasis have chronic sinusitis.

If the disease is not treated, you may experience an increasing shortness of breath, rounding at the tips of the fingers (clubbing) from lack of adequate oxygen and right-sided heart failure.

How Is It Diagnosed?

The evaluation for bronchiectasis usually includes:

- A complete medical history and physical exam.

- A chest X-ray.

- Breathing tests, called pulmonary function tests, determine abnormality with air flow to and from the lungs.

- A CAT scan (a specialized X-ray) of the lungs.

- In rare cases, a clinician may request a bronchogram. This is an X-ray procedure that tracks the distribution of dye introduced into the airways, assessing the location and amount of lung involvement.

What Is the Treatment?

Bronchiectasis can be treated in a number of ways. Your clinician will evaluate your case and recommend the best treatment for you.

Treatment of Sinusitis

Saline nasal washes help control sinusitis, which causes drainage into the airways and subsequent infections. A prescription corticosteroid nasal spray can decrease swelling and mucus production. A nasal spray containing cromolyn sodium may be helpful if allergies cause your nasal symptoms.

Treatment of Gastroesophageal Reflux

Elevate the head of your bed six to eight inches and avoid consuming food, alcohol, coffee, cola or tea for several hours before bedtime. You may need antacids or other medications to control heartburn because stomach acids can irritate the lungs. If your case is severe, you may need surgery to tighten the sphincter at the base of the esophagus.

Antibiotics

Sometimes continuous treatment with an antibiotic can help bronchiectasis, but drug-resistant organisms can develop in the lung. Therefore, your doctor will prescribe an antibiotic based on your individual signs and symptoms. For example, you may need an antibiotic only when you experience increased shortness of breath, cough, blood in the mucus or an increase in the amount and thickness of the mucus.

Other Medications

A bronchodilator medication, which opens the airways, is recommended only if lung tests show improvement with its use. This type of medication is available as an inhaler, nebulizer solution and/or tablet. Commonly used inhaled bronchodilators include: albuterol (Proventil, Ventolin), pirbuterol (Maxair and terbutaline (Brethaire). Theophylline is an oral (tablet or syrup) bronchodilator which acts by relaxing the smooth muscle of the airways. A corticosteroid medication, such as the tablet prednisone or methylprednisolone, can reduce inflammation in the airways and may be helpful for some people. An oral corticosteroid should only be used over a long period of time if the benefit outweighs the risk of possible side effects.

Chest Physiotherapy

Your clinician may recommend this procedure if you are producing an abnormally large amount of mucus or if you are having recurrent infections. This procedure uses gravity to promote drainage of mucus from all areas of the lung and decrease the risk of infection. As demonstrated by your clinician, an assistant can help loosen the mucus by clapping on your back in a certain manner. Your clinician may prescribe an electric vibrator to assist you in performing this procedure. Any specific condition contributing to bronchiectasis should be treated as indicated:

- Prompt removal of any foreign object in the lung.

- Treatment of immune deficiency disorder with gamma globulin as appropriate.

- Treatment of allergic aspergillosis with corticosteroids.

- Surgery may be indicated if bronchiectasis is very localized in the lung and medical treatment and other therapies are not effective.

What Are Your Responsibilities in Managing Bronchiectasis?

- Stop smoking and avoid exposure to passive smoke.

- Get a flu shot yearly and a pneumococcal vaccine as recommended by your clinician.

- Exercise regularly as directed by your clinician as this helps you breathe easier by improving your muscle strength and tone.

- Eat a well-balanced diet and drink plenty of fluids to help hydrate and thin mucus.

Chapter 12

Bronchitis

What Is Chronic Bronchitis?

Chronic bronchitis is an inflammation, or irritation, of the airways in the lungs. Airways are tubes in your lungs that air passes through. They are also called bronchial tubes. When the airways are irritated, thick mucus gets into the tubes. The tubes get plugged up with mucus. The mucus blocks the airways and makes it hard for you to get air into your lungs. Symptoms of chronic bronchitis include a cough that makes mucus (sometimes called sputum), troubled breathing and a feeling of tightness in your chest. Chronic bronchitis is a form of chronic obstructive pulmonary disease (which is often called COPD). Another type of COPD is emphysema. Mucus is not the main problem in emphysema.

What Causes Chronic Bronchitis?

Cigarette smoking is the main cause of chronic bronchitis. When tobacco smoke is breathed into the lungs, it irritates the airways and causes mucus production. Sometimes people who don't smoke get chronic bronchitis. People who have been exposed for a long time to things that irritate their lungs, like chemical fumes, dust and other substances, can also get chronic bronchitis.

Reprinted with permission from http://www.familydoctor.org/handouts/ 280.html. AAFP © 1999. All rights reserved.

What Tests Might Be Done If My Doctor Thinks I Have Chronic Bronchitis?

Before you have tests, your doctor will ask you about your symptoms:

- Are you coughing up mucus?
- Are you having trouble breathing?
- Does your chest feel tight?
- Do you smoke cigarettes?
- How many cigarettes do you smoke each day?
- How many years have you been smoking?
- Have you been breathing in other things that can irritate your lungs?

If your doctor thinks you have chronic bronchitis, you may be tested to find out if your lungs are damaged. You might have a pulmonary function test to see how well your lungs are working: you breathe into a machine that measures the amount of air in your lungs. Your doctor may also order blood tests and a chest x-ray.

What Can Be Done to Improve My Breathing and Reduce My Coughing?

If you smoke, the most important thing you can do is to stop smoking. The more smoke you breathe into your lungs, the more lung damage you'll have. Ask your doctor to help you stop smoking. If you stop smoking, you'll breathe better and your lungs will begin to heal. You'll also have less chance of getting lung cancer.

It's important to try to avoid other things that can irritate your lungs. It's best if you don't breathe in aerosol products, like hairspray, spray deodorant and spray paint. Also avoid breathing in dust or chemical fumes. To protect your lungs, wear a filtering mask over your nose and mouth if you are using something that can irritate your lungs, such as paint remover, varnish, paint or anything else with strong fumes.

Can Medicine Treat Chronic Bronchitis?

Yes, your doctor may prescribe several medicines, called bronchodilators, to treat your chronic bronchitis. The medicine opens, or dilates, the airways in your lungs and helps you breathe better. Medicine for chronic bronchitis is usually inhaled (breathed in) rather than taken as a pill. An inhaler is used to get the medicine into your lungs. It's important to use your inhaler the right way, so you get the most benefit from the medicine. Ask your doctor to show you how to use the inhaler. Then, show your doctor how you are using the inhaler so you can be sure you're using it the right way. Your doctor may also prescribe medicines for you to take as pills. Theophylline is one kind of medicine that is taken as a pill for chronic bronchitis. It's the same medicine that is used by people with asthma.

If your symptoms don't get better with these medicines, your doctor may prescribe steroids. You can take steroids either with an inhaler or in pills.

Will Antibiotics Help Chronic Bronchitis?

In general, antibiotics don't help chronic bronchitis. But antibiotics may be helpful if you get a lung infection along with your chronic bronchitis. If you have a lung infection, the amount of mucus you cough up may increase. This mucus might be yellow or dark green. You also may have a fever. Your shortness of breath might get worse.

Because chronic bronchitis increases your risk of getting lung infections, be sure to get a flu shot every year. Also, get a pneumococcal vaccination to protect yourself against pneumonia.

What about Oxygen Therapy?

Because of the damage from chronic bronchitis, your lungs may not be able to get enough oxygen into your body. Your doctor may prescribe oxygen if your chronic bronchitis is severe and medicine doesn't help you feel better. If your doctor prescribes oxygen for you, be sure to use it day and night to get the most benefit from it. Oxygen can help you breathe better and live longer.

Can I Do Anything Else to Help My Lungs?

Yes. Exercising regularly can strengthen the muscles that help you breathe. Try to exercise at least three times a week. Start by exercising slowly and for just a little while. Then slowly increase the amount of time you exercise each day and how fast you exercise. For example, you might begin exercising by walking slowly for 15 minutes three times a week. Then, as you get in better shape, you can increase your walking speed. You can also increase the length of time you walk to 20 minutes, then 25 minutes, then 30 minutes.

You could ask your doctor about an exercise program called pulmonary rehabilitation to help you improve your breathing. Pulmonary rehabilitation is often given by a respiratory therapist (a health care professional who knows about lung treatments). Your doctor may refer you to the pulmonary rehabilitation program at your local hospital.

A breathing method called "pursed-lip breathing" may help you: take a deep breath and then breathe out slowly through your mouth while you hold your lips as if you're going to kiss someone. Pursed-lip breathing slows down the fast breathing that goes with chronic bronchitis. It may help you feel better.

This information provides a general overview of chronic bronchitis and may not apply to everyone. Talk with your family doctor to find out if this information applies to you and to get more information on this subject.

Chapter 13

Bronchopulmonary Dysplasia (BPD)

Introduction

Your baby has been diagnosed with bronchopulmonary dysplasia (BPD). BPD is a chronic lung disease of newborn infants marked by inflammation of the airways. The lungs of babies with BPD are immature or have not developed normally. Their lungs are therefore unable to perform gas exchange. Gas exchange is the primary function of the lungs. This term is used for the process by which lungs transfer oxygen from inhaled air into the bloodstream in exchange for carbon dioxide from the blood to be exhaled. Inhaled air travels to the alveoli (tiny air sacs located at the end of the conducting airways of the lungs) where it comes in contact with blood containing carbon dioxide.

The blood travels through a fine network of pulmonary vessels called capillaries. Gas exchange occurs instantaneously in normal infants as the red blood cells pass through the capillaries. It does not occur adequately in BPD infants because their alveoli and capillaries are not fully developed.

What Is BPD?

BPD is a serious, chronic lung disease of infants. The dictionary defines BPD as abnormal development or growth (dysplasia) of the lungs and air passages.

Text in this chapter is from an undated fact sheet from the National Heart, Lung, and Blood Institute (NHLBI), available online at http://www.nhlbi.nih.gov/health/public/lung/other/bpd; cited October 2001.

BPD was first described in 1967 by William Northway, a radiologist at Stanford University, as a chronic lung disease that occurred in premature babies who needed intensive oxygen therapy to survive respiratory distress syndrome (RDS). Northway noted that the symptoms and chest x-rays of these babies were different than those seen in newborns with other lung diseases.

BPD develops most commonly during the first 4 weeks after birth. Although it is seen most often in premature babies, it can also occur in full-term babies who have respiratory problems during their first days of life. Babies who are still dependent on a respirator for oxygen at 28 days of age and whose chest x-rays are typical of BPD are considered to have the disorder.

BPD can occur when a baby's lungs which have not fully developed at birth have to begin breathing immediately and also adjust to adverse conditions outside the mother's womb. Among the adverse conditions which injure the lungs and cause BPD are oxygen under high pressure and infectious agents such as bacteria or viruses.

How Common Is BPD?

BPD is a worldwide problem. BPD and RDS together are probably responsible for most of the infant morbidity and mortality in developed countries. BPD ranks with cystic fibrosis and asthma among the most common chronic lung diseases in infants in the United States. Approximately 5,000 to 10,000 new cases of BPD (20 to 30 percent of infants surviving RDS) occur each year.

Development of BPD is not limited to RDS survivors. Any newborn infant who has serious respiratory problems in its first few days after birth is at risk of developing BPD. Although BPD is most common in premature babies, it can occur in full-term infants who need mechanical ventilation and oxygen under pressure for problems such as neonatal pulmonary hypertension.

Ninety percent of the infants who develop BPD are premature and weigh less than 1500 grams (3.5 pounds). In very premature infants (weighing 1 to 1.5 pounds or born after less than 22 weeks of gestation) BPD sometimes develops even in the absence of acute respiratory problems.

The risk of BPD increases with decreasing birth weight and gestation period. BPD occurs in 5 percent of infants whose birth weight is over 1,500 grams; the incidence rises to 85 percent in surviving newborns weighing between 500 and 700 grams (1 to 1.5 pounds).

Male gender and non-African ethnicity seem to be additional risk factors. Genetic factors also may have a role.

In the late 1960s, infants with BPD who survived past 4 weeks of age were an average of 6 weeks premature and their average weight was 2,234 grams (a little more than 4.5 pounds). Improved and more sophisticated neonatal critical care now makes it possible for the majority of infants weighing at least 500 grams to survive. This increased survival of very low birth weight infants is a major factor contributing to the growing incidence of BPD.

What Causes BPD?

BPD does not develop in all infants for the same reason. When it was first described, doctors thought that BPD was a result of lung injury from the mechanical ventilation and supplemental oxygen provided as therapy for RDS.

Today the specialists who treat BPD believe that, although RDS and premature birth play a role in the development of the disorder, these are not the only factors. Rather, BPD appears to reflect the limited ability of the baby's lungs during its first hours and days after birth to respond to adverse situations. These challenges may include oxygen toxicity, mechanical lung trauma, infections, or pneumonia. The state of immaturity of the lung at birth and the type of lung injury probably determine how the newborn's lungs respond and whether or not BPD actually develops.

What Are the Signs and Symptoms of BPD?

The signs and symptoms of BPD and how severe they are vary from infant to infant. They reflect differences in lung maturity and in the severity of disease. Respiratory signs include:

- rapid shallow breathing (tachypnea), sucked-in ribs and chest (retraction), and cough;
- movement of the chest and abdomen in opposite directions with every breath (paradoxical or see-saw respiration); and
- wheezing.

The BPD infant's struggle to breathe is reflected in an abnormal posture of its neck, shoulders, and trunk. These babies also crane their necks as they use their neck muscles to try to get as much air as possible into their lungs.

Many of the symptoms of BPD are seen with other breathing problems, for example, severe asthma. If an infant shows any of these symptoms, the doctor will conduct tests to find the cause.

How Is BPD Diagnosed?

Although BPD may begin as early as 1 week of age, it is difficult to diagnose until a baby is 14 to 30 days old. A diagnosis of BPD is based on:

- a history of lung injury in the first days after birth, (Pulmonary injury can result when a respirator must be used to provide oxygen under pressure for a minimum of 3 days during the first 2 weeks of life.)

- a continuing need for supplemental oxygen at age 28 days, and

- persistence of the clinical signs of respiratory difficulty beyond 28 days of age.

An x-ray of the infant's chest is also taken to help diagnose BPD. However, the most important functional criterion for the diagnosis of BPD is the need for supplemental oxygen beyond the 28th day of life.

The criteria used for a diagnosis of BPD vary among neonatologists. They include how long respiratory distress exists and how long the baby needs to be on a respirator. Many doctors make a diagnosis of BPD in the second or third week of life. However, some doctors defer a diagnosis until the baby is at least 28 days old.

What Is the Outcome for Babies with BPD?

Most infants over 1,500 grams birth weight (3.5 pounds) who develop BPD have severe respiratory failure in the first week of life which may continue for several weeks. Extremely premature infants (those weighing less than 1,500 grams at birth, and especially those weighing less than 1,000 grams), seem to have minimal lung disease or acute lung disease that has apparently resolved, and then symptoms of BPD begin in the second week of life.

As BPD develops and progresses, the infants become increasingly dependent on oxygen and artificial ventilation. They typically display recurrent blueing or cyanotic episodes, and asthma-like symptoms. They may develop life-threatening bronchiolitis and other pulmonary complications. They may also develop serious medical complications of the heart, kidney, gastrointestinal tract, brain, or retina. In severe cases, the baby may die. Most of these deaths occur during the baby's first hospital stay. They are due to progressive respiratory failure, or its complications.

Most BPD infants will show continued slow improvement, but some may require extra weeks and months of care in the neonatal intensive care unit (NICU). It is estimated that infants with BPD require intensive in-hospital care for an average of 120 days.

At 36 weeks after conception (4 weeks before the baby's original due date), nearly a third of the infants with BPD no longer require supplemental oxygen therapy. Those who continue to require supplemental oxygen are usually otherwise growing and improving. Even if they continue to require supplemental oxygen, BPD infants may be discharged from the hospital if they are in stable condition on medication and if the family and the baby's doctor agree that providing continuing care at home is best for the baby.

How Is BPD Treated?

There is no treatment that is specific for BPD. In the NICU supportive measures and symptomatic treatment are provided to help BPD babies breathe and give their lungs time to mature. The baby's lungs improve gradually through normal repair processes.

The treatment of BPD includes three components: therapy for RDS before BPD is confirmed, therapy after BPD is diagnosed, and home care. For infants who show signs and symptoms of RDS but who are not yet diagnosed with BPD treatment may include:

- surfactant administration to improve lung aeration,

- mechanical ventilators to make up for respiratory failure,

- supplemental oxygen to insure that the baby has enough oxygen in its blood,

- careful control of fluids to avoid pulmonary edema (accumulation of fluid in the lungs),

- treatment for patent ductus arteriosus, a circulatory problem sometimes found in premature infants.

- giving the baby medicines that improve air flow in and out of the lungs, and

- feedings and appropriate supplemental formula to prevent malnutrition.

Once the diagnosis of BPD is confirmed the following treatments are continued in the NICU:

- continued mechanical ventilation and supplemental oxygen to overcome respiratory failure and maintain blood oxygen levels,

- bronchodilator medications to improve airflow in the lungs,

- corticosteroids and other medicines to reduce swelling and inflammation of airways,

- fluid restriction and diuretics to decrease water accumulation in the lungs

- antibiotics to control infections,

- intravenous feeding of needed nutrients, and

- physical therapy to improve muscle performance and to help the lungs expel mucus.

Scientists are working to develop new drugs and methods to prevent, lessen, or repair the lung injury that is seen with BPD. Some of the areas of research include:

- improving respirators so that fewer complications of positive pressure ventilation occur,

- using drugs to protect premature lungs from injury, or speed healing, and

- developing new drugs that improve lung function.

The best place for the baby's growth and development is at home with the family. It is important that the parents be loving and well-informed about the symptoms and treatment of BPD. These babies continue to have some respiratory symptoms for varying periods after leaving the hospital, and they remain in fragile health. A primary care pediatrician should be available to provide acute, long-term, and preventive health care. In addition, nurses, respiratory and physical therapists, and social services may be needed.

What Are the Short- and Long-Term Consequences of BPD?

The symptoms that persist after the infant is discharged from the hospital vary. Babies with a history of BPD are more susceptible to respiratory infections and may continue to need low levels of supplemental oxygen. Some may remain dependent on a mechanical ventilator throughout early childhood.

BPD survivors are at higher risk of complications after the usual childhood infections. As a precaution, hospital care may be recommended when a BPD baby becomes ill with a respiratory infection.

Babies who survive BPD grow more slowly than normal. This delayed growth continues into their second year of life. They usually remain smaller than normal children of the same age. Their lung growth is almost complete at 8 years of age as in all children, but they may continue to have some problems with their lung function even when they are adults.

The outlook for growth and development of babies with BPD varies. It depends more on the effects of prematurity and acute respiratory failure, rather than BPD itself. In very severe cases there may be some long-term limitations. These might include abnormalities in coordination, gait and muscle tone, inability to tolerate exercise, vision and hearing problems, and learning disabilities. The risk of these problems varies greatly among individual patients but is actually quite small. Parents of BPD infants need not assume that their child has a high risk of such developmental handicaps. If they should occur, however, parents and families can obtain information about these problems from their baby's doctors.

Living with BPD

An infant with BPD may spend several weeks or months in the NICU. This is a stressful period for the parents and the family. While the baby remains in the hospital the parents should visit as frequently as possible, to bond with the baby and help the infant recognize the voices and touch of its parents.

Social service agency personnel may be needed to teach parents of a baby with BPD how to play with and care for their infant. It is not uncommon for concern about the baby's medical condition to interfere with the parents care-giving abilities. Continued monitoring of the BPD survivor's growth and nutritional needs throughout infancy and childhood by a pediatric nutritionist can be reassuring to parents.

The parents of BPD infants can take a number of other steps to help their infants recover and grow as normally as possible. These include:

- seeking medical help when the child shows any signs of respiratory infection, for example, irritability, fever, nasal congestion, cough, changes in breathing pattern, wheezing;

- limiting the exposure of the infant to infections by avoiding the use of large day-care settings and crowds;

- protecting the baby from exposure to cigarette smoke and other respiratory irritants in the air; and

- making sure that the baby and its siblings receive all routine immunizations. Some doctors now recommend shots to protect against infection with RSV (respiratory syncytial virus) which causes bronchiolitis.

Can BPD Be Prevented?

At present, the only practical way to prevent BPD is to eliminate high risk pregnancies that result in low birth weight babies. Programs of regular prenatal care for women at high risk of early delivery have been shown to lower the incidence of premature babies.

Scientists are studying ways to better understand the processes involved in premature labor and its prevention. In addition, research is being conducted on how to prevent or lessen the adverse effects that result when birth occurs before the lungs are mature. Ways are being sought to accelerate the process of lung maturation in infants at high risk of developing RDS and BPD. Providing corticosteroids to women at risk of premature delivery reduces infant mortality and decreases the incidence of RDS.

What Are the Healthcare Costs of BPD?

Infants with BPD need intensive hospital care for an average of 120 days. In 1990, the cost of caring for these infants was more than $170,000. These infants may also require home oxygen therapy for an average of 92 days. This cost is estimated to be more than $5,000 per child per year (1990 costs). However, if the infant were hospitalized during this period, the comparable cost would be $45,000 to $50,000. The overall costs of treating infants with BPD in the United States are estimated to be $2.4 billion. This amount is second only to the costs for treating asthma and far exceeds the cost of treating cystic fibrosis.

Chapter 14

Chronic Obstructive Pulmonary Disease (COPD)

Chronic obstructive pulmonary disease (COPD), also called chronic obstructive lung disease, is a term that is used for two closely related diseases of the respiratory system: chronic bronchitis and emphysema. In many patients these diseases occur together, although there may be more symptoms of one than the other. Most patients with these diseases have a long history of heavy cigarette smoking.

COPD gets gradually worse over time. At first there may be only a mild shortness of breath and occasional coughing. Then a chronic cough develops with clear, colorless sputum. As the disease progresses, the cough becomes more frequent and more and more effort is needed to get air into and out of the lungs. In later stages of the disease, the heart may be affected. Eventually death occurs when the function of the lungs and heart is no longer adequate to deliver oxygen to the body's organs and tissues.

Cigarette smoking is the most important risk factor for COPD; it would probably be a minor health problem if people did not smoke. Other risk factors include age, heredity, exposure to air pollution at work and in the environment, and a history of childhood respiratory infections. Living in low socioeconomic conditions also seems to be a contributing factor.

More than 13.5 million Americans are thought to have COPD. It is the fifth leading cause of death in the United States. Between 1980

Text in this chapter is from an undated fact sheet produced by the National Heart, Lung, and Blood Institute (NHLBI), available online at http://www.nhlbi.nih.gov; cited October 2001.

and 1990, the total death rate from COPD increased by 22 percent. In 1990, it was estimated that there were 84,000 deaths due to COPD, approximately 34 per 100,000 people. Although COPD is still much more common in men than women, the greatest increase in the COPD death rate between 1979 and 1989 occurred in females, particularly in black females (117.6 percent for black females vs. 93 percent for white females). These increases reflect the increased number of women who smoke cigarettes.

COPD attacks people at the height of their productive years, disabling them with constant shortness of breath. It destroys their ability to earn a living, causes frequent use of the health care system, and disrupts the lives of the victims' family members for as long as 20 years before death occurs.

In 1990, COPD was the cause of approximately 16.2 million office visits to doctors and 1.9 million hospital days. The economic costs of this disease are enormous. In 1989, an estimated $7 billion was spent for care of persons with COPD and another $8 billion was lost to the economy by lost productivity due to morbidity and mortality from COPD.

What Are Chronic Bronchitis and Emphysema?

Chronic bronchitis, one of the two major diseases of the lung grouped under COPD, is diagnosed when a patient has excessive airway mucus secretion leading to a persistent, productive cough. An individual is considered to have chronic bronchitis if cough and sputum are present on most days for a minimum of 3 months for at least 2 successive years or for 6 months during 1 year. In chronic bronchitis, there also may be narrowing of the large and small airways making it more difficult to move air in and out of the lungs. An estimated 12.1 million Americans have chronic bronchitis.

People with familial emphysema have a hereditary deficiency of a blood component called alpha-1-antitrypsin resulting in the loss of a lung structural protein, elastin.

In emphysema there is permanent destruction of the alveoli, the tiny elastic air sacs of the lung, because of irreversible destruction of a protein in the lung called elastin that is important for maintaining the strength of the alveolar walls. The loss of elastin also causes collapse or narrowing of the smallest air passages, called bronchioles, which in turn limits airflow out of the lung. The number of individuals with emphysema in the United States is estimated to be 2 million.

In the general population, emphysema usually develops in older individuals with a long smoking history. However, there is also a form of emphysema that runs in families. People with familial emphysema have a hereditary deficiency of a blood component, alpha-l-protease inhibitor, also called alpha-l-antitrypsin (AAT). The number of Americans with this genetic deficiency is quite small, probably no more than 70,000. It is estimated that 1 in 3,000 newborns have a genetic deficiency of AAT, and 1 to 3 percent of all cases of emphysema are due to AAT deficiency.

The destruction of elastin that occurs in emphysema is believed to result from an imbalance between two proteins in the lung—an enzyme called elastase which breaks down elastin, and AAT which inhibits elastase. In the normal individual, there is enough AAT to protect elastin so that abnormal elastin destruction does not occur. However, when there is a genetic deficiency of AAT, the activity of the elastase is not inhibited and elastin degradation occurs unchecked. If individuals with a severe genetic deficiency of alpha-l-protease inhibitor smoke, they usually have symptoms of COPD by the time they reach early middle age. Deficiency of alpha-l-protease inhibitor can be detected by blood tests available through hospital laboratories. People from families in which relatives have developed emphysema in their thirties and forties should be tested for AAT deficiency. If a deficiency is found, it is critical for these people not to smoke.

Some scientists believe that nonfamilial emphysema, usually called "smoker's emphysema," also results from an imbalance between elastin-degrading enzymes and their inhibitors. The elastase-AAT imbalance is thought to be a result of the effects of smoking, rather than inherited as in familial emphysema. Some evidence for this theory comes from studies on the effect of tobacco smoke on lung cells. These studies showed that tobacco smoke stimulates excess release of elastase from cells normally found in the lung. The inhaled smoke also stimulates more elastase-producing cells to migrate to the lung which in turn causes the release of even more elastase. To make matters worse, oxidants found in cigarette smoke inactivate a significant portion of the elastase inhibitors that are present, thereby decreasing the amount of active antielastase available for protecting the lung and further upsetting the elastase-antielastase balance.

Scientists believe that, in addition to smoking-related processes, there must be other factors that cause emphysema in the general population since only 15 to 20 percent of smokers develop emphysema. The nature and role of these other factors in smokers' emphysema are not yet clear.

What Goes Wrong with the Lungs and Other Organs in Chronic Obstructive Pulmonary Disease?

The most important job that the lungs perform is to provide the body with oxygen and to remove carbon dioxide. This process is called gas exchange, and the normal anatomy of the lungs serves this purpose well. The lungs contain 300 million alveoli whose ultra thin walls form the gas exchange surface. Enmeshed in the wall of each of these air sacs is a network of tiny blood vessels, the capillaries, which bring blood to the gas exchange surface. When a person inhales, air flows from the nose and mouth through large and small airways into the alveoli. Oxygen from this air then passes through the thin walls of the inflated alveoli and is taken up by the red blood cells for delivery to the rest of the body. At the same time, carbon dioxide leaves the blood and passes through the alveolar walls into the alveoli. During exhalation, the lung pushes the used air out of the alveoli and through the air passages until it escapes from the nose or mouth.

Gas Exchange

Inhaled air travels through the airways to the alveoli. Blood is pumped out of the heart through the pulmonary arteries to a network of capillaries that surround the alveoli. The oxygen of the inhaled air diffuses out of the alveoli into the blood while carbon dioxide in the blood moves into the alveoli to be exhaled. The oxygen-rich blood is returned to the heart through the pulmonary veins.

When COPD develops, the walls of the small airways and alveoli lose their elasticity. The airway walls thicken, closing off some of the smaller air passages and narrowing larger ones. The passageways also become plugged with mucus. Air continues to get into alveoli when the lung expands during inhalation, but it is often unable to escape during exhalation because the air passages tend to collapse during exhalation, trapping the "stale" air in the lungs. These abnormalities create two serious problems which affect gas exchange:

- Blood flow and air flow to the walls of the alveoli where gas exchange takes place are uneven or mismatched. In some alveoli there is adequate blood flow but little air, while in others there is a good supply of fresh air but not enough blood flow. When this occurs, fresh air cannot reach areas where there is good blood flow and oxygen cannot enter the bloodstream in normal quantities.

- Pushing the air through narrowed obstructed airways becomes harder and harder. This tires the respiratory muscles so that they are unable to get enough air to the alveoli. The critical step for removing carbon dioxide from the blood is adequate alveolar airflow. If airflow to the alveoli is insufficient, carbon dioxide builds up in the blood and blood oxygen diminishes. Inadequate supply of fresh air to the alveoli is called hypoventilation. Breathing oxygen can often correct the blood oxygen levels, but this does not help remove carbon dioxide. When carbon dioxide accumulation becomes a severe problem, mechanical breathing machines called respirators, or ventilators, must be used.

Pulmonary function studies of large groups of people show that lung function—the ability to move air into and out of the lungs—declines slowly with age even in healthy nonsmokers. Because healthy nonsmokers have excess lung capacity, this gradual loss of function does not lead to any symptoms. In smokers, however, lung function tends to worsen much more rapidly. If a smoker stops smoking before serious COPD develops, the rate at which lung function declines returns to almost normal. Unfortunately, because some lung damage cannot be reversed, pulmonary function is unlikely to return completely to normal.

COPD also makes the heart work much harder, especially the main chamber on the right side (right ventricle) which is responsible for pumping blood into the lungs. As COPD progresses, the amount of oxygen in the blood decreases which causes blood vessels in the lung to constrict. At the same time many of the small blood vessels in the lung have been damaged or destroyed as a result of the disease process. More and more work is required from the right ventricle to force blood through the remaining narrowed vessels. To perform this task, the right ventricle enlarges and thickens. When this occurs the normal rhythm of the heart may be disturbed by abnormal beats.

This condition, in which the heart is enlarged because of lung problems, is called cor pulmonale. Patients with cor pulmonale tire easily and have chest pains and palpitations. If an additional strain is placed on the lungs and heart by a normally minor illness such as a cold, the heart may be unable to pump enough blood to meet the needs of other organs. This results in the inability of the liver and kidneys to carry out their normal functions which leads to swelling of the abdomen, legs, and ankles.

Another adjustment the body makes to inadequate blood oxygen is called secondary polycythemia, an increased production of oxygen-carrying red blood cells. The larger than normal number of red blood cells is helpful up to a point; however, a large overpopulation of red cells thickens the blood so much that it clogs small blood vessels causing a new set of problems. People who have poor supply of oxygen usually have a bluish tinge to their skin, lips, and nailbeds, a condition called cyanosis.

Too little oxygen and too much carbon dioxide in the blood also affect the nervous system, especially the brain, and can cause a variety of problems including headache, inability to sleep, impaired mental ability, and irritability.

What Is the Course of Chronic Obstructive Pulmonary Disease?

Daily morning cough with clear sputum is the earliest symptom of COPD. During a cold or other acute respiratory tract infection, the coughing may be much more noticeable and the sputum often turns yellow or greenish. Periods of wheezing are likely to occur especially during or after colds or other respiratory tract infections. Shortness of breath on exertion develops later and progressively becomes more pronounced with severe episodes of breathlessness (dyspnea) occurring after even modest activity.

A typical course of COPD might proceed as follows. For a period of about 10 years after cigarette smoking begins, symptoms are usually not very noticeable. After this, the patient generally starts developing a chronic cough with the production of a small amount of sputum. It is unusual to develop shortness of breath during exertion below the age of 40, after which it becomes more common and may be well developed by the age of 50. However, although all COPD patients have these symptoms, not all cigarette smokers develop a notable cough and sputum production, or shortness of breath.

Most patients with COPD have some degree of reversible airways obstruction. It is therefore likely that, at first, treatment will lead to some improvement or stability in lung function. But as COPD progresses, almost all signs and symptoms except cough and sputum production tend to show a gradual worsening. This trend can show fluctuations, but over the course of 4 or 5 years, a slow deterioration becomes evident.

Repeated bouts of increased cough and sputum production disable most patients and recovery from coughing attacks may take a long time. Patients with severe lung damage sleep in a semi-sitting position because they are unable to breathe when they lie down. They often complain that they awaken during the night feeling "choked-up," and they need to sit up to cough.

Survival of patients with COPD is closely related to the level of their lung function when they are diagnosed and the rate at which they lose this function. Overall, the median survival is about 10 years for patients with COPD who have lost approximately two-thirds of their normally expected lung function at diagnosis.

How Is Chronic Obstructive Pulmonary Disease Detected?

Researchers are still looking for accurate methods to predict a person's chances of developing airway obstruction. None of the current ways used to diagnose COPD detects the disease before irreversible lung damage occurs. While many measures of lung function have been developed, those most commonly used determine:

1. air-containing volume of the lung (lung volume),

2. the ability to move air into and out of the lung,

3. the rate at which gases diffuse between the lung and blood, and

4. blood levels of oxygen and carbon dioxide.

Lung volumes are measured by breathing into and out of a device called a spirometer. Some types of spirometers are very simple mechanical devices which record volume changes as air is added to or removed from them. Other kinds are more sophisticated and use various types of electronic equipment to determine and record the volume of air moved into and out of the lungs.

The three volume measures most relevant to COPD are forced vital capacity (FVC), residual volume (RV), and total lung capacity (TLC). The forced vital capacity is the maximum volume of air which can be forcibly expelled after inhaling as deeply as possible. Not all of the air in the lungs is removed when measuring the vital capacity. The amount remaining is called the residual volume. The total lung capacity is the combination of the forced vital capacity and residual volume. While most of the measured lung volumes or capacities change to some degree with COPD, residual volume usually increases quite markedly. This increase is the result of the weakened airways collapsing before all the normally expired air can leave the lungs. The increased residual volume makes breathing even more difficult and labored.

Because COPD results in narrowed air passages, a measure of the rate at which air can be expelled from the lungs can also be used to determine how severe the narrowing has become. In this test, the forced vital capacity maneuver, the patient is asked to inhale as deeply as possible, and on signal, exhale as completely and as rapidly as possible. The volume of air exhaled within 1 second is then measured. This value is referred to as the forced expiratory volume in 1 second (FEV1). When FEV1 is used as an indicator of lung function, the average rate of decline in patients with chronic obstructive lung disease is observed to be two to three times the normal rate of 20-30 milliliters per year. This volume may also be expressed in terms of the percent of the vital capacity which can be expelled in 1 second. As COPD progresses, less air can be expelled in 1 second. A greater than expected annual fall in FEV1 is the most sensitive test for COPD and a fairly good predictor of disability and early death.

Another measure of lung function is called diffusing capacity. For this, a more complicated test determines the amount of gas which can move in a given period of time from the alveolar side of the lung into the blood. A number of conditions can cause the diffusing capacity to decrease. However, in COPD the decrease is the result of the destruction of alveolar walls which leads to a significant decrease in surface area for diffusion of oxygen into the blood.

Because the primary function of the lung is to remove carbon dioxide from the blood and add oxygen, another indicator of pulmonary function is the blood levels of oxygen and carbon dioxide. As chronic obstructive pulmonary disease progresses, the amount of oxygen in the blood decreases and carbon dioxide increases.

In most cases, it is necessary to compare the results of several different tests in order to make the correct diagnosis, and to repeat some tests at intervals to determine the rate of disease progression or improvement. Measurement of FEV1 and FEV1/FVC ratio should be a routine part of the physical examination of every COPD patient. It is hoped that current research will result in more accurate and earlier measures for detecting lung destruction and diminished function.

How Is Chronic Obstructive Pulmonary Disease Treated?

Although there is no cure for COPD, the disease can be prevented in many cases. And, in almost all cases the disabling symptoms can be reduced. Because cigarette smoking is the most important cause of COPD, not smoking almost always prevents COPD from developing, and quitting smoking slows the disease process.

If the patient and medical team develop and adhere to a program of complete respiratory care, disability can be minimized, acute episodes prevented, hospitalizations reduced, and some early deaths avoided. On the other hand, none of the therapies has been shown to slow the progression of the disease, and only oxygen therapy has been shown to increase the survival rate.

Home oxygen therapy can improve survival in patients with advanced COPD who have hypoxemia, low blood oxygen levels. This treatment can improve a patient's exercise tolerance and ability to perform on psychological tests which reflect different aspects of brain function and muscle coordination. Increasing the concentration of oxygen in blood also improves the function of the heart and prevents the development of cor pulmonale. Oxygen can also lessen sleeplessness, irritability, headaches, and the overproduction of red blood cells. Continuous oxygen therapy is recommended for patients with low oxygen levels at rest, during exercise, or while sleeping. Many oxygen sources are available for home use; these include tanks of compressed gaseous oxygen or liquid oxygen and devices that concentrate oxygen from room air. However, oxygen is expensive with the cost per patient running into several hundred dollars per month, depending on the type of system and on the locale.

Medications frequently prescribed for COPD patients include:

- Bronchodilators help open narrowed airways. There are three main categories:

  sympathomimetics (isoproterenol, metaproterenol, terbutaline, albuterol) which can be inhaled, injected, or taken by mouth;

  parasympathomimetics (atropine, ipratropium bromide); and

  methylxanthines (theophylline and its derivatives) which can be given intravenously, orally, or rectally.

- Corticosteroids or steroids (beclomethasone, dexamethasone, triamcinolone, flunisolide) lessen inflammation of the airway walls. They are sometimes used if airway obstruction cannot be kept under control with bronchodilators, and lung function is shown to improve on this therapy. Inhaled steroids given regularly may be of benefit in some patients and have few side effects.

- Antibiotics (tetracycline, ampicillin, erythromycin, and trimethoprim-sulfamethoxazole combinations) fight infection. They are frequently given at the first sign of a respiratory infection such as increased sputum production with a change in color of sputum from clear to yellow or green.

- Expectorants help loosen and expel mucus secretions from the airways.

- Diuretics help the body excrete excess fluid. They are given as therapy to avoid excess water retention associated with right-heart failure. Patients taking diuretics are monitored carefully because dehydration must be avoided. These drugs also may cause potassium imbalances which can lead to abnormal heart rhythms.

- Digitalis (usually in the form of digoxin) strengthens the force of the heartbeat. It is used very cautiously in patients who have COPD, especially if their blood oxygen tensions are low, because they are vulnerable to abnormal heart rhythms when taking this drug.

- Other drugs sometimes taken by patients with COPD are tranquilizers, pain killers (meperidine, morphine, propoxyphene, etc.), cough suppressants (codeine, etc.), and sleeping pills (barbiturates, etc.). All these drugs depress breathing to some extent; they are avoided whenever possible and used only with great caution.

A number of combination drugs containing various assortments of sympathomimetics, methylxanthines, expectorants, and sedatives are marketed and widely advertised. These drugs are undesirable for COPD patients for several reasons. It is difficult to adjust the dose of methylxanthines without getting interfering side effects from the other ingredients. The sympathomimetic drug used in these preparations is ephedrine, a drug with many side effects and less bronchodilating effect than other drugs now available. The combination drugs often contain sedatives to combat the unpleasant side effects of ephedrine. They also contain expectorants which have not been proven to be effective for all patients and may have some side effects.

Bullectomy, or surgical removal of large air spaces called bullae that are filled with stagnant air, may be beneficial in selected patients. Recently, use of lasers to remove bullae has been suggested.

Lung transplantation has been successfully employed in some patients with end-stage COPD. In the hands of an experienced team, the 1-year survival in patients with transplanted lungs is over 70 percent.

Pulmonary rehabilitation programs, along with medical treatment, are useful in certain patients with COPD. The goals are to improve overall physical endurance and generally help to overcome the conditions which cause dyspnea and limit capacity for physical exercise and activities of daily living. General exercise training increases performance, maximum oxygen consumption, and overall sense of well-being. Administration of oxygen and nutritional supplements when necessary can improve respiratory muscle strength. Intermittent mechanical ventilatory support relieves dyspnea and rests respiratory muscles in selected patients. Continuous positive airway pressure (CPAP) is used as an adjunct to weaning from mechanical ventilation to minimize dyspnea during exercise. Relaxation techniques may also reduce the perception of ventilatory effort and dyspnea. Breathing exercises and breathing techniques, such as pursed lips breathing and relaxation, improve functional status.

Keeping air passages reasonably clear of secretions is difficult for patients with advanced COPD. Some commonly used methods for mobilizing and removing secretions are the following:

- Postural bronchial drainage helps to remove secretions from the airways. The patient lies in prescribed positions that allow gravity to drain different parts of the lung. This is usually done after inhaling an aerosol. In the basic position, the patient lies on a bed with his chest and head over the side and his forearms resting on the floor.

- Chest percussion or lightly clapping the chest and back, may help dislodge tenacious or copious secretions.

- Controlled coughing techniques are taught to help the patient bring up secretions.

- Bland aerosols, often made from solutions of salt or bicarbonate of soda, are inhaled. These aerosols thin and loosen secretions. Treatments usually last 10 to 15 minutes and are taken three or four times a day. Bronchodilators are sometimes added to the aerosols.

How Can Patients with Chronic Obstructive Pulmonary Disease Cope Best with Their Illness?

In most instances of COPD, some irreversible damage has already occurred by the time the doctor diagnoses the disease. At this point, the patient and the family should learn as much as possible about the disease and how to live with it. The goals, limitations, and techniques of treatment must be understood by the patient so that symptoms can be kept under control, and daily living can proceed as normally as possible. The doctor and other health care providers are good sources of information about COPD education programs. Patients and family members can usually take part in educational programs offered at a hospital or by a local branch of the American Lung Association.

Patients with COPD can help themselves in many ways. They can:

- Stop smoking. Many programs are available to help smokers quit smoking and to stay off tobacco. Some programs are based on behavior modification techniques; others combine these methods with nicotine gum or nicotine patches as aids to help smokers gradually overcome their dependence on nicotine.

- Avoid work-related exposures to dusts and fumes.

- Avoid air pollution, including cigarette smoke, and curtail physical activities during air pollution alerts.

- Refrain from intimate contact with people who have respiratory infections such as colds or the flu and get a one-time pneumonia vaccination (polyvalent pneumococcal vaccination) and yearly influenza shots.

- Avoid excessive heat, cold, and very high altitudes. (Note: Commercial aircraft cruise at high altitudes and maintain a cabin pressure equal to that of an elevation of 5,000 to 10,000 feet. This can result in hypoxemia for some COPD patients. However, with supplemental oxygen, most COPD patients can travel on commercial airlines.)

- Drink a lot of fluids. This is a good way to keep sputum loose so that it can be brought up by coughing.

- Maintain good nutrition. Usually a high protein diet, taken as many small feedings, is recommended.

- Consider "allergy shots." COPD patients often also have allergies or asthma which complicate COPD.

Of all the avoidable risk factors for COPD, smoking is by far the most significant. Cessation of smoking is the best way to decrease one's risk of developing COPD.

What Types of Research on Chronic Obstructive Pulmonary Disease Is the NHLBI Supporting?

The National Heart, Lung, and Blood Institute (NHLBI) is supporting a number of research programs on COPD with the following objectives:

1. to understand its underlying causes,
2. to develop methods of early detection,
3. to improve treatment, and
4. to help patient's and their families better manage the disease.

A study completed several years ago examined the use of oxygen therapy for people who, because of COPD, cannot get enough oxygen into their blood by breathing air. This study has determined that continuous oxygen therapy is more beneficial in extending life than giving oxygen only for 12 hours at night.

Another clinical study compared inhalation therapy using a machine which administers medication to the lungs by intermittent positive pressure breathing (IPPB) with one that delivers the medicine by relying on the patient's own breathing. Although home use of IPPB machines is widespread, previous studies had not been able to show conclusively whether they were effective. In this study, 985 ambulatory patients with COPD were randomly assigned to a treatment group which received a bronchodilator aerosol solution by IPPB, or to a control group which received the medication via a compressor nebulizer. The only difference between the two groups was the positive pressure applied by the IPPB. There was no statistically significant difference between the two treatment groups in numbers of deaths, frequency and length of hospitalization, change in lung function tests, or in measurements of quality of life. This study suggests that the use of IPPB devices may be unnecessary.

An intervention trial called the Lung Health Study, which began in 1983, has enrolled approximately 6,000 smokers in a study to determine whether an intervention program incorporating smoking cessation and use of inhaled bronchodilators (to keep air passages open) in men and women at high risk of developing COPD can slow the decline in pulmonary function compared to a group receiving usual care. When this study is completed, it should help to determine the extent to which identification and treatment of asymptomatic subjects with early signs of obstructive lung disease would be useful as a preventive health measure. In addition, the study will test some of the current theories about behavior and smoking cessation. Early results indicate that cigarette smoking may be more harmful to women than to men. Furthermore, smoking cessation results in greater weight gain in women than in men, and to avoid weight gain women are less likely to quit smoking and more likely to revert to their smoking habit.

Because familial emphysema results from a deficiency of AAT in affected individuals, efforts to minimize the risk of emphysema have been directed at increasing the circulating AAT levels either by promoting or increasing the production of AAT within the individual, or augmenting it from the outside. One strategy for improving the production of AAT is by pharmacological means (e.g., by administration of drugs such as danazol or estrogen/progesterone combinations), but this has not been found to be effective. Genetic engineering to correct the defective gene or introduce the functional gene in the deficient individuals is being attempted by several NHLBI-supported investigators. The normal gene for AAT as well as the mutant genes causing AAT deficiency have been characterized and cloned, and animal models carrying the mutant gene have been developed. The resulting animals displayed many of the physical and histologic changes seen in human neonatal AAT deficiency. These studies should provide the groundwork for future development of gene replacement therapy for AAT deficiency.

In the meantime, attention is being focused on AAT augmentation therapy for familial emphysema. Studies have shown that intravenous infusion of AAT fractionated from blood is safe and biochemically effective, that is, the needed blood levels of AAT can be maintained by the continued administration of AAT at appropriate intervals.

Because of the practical and fiscal limitations to mounting a clinical trial for establishing the clinical efficacy of AAT augmentation therapy for emphysema, the NHLBI sponsored a national registry of patients with AAT deficiency to assess the natural history of severe AAT deficiency and to examine whether the disease course is altered by the augmentation therapy. This program is enrolling, at various medical centers both in the U.S. and Europe, at least 1,000 adult patients with AAT deficiency satisfying certain other eligibility criteria. The patients will be followed for 3 to 5 years (chest x rays, lung function, blood and urine analysis, etc.) at one of 37 participating clinical centers. The evaluation of the data and the release of the conclusions are expected by early 1995.

Methods to treat emphysema before it becomes disabling remain an important research objective of programs supported by NHLBI. Since it is believed that either excess protease (elastase), or too little useful antiprotease, can lead to development of the disease, scientists have also been attempting to use other approaches to develop animal models which will mimic the human condition of inherited alpha-1-protease inhibitor deficiency and using such models to test if natural or synthetic antiproteases can be used safely to prevent development of emphysema-like lesions in these animals. If found safe and effective in animals, these agents can be tried in humans.

Chapter 15

Colds

What Is a Cold?

A cold is a minor infection of the nose and throat that lasts from a few days to a few weeks. Five different families of viruses cause colds. The Rhinovirus family causes nearly half of all colds and over 100 different varieties of Rhinovirus have been discovered. (Rhino means nose in Greek.) Because so many different viruses can cause this infection, it is unlikely that there will ever be a vaccine to protect people from catching a cold.

How Often Do People Get Colds?

Colds are common. In fact, colds are the leading cause of visits to the doctor in the United States. Adults have an average of two to four colds per year, and young children have an average of six to eight. In general, people experience far more colds between the months of September and May. Summer colds are relatively rare.

No Virus, No Cold

In order for a person to catch a cold, a cold-causing virus must first come in contact with the lining of their nose. Viruses that touch the lining of the eyes or mouth can make their way to the nose.

In some cases, the virus can travel through the air: a person with a cold sneezes, propelling droplets of mucus and virus particles into the air, and then a second person breathes this air in, allowing the virus to become attached to the lining of the nose.

However, the more likely path of transmission for these viruses is by direct contact. For example, a young child with a cold touches his face, spreading some mucus (and virus particles) to his fingers. These fingers eventually touch a mother's hands, transferring the virus to her skin. This woman then touches her nose or eyes or lips, allowing the virus into her body.

Cold viruses can also be picked up from the surfaces of objects. So touching an object that has been handled by someone with a cold and then touching one's face could also lead to a cold.

Symptoms

Almost everyone is familiar with cold symptoms. These symptoms usually develop anywhere from one to three days after the virus enters the body. The symptoms of the average cold last about one week. However, in roughly one out of every four cases, the illness lasts up to two weeks. In general, cold symptoms—especially the cough—tend to be worse in smokers.

- People generally complain of increased nasal discharge (a runny nose), difficulty breathing through the nose, sneezing, a scratchy throat, and cough.

- The ability to taste and to smell may be affected, hoarseness may develop, and the voice often develops a nasal quality.

- Adults may experience a slight fever, while infants and young children may develop a higher temperature.

Cold symptoms result from the virus invading the lining of the nose and throat, and from the reaction of the body's immune system. Mucus production increases, causing the nose to "run." The blood vessels in the lining of the nose swell, leading to clogged breathing passages. Sneezing is a protective reflex, triggered by irritation within the nose. Cough is also a protective reflex, triggered by irritation of the throat and by mucus dripping down from the nose (commonly referred to as a "post-nasal drip").

Cold Prevention

Colds are so common that it is nearly impossible to completely avoid catching one. However, there are a number of steps you can take to lower your risk:

- If possible, avoid close contact with people who have a cold, especially during the first three days when they are most likely to spread the infection.

- Wash your hands after touching the skin of someone who has a cold, or after touching an object that they have touched.

- Keep your fingers away from your nose and your eyes.

To avoid spreading a cold to others, take these specific steps:

- Cover your nose and mouth with disposable tissues when you cough or sneeze.

- Wash your hands after coughing or sneezing.

- If possible, stay away from people with asthma or chronic lung disease when you have a cold, especially during the first three days when you are most contagious.

Treatment

It's important to drink adequate quantities of liquids, water or juices. Staying well-hydrated helps prevent the drying of the lining of the nose and throat, and thereby helps keep the mucus moist and flowing out of the body. Avoid caffeinated beverages such as coffee, tea and colas, as caffeine can lead to dehydration.

There is no cure for a cold. While some medications are available to treat specific viruses, none have yet been developed to treat the viruses that cause colds. Antibiotics are not useful for colds, because they are used to treat infections caused by bacteria, not viruses. And, because of the risk of side effects, antibiotics could possibly be harmful.

While there is no cure, many medications can help relieve cold symptoms. These products will not make the cold go away faster, but they can lessen the discomfort caused by the infection, making the illness more bearable.

There are literally hundreds of products available to treat cold symptoms. The sheer number of remedies has led to confusion about what to take, when, and for which symptoms.

Current scientific evidence about cold remedies supports the following general recommendations:

- Early treatment is best: treatment should begin as soon as one feels cold symptoms developing. If possible, use medications regularly in order to prevent sneezing or coughing from getting out of control.

- Don't smoke, and avoid being around other people who are smoking. Inhaled smoke can further irritate the throat, worsening a cough.

- The preferred medication to relieve the discomfort associated with colds is acetaminophen (e.g., TYLENOL). Acetaminophen is less likely to upset the stomach than aspirin and other non-steroidal anti-inflammatory drugs (NSAIDs) such as ibuprofen (e.g., Motrin IB or Advil).

  Asthmatics and people with a history of peptic ulcer disease should not take any medication that contains aspirin or other NSAIDs without the advice of their doctor.

- For other symptoms, such as congestion, cough or nasal discharge, a combination of products may be used. Blocked nasal passages, nasal discharge and post-nasal drip are best treated with both a decongestant and an antihistamine. There are many over-the-counter cold remedies that contain both of these ingredients.

- The newer, non-sedating antihistamines do not appear to be as effective in relieving cold symptoms as the older medications in this class. While these older antihistamines, such as diphenhydramine (e.g.,Benadryl) and chlorpheniramine (e.g.,Chlor-Trimeton) tend to cause drowsiness, they are more likely to relieve nasal congestion and cough.

- Follow dosage instructions on all product labels.

Complications

Colds are self-limited. In other words, they always get better, with or without medication, within a few weeks. However, the cold viruses can affect the lining of the upper respiratory system in a way that leads to other infections, such as sinusitis, ear infections or bronchitis.

For these reasons, if any of the following occur, one should consult a physician for evaluation:

- Cold symptoms are unusually severe or associated with high fever

- Sinus pain or a toothache develops

- Ear pain develops

- A cough gets worse, rather than better, as the cold symptoms improve

Asthma (reversible narrowing of the airways) and bronchitis (prolonged inflammation of the airways, with cough) can be triggered by a cold. In addition, people who already have asthma, chronic bronchitis or emphysema are likely to suffer worsening of their symptoms for many weeks after they recover from a cold.

Colds in Children

Nearly all young children develop colds frequently—an average of six to eight times a year. After age six, colds become less frequent. Teenagers develop colds about as often as adults do—two to four times a year.

Any infant with a fever and cold symptoms should be seen by a physician. In both infants and children, the main goals of treatment are to make the child as comfortable as possible and to relieve nasal congestion. A vaporizer or humidifier should be used to prevent the mucus in the nose from becoming dry and hard. In young infants, saline nasal drops and gentle suction with a bulb syringe can help keep the nasal passages clear.

As in adults, acetaminophen (e.g., Children's TYLENOL) is preferred for treating fever and pain in children. Pediatric ibuprofen (e.g., Children's Motrin or Children's Advil) can also be used for this purpose. Aspirin should not be used, as it has been associated with a serious complication known as Reye syndrome when given to children with influenza (and it can be hard to differentiate colds from influenza in young children).

Cold Facts and Fallacies

- Large doses of Vitamin C have not been proven to effectively prevent or cure colds. It is important, however, to take the minimum daily requirement.

- Zinc lozenges may help people recover from colds more quickly—or they may not. The evidence from studies completed so far has been inconclusive.

- "Put on a coat or you'll catch a cold!"...Unlikely. Research shows that exposure to extreme cold can lead to pneumonia, not to cold or flu. But it's important to dress warmly anyway—pneumonia is something to be avoided.

- Working on a cold. Going to work or school with a cold probably won't prolong the symptoms. But it does pose a risk of passing the cold on to others. If you do venture out, wash your hands often and use disposable tissues.

- "Starve a cold and feed a fever" is not good advice. Your intake of fluids, such as water and juices, should be increased when you have a cold or fever. Hot fluids can help treat a cough. In general, you should eat enough to satisfy your appetite.

- Herbal treatments, such as echinacea, are widely touted as an alternative therapy for colds. However, there is no significant clinical evidence that this, or other types of herbal treatments, are effective.

- Alcohol toddies. Alcohol should be avoided when one has a cold.

- Chicken soup is a good source of hot liquids, but does not have special curative effects.

Chapter 16

Cystic Fibrosis

What Is Cystic Fibrosis

Cystic fibrosis (CF) is a chronic, progressive, and frequently fatal genetic (inherited) disease of the body's mucus glands. CF primarily affects the respiratory and digestive systems in children and young adults. The sweat glands and the reproductive system are also usually involved. On the average, individuals with CF have a lifespan of approximately 30 years.

CF-like disease has been known for over two centuries. The name, cystic fibrosis of the pancreas, was first applied to the disease in 1938.

How Common Is CF?

According to the data collected by the Cystic Fibrosis Foundation, there are about 30,000 Americans, 3,000 Canadians, and 20,000 Europeans with CF. The disease occurs mostly in whites whose ancestors came from northern Europe, although it affects all races and ethnic groups.

Accordingly, it is less common in African Americans, Native Americans, and Asian Americans. Approximately 2,500 babies are born with CF each year in the United States. Also, about 1 in every 20 Americans is an unaffected carrier of an abnormal "CF gene." These 12 million people are usually unaware that they are carriers.

National Heart, Lung, and Blood Institute (NHLBI), NIH Publication Number 95-3650, 1997.

What Are the Signs and Symptoms of CF?

CF does not follow the same pattern in all patients but affects different people in different ways and to varying degrees. However, the basic problem is the same—an abnormality in the glands, which produce or secrete sweat and mucus. Sweat cools the body; mucus lubricates the respiratory, digestive, and reproductive systems, and prevents tissues from drying out, protecting them from infection.

People with CF lose excessive amounts of salt when they sweat. This can upset the balance of minerals in the blood, which may cause abnormal heart rhythms. Going into shock is also a risk.

Mucus in CF patients is very thick and accumulates in the intestines and lungs. The result is malnutrition, poor growth, frequent respiratory infections, breathing difficulties, and eventually permanent lung damage. Lung disease is the usual cause of death in most patients.

CF can cause various other medical problems. These include sinusitis (inflammation of the nasal sinuses, which are cavities in the skull behind, above, and on both sides of the nose), nasal polyps (fleshy growths inside the nose), clubbing (rounding and enlargement of fingers and toes), pneumothorax (rupture of lung tissue and trapping of air between the lung and the chest wall), hemoptysis (coughing of blood), cor pulmonale (enlargement of the right side of the heart), abdominal pain and discomfort, gassiness (too much gas in the intestine), and rectal prolapse (protrusion of the rectum through the anus). Liver disease, diabetes, inflammation of the pancreas, and gallstones also occur in some people with CF.

When Should You Suspect That a Child May Have CF?

CF symptoms vary from child to child. A baby born with the CF genes usually has symptoms during its first year. Sometimes, however, signs of the disease may not show up until adolescence or even later. Infants or young children should be tested for CF if they have persistent diarrhea, bulky foul-smelling and greasy stools, frequent wheezing or pneumonia, a chronic cough with thick mucus, salty-tasting skin, or poor growth. CF should be suspected in babies born with an intestinal blockage called meconium ileus.

How Is CF Diagnosed?

The most common test for CF is called the sweat test. It measures the amount of salt (sodium chloride) in the sweat. In this test, an area of the skin (usually the forearm) is made to sweat by using a chemical called pilocarpine and applying a mild electric current. To collect the sweat, the area is covered with a gauze pad or filter paper and wrapped in plastic. After 30 to 40 minutes, the plastic is removed, and the sweat collected in the pad or paper is analyzed. Higher than normal amounts of sodium and chloride suggest that the person has cystic fibrosis.

Autosomal Recessive Inheritance

The presence of two mutant genes is needed for CF to appear. Each parent carries one defective gene and one normal gene. The single normal gene is sufficient for normal function of the mucus glands, and the parents are therefore CF-free. Each child has a 25 percent risk of inheriting two defective genes and getting CF, a 25 percent chance of inheriting two normal genes, and a 50 percent chance of being an unaffected carrier like the parents.

The sweat test may not work well in newborns because they do not produce enough sweat. In that case, another type of test, such as the immunoreactive trypsinogen test (IRT), may be used. In the IRT test, blood drawn 2 to 3 days after birth is analyzed for a specific protein called trypsinogen. Positive IRT tests must be confirmed by sweat and other tests.

Also, a small percentage of people with CF have normal sweat chloride levels. They can only be diagnosed by chemical tests for the presence of the mutated gene. Some of the other tests that can assist in the diagnosis of CF are chest x-rays, lung function tests, and sputum (phlegm) cultures. Stool examinations can help identify the digestive abnormalities that are typical of CF.

What Makes CF a Genetic Disease?

Genes are the basic units of heredity. They are located on structures within the cell nucleus called chromosomes. The function of most genes is to instruct the cells to make particular proteins, most of which have important life-sustaining roles.

Every human being has 46 chromosomes, 23 inherited from each parent. Because each of the 23 pairs of chromosomes contains a complete set of genes, every individual has two sets (one from each parent) of genes for each function. In some individuals, the basic building blocks of a gene (called base pairs) are altered (mutated). A mutation can cause the body to make a defective protein or no protein at all.

The result is a loss of some essential biological function and that leads to disease. Children may inherit altered genes from one or both parents.

Diseases such as CF that are caused by inherited genes are called genetic diseases. In CF, each parent carries one abnormal CF gene and one normal CF gene but shows no evidence of the disease because the normal CF gene dominates or "recesses" the abnormal CF gene. To have CF, a child must inherit two abnormal genes—one from each parent. The recessive CF gene can occur in both boys and girls because it is located on non-sex-linked chromosomes called autosomal chromosomes. CF is therefore called an autosomal recessive genetic disease.

Each child, whether male or female, has a 25 percent risk of inheriting a defective gene from each parent and of having CF. A child born to two CF patients (an unlikely event) would be at a 100 percent risk of developing CF.

How Is CF Treated?

Since CF is a genetic disease, the only way to prevent or cure it would be with gene therapy at an early age. Ideally, gene therapy could repair or replace the defective gene. Another option for treatment would be to give a person with CF the active form of the protein product that is scarce or missing.

At present, neither gene therapy nor any other kind of treatment exists for the basic causes of CF, although several drug-based approaches are being investigated. In the meantime, the best that doctors can do is to ease the symptoms of CF or slow the progress of the disease so the patient's quality of life is improved. This is achieved by antibiotic therapy combined with treatments to clear the thick mucus from the lungs. The therapy is tailored to the needs of each patient. For patients whose disease is very advanced, lung transplantation may be an option.

CF was once always fatal in childhood. Better treatment methods developed over the past 20 years have increased the average lifespan of CF patients to nearly 30 years.

Management of Lung Problems

A major focus of CF treatment is the obstructed breathing that causes frequent lung infections. Physical therapy, exercise, and medications are used to reduce the mucus blockage of the lung's airways.

Chest therapy consists of bronchial, or postural, drainage, which is done by placing the patient in a position that allows drainage of the mucus from the lungs. At the same time, the chest or back is clapped (percussed) and vibrated to dislodge the mucus and help it move out of the airways.

This process is repeated over different parts of the chest and back to loosen the mucus in different areas of each lung. This procedure has to be done for children by family members but older patients can learn to do it by themselves. Mechanical aids that help chest physical therapy are available commercially. Exercise also helps to loosen the mucus, stimulate coughing to clear the mucus, and improve the patient's overall physical condition.

Medications used to help breathing are often aerosolized (misted) and can be inhaled. These medicines include bronchodilators (which widen the breathing tubes), mucolytics (which thin the mucus), and decongestants (which reduce swelling of the membranes of the breathing tubes). A recent advance, approved by the Food and Drug Administration, is an inhaled aerosolized enzyme that thins the mucus by digesting the cellular material trapped in it. Antibiotics to fight lung infections also are used and may be taken orally or in aerosol form, or by injection into a vein.

Management of Digestive Problems

The digestive problems in CF are less serious and more easily managed than those in the lungs. A well-balanced, high-caloric diet, low in fat and high in protein, and pancreatic enzymes (which help digestion) are often prescribed. Supplements of vitamins A, D, E, and K are given to ensure good nutrition. Enemas and mucolytic agents are used to treat intestinal obstructions.

How Does the Gene Mutation Cause CF?

The CF gene was identified in 1989. Since then, a great deal has been learned about this gene and its protein product. The biochemical abnormality in CF results from a mutation in a gene that produces a protein responsible for the movement through the cell membranes of chloride ions (a component of sodium chloride, or common table salt). The protein is called CFTR—cystic fibrosis transmembrane regulator.

CFTR is present in cells that line the passageways of the lungs, pancreas, colon, and genitourinary tract. When this protein is abnormal, two of the hallmarks of CF result—blockage of the movement of chloride ions and water in the lung and other cells and secretion of abnormal mucus.

The mutation involved in CF causes the deletion of three of the base pairs in the gene. This in turn, causes a loss in the CFTR protein of an amino acid (the building blocks of proteins). Because phenyla-lanine is located in position 508 of the protein chain, this mutant pro-tein is called deltaF508 CFTR.

However, deltaF508 CFTR accounts for only 70-80 percent of all CF cases. Various other mutations—over 400 at the last count—seem to be responsible for the remaining CF cases. Differences in disease patterns seen in individuals and families probably result from the combined effects of the particular mutation and various, but still un-known, factors in the CF patient and his or her environment.

Gene Therapy—The Future of CF Treatment?

Gene therapy for CF is not yet possible but impressive progress is being made in developing ways to treat the gene abnormality that causes CF. In the laboratory, scientists have been able to grow cells from the nasal passages of CF patients. By introducing the normal gene into these cells, researchers corrected the cells' chloride trans-port abnormality. The chloride defect has also been corrected in small regions in the nasal passages themselves by giving CF patients the normal gene in nose drops.

Scientists are still looking for answers to many questions about gene therapy. Some of these questions are:

- How should the gene be packaged?
- What are the best ways to get the gene-containing package into the patient's lungs?
- What will the long-term results of this treatment be?
- Can the abnormal chloride transport be corrected in other parts of the body?
- How long will the correction last?
- And, most importantly, can gene therapy cure or prevent the lung disease in CF?

Is It Possible to Detect CF in an Unborn Baby?

Finding out whether a baby is likely to have CF is possible using prenatal genetic tests. However, the tests cannot detect all of the CF gene mutations. Also, because these tests are very expensive and have certain risks to the mother, they are not used for all pregnant women. If there is another child with CF in the family, the expectant mother may request a prenatal test to see if the fetus has CF genes from both parents, is a carrier for one gene, or is altogether free of the CF genes.

There are two special prenatal tests that can be done—either an amniocentesis or chorionic villus biopsy will be performed. In amniocentesis, cells from the fluid surrounding the baby in the mother's womb (called the amniotic fluid) are tested to see if the CF genes common to the parents are present. In chorionic villus biopsy, cells from the tissue that will eventually form the placenta are tested for the CF gene.

Can CF Be Prevented?

At this time, preventing CF is not possible. In babies with two abnormal CF genes, the disease is already present at birth in some organs, such as the pancreas and liver, but develops only after birth in the lungs. Someday, gene therapy may be used to prevent the lung disease from developing.

Yet, CF might be prevented in the future. Since CF occurs only when both parents pass on a CF gene to a child, it could be prevented by identifying all carriers of CF genes. Genetic counselors might then persuade couples who are carriers not to have children. However, as noted, current tests can detect only some of the more than 400 gene mutations and so the tests are only 80-85 percent accurate.

Yet, progress in gene therapy and the realization that not all CF mutations are life-threatening should reassure couples. Potential parents who carry the defective gene may choose to have children.

How Can Patients and Their Families and Friends Be Helped to Cope with CF?

CF education helps patients and their families face the physical and emotional effects of the disease and encourages CF patients to lead active, fulfilling lives. Educational programs and materials suitable for both patients of various ages and their parents are available from local CF centers and from local chapters of the CF Foundation.

Patients and their families and friends should know that:

- CF parents should not feel guilty or responsible for causing their child's disease; they could not have prevented it.

- Parents should treat their children with CF as normally as possible. They shouldn't be over-protective but should encourage them to be active and self-reliant.

- Family and friends should remember that CF is not contagious; nobody can get it from a patient.

- In families with CF, brothers, sisters, and first cousins of the CF patient should be tested to see if they carry a defective gene, especially if they seem to have a chronic lung or digestive problem. Carriers of the abnormal gene should get genetic counseling.

- Individuals with CF have normal sexual development and can expect to have a normal sex life. However, most, but not all, men are infertile because of a mechanical blockage of sperm and cannot have children. Women with CF can have children, although they may be less fertile   than women without CF.

- Patients and families should work closely with doctors and other medical specialists to develop self-management skills that can improve their quality of life.

Above all, CF patients and their families should keep a positive attitude. Scientists continue to make significant advances in understanding the genetic and physiological disturbances in CF and in developing new treatment approaches such as gene therapy. The outlook is bright for further improvements in the care of CF patients and even for the discovery of a cure.

For More Information

Additional information about CF can be obtained from the following organizations:

National Heart, Lung, and Blood Institute (NHLBI)
Information Center
P.O. Box 30105
Bethesda, MD 20824-0105
Tel: 301-592-8573

National Diabetes Information Clearinghouse
1 Information Way
Bethesda, MD 20892-3560
Toll Free: 800-891-5388
Tel: 301-654-3327

The Cystic Fibrosis Foundation
6931 Arlington Road, #200
Bethesda, MD 20814
Toll Free: 800-344-4823
Tel: 301-951-4422

Chapter 17

Emphysema

What Is Emphysema?

Emphysema is a condition in which there is over-inflation of structures in the lungs known as alveoli or air sacs. This over-inflation results from a breakdown of the walls of the alveoli, which causes a decrease in respiratory function (the way the lungs work) and often, breathlessness.

Early symptoms of emphysema include shortness of breath and cough. Emphysema and chronic bronchitis together comprise chronic obstructive pulmonary disease (COPD).

How Serious Is Emphysema?

Emphysema is a widespread disease of the lungs. Currently there are about 2.0 million Americans in the U.S. who have emphysema.

Emphysema ranks 15th among chronic conditions that contribute to activity limitations: almost 44 percent of individuals with emphysema report that their daily activities have been limited by the disease.

Many of the people with emphysema are older men, but the condition is increasing among women. Males with emphysema outnumber females by more than 54 percent.

Causes of Emphysema

It is known from scientific research that the normal lung has a remarkable balance between two classes of chemicals with opposing action. The elastic fibers in the lung allow the lungs to expand and contract. When the chemical balance is altered, the lungs lose the ability to protect themselves against the destruction of these elastic fibers. This is what happens in emphysema.

There are a number of reasons this chemical imbalance occurs. Smoking is responsible for 82 percent of COPD (chronic obstructive pulmonary disease), including emphysema.

It is estimated that 50,000 to 100,000 Americans living today were born with a deficiency of a protein known as alpha 1-antitrypsin (AAT) which can lead to an inherited form of emphysema called alpha 1-antitrypsin (AAT) deficiency-related emphysema.

How Does Emphysema Develop?

Emphysema begins with the destruction of air sacs (alveoli) in the lungs where oxygen from the air is exchanged for carbon dioxide in the blood. The walls of the air sacs are thin and fragile. Damage to the air sacs is irreversible and results in permanent "holes" in the tissues of the lower lungs.

As air sacs are destroyed, the lungs are able to transfer less and less oxygen to the bloodstream, causing shortness of breath. The lungs also lose their elasticity. The patient experiences great difficulty exhaling.

Emphysema doesn't develop suddenly, it comes on very gradually. Years of exposure to the irritation of cigarette smoke usually precede the development of emphysema.

A person may initially visit the doctor because he or she has begun to feel short of breath during activity or exercise. As the disease progresses, a brief walk can be enough to bring on difficulty in breathing. Some people may have had chronic bronchitis before developing emphysema.

Treatment for Emphysema

Doctors can help persons with emphysema live more comfortably with their disease. The goal of treatment is to provide relief of symptoms and prevent progression of the disease with a minimum of side effects. The doctor's advice and treatment may include:

- *Quitting smoking:* the single most important factor for maintaining healthy lungs.

- *Bronchodilator drugs* (prescription drugs that relax and open air passages in the lungs): may be prescribed to treat emphysema if there is a tendency toward airway constriction or tightening. These drugs may be inhaled as aerosol sprays or taken orally.

- *Antibiotics:* if you have a bacterial infection, such as pneumococcal pneumonia.

- *Exercise:* including breathing exercises to strengthen the muscles used in breathing as part of a pulmonary rehabilitation program to condition the rest of the body.

- *Treatment:* with Alpha 1-Proteinase Inhibitor (A1PI) only if a person has AAT deficiency-related emphysema. A1PI is not recommended for those who develop emphysema as a result of cigarette smoking or other environmental factors.

- *Lung transplantation:* Recent reports have been encouraging.

Lung volume reduction surgery is a new modification of a surgical procedure in which the most severely diseases portions of the lung are removed to allow the remaining lung and breathing muscles to work better. Studies are promising.

Prevention of Emphysema

Continuing research is being done to find answers to many questions about emphysema, especially about the best ways to prevent the disease.

Researchers know that quitting smoking can prevent the occurrence and decrease the progression of emphysema. Other environmental controls can also help prevent the disease.

If an individual has emphysema, the doctor will work hard to prevent the disease from getting worse by keeping the patient healthy and clear of any infection. The patient can participate in this prevention effort by following these general health guidelines:

- DON'T SMOKE. The majority of those who get emphysema are smokers. Continued smoking makes emphysema worse, especially for those who have AAT deficiency, the inherited form of emphysema.

- Maintain overall good health habits, which include proper nutrition, adequate sleep, and regular exercise to build up your stamina and resistance to infections.

- Reduce your exposure to air pollution, which may aggravate symptoms of emphysema. Refer to radio or television weather reports or your local newspaper for information about air quality. On days when the ozone (smog) level is unhealthy, restrict your activity to early morning or evening. When pollution levels are dangerous, remain indoors and stay as comfortable as possible.

- Consult your doctor at the start of any cold or respiratory infection because infection can make your emphysema symptoms worse. Ask about getting vaccinated against influenza and pneumococcal pneumonia.

Chapter 18

Inherited Emphysema

Chronic obstructive pulmonary disease or COPD for short, is a progressive lung disease that affects millions of people each year. COPD is a general term used to describe specific diseases such as emphysema and chronic bronchitis. Emphysema involves destruction of the walls of the air sacs (alveoli) in the lungs.

What Is Inherited Emphysema?

Most cases of emphysema are caused by smoking or other environmental factors. However, in a small number of cases of emphysema, there is a hereditary basis for the disease. Emphysema is characterized by progressive shortness of breath (dyspnea) and cough. This disease can cause air to become trapped in the lung, which is called hyperinflation.

The inherited form of emphysema is called alpha-1 proteinase inhibitor deficiency or "alpha-one" for short. People with this disease have a deficiency in a major protein, alpha-1 proteinase inhibitor. [Please see Chapter 6 for more information about alpha-1 antitrypsin deficiency.] Although there are many different genetic variations of this disorder, only some will cause lung disease. It is more commonly seen in individuals of northern African and northern European descent, especially Scandinavians.

What Does the Alpha-1 Protein Do in the Body?

Alpha-1 proteinase inhibitor is a major protein in the blood. It is produced primarily in the liver cells but also by some white blood cells. It protects the lung by blocking the effects of powerful enzymes called elastases. Elastase is normally carried in white blood cells and protects the delicate tissue of the lung by killing bacteria and neutralizing tiny particles inhaled into the lung. Once the protective work of this enzyme is finished, further action is blocked by the alpha-1 proteinase inhibitor. Without alpha-1 proteinase inhibitor, elastase can destroy the air sacs of the lung.

How Is the Diagnosis Made?

Because inherited emphysema is one of the chronic obstructive lung diseases, the diagnosis is made by the same methods. These methods include a complete medical history and physical examination, a family history of lung disease, a chest x-ray and may include other special x-rays (computerized tomography or CT scan) and pulmonary function tests (breathing tests).

Two specific blood tests determine the diagnosis of inherited emphysema. The first test measures the concentration of alpha-1 antiproteinase inhibitor in the plasma or serum. A second blood test can be done to determine the actual gene in both the person with the disease and in family members. Healthy individuals have an MM genetic pattern which leads to normal levels of alpha-1antiproteinase inhibitor in the blood. The most common abnormal genetic pattern associated with inherited emphysema is ZZ. Some persons may inherit a single gene for inherited emphysema, this may be MZ. It is unclear whether this abnormal gene leads to emphysema.

How Is Inherited Emphysema Managed?

A new therapy has been available for inherited emphysema since 1987, a special medication called Prolastin. This medicine replaces the alpha-1 protein in the blood. It is given intravenously and the dose is dependent on body weight. This treatment is usually given once a month. Long term studies are being conducted to determine the effectiveness of Prolastin in preventing further lung destruction.

In addition to medications, the management of inherited emphysema includes exercise and a healthy lifestyle, avoidance of infection, bronchial hygiene, oxygen therapy and pulmonary rehabilitation. For more information, ask your health care professional for information on any of these topics. Smoking cessation and avoidance of secondhand smoke is extremely important, since smoking can accelerate or speed the development of the disease and shorten the life span. Genetic counseling is important for family members of the person diagnosed with inherited emphysema to address family planning issues and early interventions, such as smoking cessation. Lung transplantation may be an option for younger persons severely affected by the disorder.

What Does the Future Hold?

Inherited emphysema is a common inherited disorder and because of this, research is constantly being done to develop new therapies. One potentially promising therapy is replacement of the abnormal gene. Doctors and researchers at National Jewish Medical and Research Center are looking for new ways to manage and treat this and other chronic lung diseases.

Chapter 19

Influenza

Influenza is a potentially life-threatening, contagious disease that is caused by a virus. When influenza attacks the lungs, the lining of the respiratory tract is damaged. The tissues temporarily become swollen and inflamed but usually heal within two or more weeks.

Influenza and pneumonia combined are the sixth leading cause of death among all Americans and the fifth leading cause of death among all Americans over the age of 65. Influenza and pneumonia together resulted in 82,727 deaths in 1996.

In 1995, there were more than 108 million estimated cases of influenza nationwide, resulting in 192.9 million bed days.

Total annual costs of influenza are estimated at $14.6 billion in the U.S. This includes $1.4 billion in direct health care costs, which are primarily hospital care, physician, and other health service costs. There were also $13.2 billion in indirect health costs comprised of lost earnings due to illness and lost future earnings due to mortality from influenza.

According to the most recent data, in 1995 there were an estimated 75.1 million work-loss days attributed to influenza (in employed persons age 18 and over).

For healthy children and adults, influenza is typically a moderately severe illness. For unhealthy people, influenza can be very dangerous.

Adults 65 years of age and older who contract influenza are much more likely to have serious complications from this illness, which can affect their health and independence.

A person can have influenza more than once because the virus that causes influenza may belong to different strains of one of three different influenza virus families, A, B, or C. Type A viruses tend to have a disproportionate effect on adults, Type B viruses have a disproportionate effect on children. Both A and B have strains that cause illness of varying severity. The influenza A family has more strains than the B family.

Influenza can be prevented with the influenza vaccine. This vaccine is produced each year so that it can be effective against influenza viruses that are expected to cause illness that year. A yearly influenza vaccination has been reported to be between 67 and 92 percent effective in preventing influenza and reducing the severity of the influenza.

In 1997, 65.5% of U.S. adults age 65 and older received an influenza vaccine during the preceding year.

Target populations for influenza vaccine include people 65 years of age and older, health care workers and people with chronic health conditions such as lung disease.

Influenza vaccines are covered by Medicare and other health insurance programs.

Most people experience little or no reaction to the vaccine. One in four people may have a swollen, red, tender area where the vaccination is given.

The best period to receive the influenza vaccine is soon after the vaccine becomes available in the fall of each year.

Influenza is a very serious illness for anyone at high risk. Certain diseases that place people at high risk include:

- chronic lung disease such as asthma, emphysema, chronic bronchitis, bronchiectasis, tuberculosis, or cystic fibrosis

- heart disease

- chronic kidney disease

- diabetes or other chronic metabolic disorder

- severe anemia

- diseases or treatments that depress immunity

Some of the symptoms associated with influenza are:

- fever

- bodily aches and pains

- chills
- sore throat/dry cough
- coughing
- loss of appetite
- weakness

Two antiviral drugs, amantadine and rimantadine are useful for treating influenza A if given as soon as possible after exposure to or onset of influenza. Both drugs are used as preventive medications, but they must be taken daily as long as influenza cases continue to occur in the community. Both may cause mild side effects.

A new drug called zanamivir (Relenza), which inhibits an influenza virus enzyme, received FDA approval in July 1999. One recent study found zanamivir was well-tolerated and effective in shortening the duration and severity of influenza symptoms, and in high-risk patients, the rate of complications. Another study found that zanamivir was 67% effective in preventing influenza infection, and 84% effective in preventing illnesses with fever. The researchers concluded that zanamivir may be useful in preventing influenza A and B. Zanamivir belongs to a class of drugs called neuraminidase inhibitors.

In 1998, researchers published a study showing that a nasal spray vaccine was highly successful in preventing influenza in a large test in children. The nasal spray vaccine has not yet been approved by the U.S. Food and Drug Administration.

Chapter 20

Histoplasmosis

What Is Histoplasmosis?

Histoplasmosis is an infectious disease caused by inhaling the spores of a fungus called *Histoplasma capsulatum*. Histoplasmosis is not contagious; it cannot be transmitted from an infected person or animal to someone else.[1]

Histoplasmosis primarily affects a person's lungs, and its symptoms vary greatly. The vast majority of infected people are asymptomatic (have no apparent ill effects), or they experience symptoms so mild they do not seek medical attention and may not even realize that their illness was histoplasmosis.[2] If symptoms do occur, they will usually start within 3 to 17 days after exposure, with an average of 10 days.[1] Histoplasmosis can appear as a mild, flu-like respiratory illness and has a combination of symptoms, including malaise (a general ill feeling), fever, chest pain, dry or nonproductive cough, headache, loss of appetite, shortness of breath, joint and muscle pains, chills, and hoarseness.[1-4] A chest X-ray can reveal distinct markings on an infected person's lungs.

Chronic lung disease due to histoplasmosis resembles tuberculosis and can worsen over months or years. Special antifungal medications are needed to arrest the disease.[1,2,5] The most severe and rarest form of this disease is disseminated histoplasmosis, which involves spreading of the fungus to other organs outside the lungs. Disseminated

Centers for Disease Control and Prevention (CDC), DHHS Publication Number 97-146, 1997.

histoplasmosis is fatal if untreated,[1,6] but death can also occur in some patients even when medical treatment is received.[5] People with weakened immune systems are at the greatest risk for developing severe and disseminated histoplasmosis. Included in this high-risk group are persons with acquired immunodeficiency syndrome (AIDS) or cancer and persons receiving cancer chemotherapy; high-dose, long-term steroid therapy; or other immuno-suppressive drugs.[2,5,7-11]

Impaired vision and even blindness develop in some people because of a rare condition called "presumed ocular histoplasmosis."[12] The factors causing this condition are poorly understood. Results of laboratory tests suggest that presumed ocular histoplasmosis is associated with hypersensitivity to *H. capsulatum* and not from direct exposure of the eyes to the microorganism. What delayed events convert the condition from asymptomatic to symptomatic are also unknown.[13]

How Is Histoplasmosis Diagnosed?

Histoplasmosis can be diagnosed by identifying *H. capsulatum* in clinical samples of a symptomatic person's tissues or secretions, testing the patient's blood serum for antibodies to the microorganism, and testing urine, serum, or other body fluids for *H. capsulatum* antigen. On occasion, diagnosis may require a transbronchial biopsy.[7]

Culturing of H. capsulatum

Culturing clinical specimens is a standard method of microbial identification, but the culturing process for isolating *H. capsulatum* is costly and time-consuming.[14] To complicate matters, positive results are seldom obtained during the acute stage of the illness, except from clinical specimens from patients with disseminated histoplasmosis.[2,5,7,14-16] Research advances in polymerase chain reaction (PCR) technology suggest that a laboratory method may soon be available that will allow direct identification of pathogenic fungi in clinical samples without the need for culturing them.[17,18]

Serologic Tests

Most cases of histoplasmosis are diagnosed serologically.[7] Because of their convenience, availability, and utility, the most widely accepted serologic tests are the immunodiffusion test and the complement-fixation test.[4,14-16] Serologic test results are useful when positive. However, sometimes test results are negative even when a person is sick with histoplasmosis, a situation that arises especially in patients with weakened immune systems.[2,7,15]

The immunodiffusion test qualitatively measures precipitating antibodies (H and M precipitin lines or bands) to concentrated histoplasmin.[4,7,19] While this test is more specific for histoplasmosis (i.e., a person who is not infected with *H. capsulatum* is unlikely to have a positive test result) than the complement-fixation test, it is less sensitive (i.e., someone who is acutely infected can have a negative test result).[4,7,14] Because the H band of the immunodiffusion test is usually present for only 4 to 6 weeks after exposure, it indicates active infection.[2,4,14] The M band is observed more frequently, appears soon after infection, and may persist up to 3 years after a patient recovers.[4,7]

The complement-fixation test, which measures antibodies to the intact yeast form and mycelial (histoplasmin) antigen, is more sensitive but less specific than the immunodiffusion test.[7] Complement-fixing antibodies may appear in 3 to 6 weeks (sometimes as early as 2 weeks19) following infection by *H. capsulatum*, and repeated tests will give positive results for months.[2,19]

The results of complement-fixation tests are of greatest diagnostic usefulness when both acute and convalescent serum specimens can be obtained. A high titer (1:32 or higher) or a fourfold increase is indicative of active histoplasmosis.[4,15,16,19] Lower titers (1:8 or 1:16), although less specific, may also provide presumptive evidence of infection,[3,14] but they can also be measured in the serum of healthy persons from regions where histoplasmosis is endemic.[16] Antibody titers will gradually decline and eventually disappear months to years after a patient recovers.[2,4,14,19]

Detection of H. capsulatum *Antigen*

A radioimmunoassay method can be used to measure *H. capsulatum* polysaccharide antigen (HPA) levels in samples of a patient's urine, serum, and other body fluids.[5,14,20,21] The test appears to meet the important need for a rapid and accurate method for early diagnosis of disseminated histoplasmosis, especially in patients with AIDS.[5,14,21] HPA is detected in body fluid samples of most patients with disseminated infection and in the urine and serum of 25% to 50% of those with less severe infections.[14]

Histoplasmin Skin Test

A person can learn from a histoplasmin skin test whether he or she has been previously infected by *H. capsulatum*. This test, similar to a tuberculin skin test, is available at many physicians' offices and medical clinics. A histoplasmin skin test becomes positive 2 to 4 weeks after a person is infected by *H. capsulatum*, and repeated tests will usually give positive results for the rest of the person's life.[15] A previous infection by *H. capsulatum* can provide partial protection against ill effects if a person is reinfected.[19] Since a positive skin test does not mean that a person is completely protected against ill effects,[19] appropriate exposure precautions should be taken regardless of a worker's skin-test status. Furthermore, while histoplasmin skin test information is useful to epidemiologists, a positive skin test does not help diagnose acute histoplasmosis, unless a previous skin test is known to have been negative.[1,2,4,7]

Where Are H. capsulatum *Spores Found?*

H. capsulatum grows in soils throughout the world.[7,22] In the United States, the fungus is endemic and the proportion of people infected by *H. capsulatum* is higher in central and eastern states, especially along the valleys of the Ohio, Mississippi, and St. Lawrence rivers, and the Rio Grande.[4,23] The fungus seems to grow best in soils having a high nitrogen content, especially those enriched with bird manure or bat droppings. The organism can be carried on the wings, feet, and beaks of birds and infect soil under roosting sites or manure accumulations inside or outside buildings. Active and inactive roosts of blackbirds (e.g., starlings, grackles, red-winged blackbirds, and cowbirds) have been found heavily contaminated by *H. capsulatum*.[19,24-36] Therefore, the soil in a stand of trees where blackbirds have roosted for 3 or more years should be suspected of being contaminated by the fungus.[28,37] Habitats of pigeons[24-26, 38-40] and bats,[24, 41-56] and poultry houses with dirt floors[24, 57-62] have also been found contaminated by *H. capsulatum*.

On the other hand, fresh bird droppings on surfaces such as sidewalks and windowsills have not been shown to present a health risk for histoplasmosis because birds themselves do not appear to be infected by *H. capsulatum*.[19,63] Rather, bird manure is primarily a nutrient source for the growth of *H. capsulatum* already present in soil.[16] Unlike birds, bats can become infected with *H. capsulatum* and consequently can excrete the organism in their droppings.[16,46,49,64]

To learn whether soil or droppings are contaminated with *H. capsulatum* spores, samples must be collected and cultured. The culturing process involves inoculating mice with small portions of a sample, sacrificing the mice after 4 weeks, and streaking agar plates with portions of each mouse's liver and spleen.[24] Then for four more weeks, the plates are watched for the growth of *H. capsulatum*. Enough samples must be collected so that small but highly contaminated areas are not overlooked. On several occasions, *H. capsulatum* has not been recovered from any of the samples collected from material believed responsible for causing illness in people diagnosed from the results of clinical tests as having histoplasmosis.[25,26,45,58,65-67]

Until a less expensive and more rapid method is available, testing field samples for *H. capsulatum* will be impractical in most situations. Consequently, when thorough testing is not done, the safest approach is to assume that the soil in regions where *H. capsulatum* is endemic and any accumulations of bat droppings or bird manure are contaminated with *H. capsulatum* and to take appropriate exposure precautions.

Who Can Get Histoplasmosis and What Jobs and Activities Put People at Risk for Exposure to H. capsulatum *Spores?*

Anyone working at a job or present near activities where material contaminated with *H. capsulatum* becomes airborne can develop histoplasmosis if enough spores are inhaled. After an exposure, how ill a person becomes varies greatly and most likely depends on the number of spores inhaled and a person's age and susceptibility to the disease. The number of inhaled spores needed to cause disease is unknown. Infants, young children, and older persons, in particular those with chronic lung disease, are at increased risk for developing symptomatic histoplasmosis.[7,68]

The U.S. Public Health Service (USPHS) and the Infectious Diseases Society of America (IDSA) have jointly published guidelines for the prevention of opportunistic infections in persons infected with the human immunodeficiency virus (HIV).[69,70] The USPHS/IDSA Prevention of Opportunistic Infections Working Group recommended that HIV-infected persons "should avoid activities known to be associated with increased risk (e.g., cleaning chicken coops, disturbing soil beneath bird-roosting sites, and exploring caves)."[70] HIV-infected persons should consult their health care provider about appropriate exposure precautions that should be taken for any activity with a risk of exposure to *H. capsulatum*.

Following is a partial list of occupations and hobbies with risks for exposure to *H. capsulatum* spores. Appropriate exposure precautions should be taken by these people and others whenever contaminated soil, bat droppings, or bird manure are disturbed.

139

- Bridge inspector or painter[47,56,67]
- Chimney cleaner[50]
- Construction worker[5,41,42,51,66,71]
- Demolition worker[3,41,57]
- Farmer[3,5,58-61,67]
- Gardener[3,62,72]
- Heating and air-conditioning system installer or service person[4,45]
- Microbiology laboratory worker[13,39,48,67]
- Pest control worker
- Restorer of historic or abandoned buildings[45,48]
- Roofer[38]
- Spelunker (cave explorer)[43,44,52-55]

If someone who engages in these activities develops flu-like symptoms days or even weeks after disturbing material that might be contaminated with *H. capsulatum*, and the illness worsens rather than subsides after a few days, medical care should be sought and the health care provider informed about the exposure.

Should Workers Who Might Be Exposed to H. capsulatum Have Pre-Exposure Skin or Blood Tests?

Workers at risk of exposure to *H. capsulatum* may learn useful information from a histoplasmin skin test. The results of skin testing would inform each worker of his or her status regarding either susceptibility to infection by *H. capsulatum* (a negative skin test) or partial protection against ill effects if reinfected (a positive skin test). However, a false-negative skin test result can be reported early in an infection or with persons with weakened immune systems.[2,4,7,15,19]

A false-positive skin test can result from cross-reactions with antigens of certain other pathogenic fungi.[4,23] One drawback to routine pre-exposure skin testing is that a person with a positive skin test might incorrectly assume a false sense of security that he or she is completely protected against ill effects if reinfected. The work practices and personal protective equipment described in this booklet are expected to protect both skin-test positive and skin-test negative persons from excessive inhalation exposures to materials that might be contaminated with *H. capsulatum*.

Although a pre-exposure serum sample could be useful in determining whether a worker's post-exposure illness is histoplasmosis, routine collection and storage of serum specimens from workers is unnecessary and impractical in most work settings. Some employers, such as public health agencies and microbiology laboratories, have facilities for long-term storage of serum and do collect pre-exposure serum specimens from those employees who might be exposed to high-risk infectious agents. If a worker is to have blood drawn for this purpose and is to receive a histoplasmin skin test, the blood sample should be drawn first because the skin test may cause a positive complement-fixation test for up to 3 months and the appearance of the M band on an immunodiffusion test for *H. capsulatum*.[1,3,4,15]

What Can Be Done to Reduce Exposures to H. capsulatum?

The best work practice is to prevent the accumulation of manure in the first place. Therefore, when a colony of bats or a flock of birds is discovered roosting in a building, immediate action should be taken to exclude the intruders by sealing all entry points. Any measure that might unnecessarily harm or kill a bat or bird should be avoided.

Before excluding a colony of bats or a flock of birds from a building, attention should be given to the possibility that flightless young may be present. In the United States, this is an especially important consideration for bats from May through August.[73]

Ultrasonic devices and chemical repellents are ineffective for eliminating bats from a roosting area.[73,74] While there may be several openings in a building, bats will typically use only one or two.[75] Therefore, after observing the bats leaving a building on several nights, all openings except the ones used by the bats should be sealed. Because some bats are so small that they can squeeze through an opening smaller than the diameter of a dime,[37] even the smallest hole should be sealed.

Exclusion valves—flaps made of polypropylene bird netting that allow bats to leave but not enter—should then be placed over the remaining openings.[73,75] If these openings are inaccessible, installing and maintaining lights in a roosting area will force bats to seek another daytime roosting site. Because of concerns for the welfare of evicted bats, constructing bat houses near former roosts has become a common practice of some pest control companies.[75]

In some buildings, extensive bat exclusion measures may be more successful in the late fall or winter months after a colony has migrated to a warmer habitat or to another location for hibernation. In some regions of the United States, bats may not migrate, but rather will hibernate in the same building. Consequently, any work on a building that might disturb such a colony should be delayed until spring. Disturbing bats during hibernation is likely to result in their death.

Excluding birds from a building also involves sealing entry points. Because their food source is usually nearby, birds prevented from re-entering a building will often complicate an exclusion by beginning to roost on window sills and ledges of the building or others nearby. Visual deterrents (e.g., balloons, flags, lights, and replicas of hawks and owls) and noises (e.g., gun shots, alarms, gas cannons, and fireworks) may scare birds away, but generally only temporarily.[76]

Nontoxic, chemical bird repellents are available as liquids, aerosols, and nondrying films and pastes. Disadvantages of these antiroosting materials are that some are messy and none are permanent. Even the most effective ones require periodic reapplication. More permanent repellents include mechanical antiroosting systems consisting of angled and porcupine wires made of stainless steel. These systems may require some occasional maintenance to clear nesting material or other debris from the wires.[76]

Live trapping of birds to relocate them is seldom effective when traps are put in a roosting site, but this method can be effective when used in a feeding area. Shooting birds, using contact poisons, and baiting with poisoned food should be used as last resorts and should only be done by qualified pest control specialists. Using such methods to kill nuisance birds may also require a special permit.

Posting Health Risk Warnings

If a colony of bats or a flock birds is allowed to live in a building or a stand of trees, their manure will accumulate and create a health risk for anyone who enters the roosting area and disturbs the material. Once a roosting site has been discovered in a building, exclusion plans should be made, and the extent of contamination should be determined. When an accumulation of bat or bird manure is discovered in a building, removing the material is not always the next step. Simply leaving the material alone if it is in a location where no human activity is likely may be the best course of action.

Areas known or suspected of being contaminated by *H. capsulatum*, such as bird roosts, attics, or even entire buildings that contain accumulations of bat or bird manure, should be posted with signs warning of the health risk. Each sign should provide the name and telephone number of a person to be contacted if there are questions about the area. In some situations, a fence may need to be built around a property or locks put on attic doors to prevent unsuspecting or unprotected individuals from entering.

Communicating Health Risks to Workers

Before an activity is started that may disturb any material that might be contaminated by *H. capsulatum*, workers should be informed in writing of the personal risk factors that increase an individual's chances of developing histoplasmosis. Such a written communication should include a warning that individuals with weakened immune systems are at the greatest risk of developing severe and disseminated histoplasmosis if they become infected. These people should seek advice from their health care provider about whether they should avoid exposure to materials that might be contaminated with *H. capsulatum*. The fact sheet in the appendix is one way of conveying information about histoplasmosis; it can be distributed to workers during their hazard communication training.

Controlling Aerosolized Dust When Removing Bat or Bird Manure from a Building

The best way to prevent exposure to *H. capsulatum* spores is to avoid situations where material that might be contaminated can become aerosolized and subsequently inhaled. A brief inhalation exposure to highly contaminated dust may be all that is needed to cause infection and subsequent development of histoplasmosis. Therefore, work practices and dust control measures that eliminate or reduce dust generation during the removal of bat or bird manure from a building will also reduce risks of infection and subsequent development of disease. For example, instead of shoveling or sweeping dry, dusty material,[25] carefully wetting it with a water spray can reduce the amount of dust aerosolized during an activity. Adding a surfactant or wetting agent to the water might reduce further the amount of aerosolized dust. Once the material is wetted, it can be collected in double, heavy-duty plastic bags, a 55-gallon drum, or some other secure container for immediate disposal.

An alternative method is use of an industrial vacuum cleaner with a high-efficiency filter to bag contaminated material. Truck-mounted or trailer-mounted vacuum systems are recommended for buildings with large accumulations of bat or bird manure. These high-volume systems can remove tons of contaminated material in a short period.

Using long, large-diameter hoses, such a system can also remove contaminated material located several stories above its waste hopper. This advantage eliminates the risk of dust exposure that can happen when bags tear accidentally or containers break during their transfer to the ground.

The removal of all material that might be contaminated by *H. capsulatum* from a building and immediate waste disposal will eliminate any further risk that someone might be exposed to aerosolized spores. Air sampling, surface sampling, or the use of any other method intended to confirm that no infectious agents remain following removal of bat or bird manure is unnecessary in most cases. However, before a removal activity is considered finished, the cleaned area should be inspected visually to ensure that no residual dust or debris remains.

Disinfecting Contaminated Material

Disinfectants have occasionally been used to treat contaminated soil and accumulations of bat manure when removal was impractical or as a precaution before a removal process was started.[27,34-36,45,51] Formaldehyde solutions are the only disinfectants proven to be effective for decontaminating soil containing *H. capsulatum*.[27,34-36] Because of the potentially serious health hazards associated with formaldehyde exposures, this chemical should be handled only by persons who know how to apply it safely.[42] If a disinfectant is applied to land known to be contaminated by *H. capsulatum*, the soil should be thoroughly saturated so that the disinfectant penetrates deeply enough to contact all the soil containing *H. capsulatum*. While *H. capsulatum* was found in a blackbird roost at a depth of more than 12 inches,[77] soil saturation to a depth of 6 to 8 inches will be sufficient for most disinfectant applications.[24,34] To ensure a disinfectant's effectiveness, soil samples should be collected before and after an application and analyzed for *H. capsulatum*. The appropriate number of samples to be collected will vary depending upon the size of the property.[24,78] Each sampling location should be flagged or marked in a way that will ensure that the same locations will be sampled after application of the disinfectant. A map of the treated area showing the approximate location of each sampling site will also be useful in the event flags or markings are lost. After a disinfectant's effectiveness has been documented—more than one application may be necessary—additional tests for *H. capsulatum* should be done periodically if the land remains idle.

Disposing of Waste

Any material that might be contaminated with *H. capsulatum* that is removed from a work site should be disposed of or decontaminated properly and safely and not merely moved to another area where it could still be a health hazard. Before an activity is started, the quantity of material to be removed should be estimated. (If the approximate volume of dry bat or bird manure in a building is known, the approximate weight can be calculated using a conversion factor of 40 pounds per cubic foot.) Requirements established by local and state authorities for the removal, transportation, and disposal of contaminated material should be followed. Arrangements should be made with a landfill operator concerning the quantity of material to be disposed of, the dates when the material will be delivered, and the disposal location. If local or state landfill regulations define material contaminated with *H. capsulatum* to be infectious waste, incineration or another decontamination method may also be required.

Controlling Aerosolized Dust During Construction, Excavation, and Demolition

Dusts containing *H. capsulatum* spores can be aerosolized during construction, excavation, or demolition. Once airborne, spores can be carried easily by wind currents over long distances. Such contaminated airborne dusts can cause infections not only in persons at a work site, but also in others nearby. Such activities were suggested as the causes of the three largest outbreaks of histoplasmosis ever recorded. All three outbreaks took place in Indianapolis, Indiana.[14,66,68] During the first outbreak, in the fall of 1978 and spring of 1979, an estimated 120,000 people were infected, and 15 people died. The second outbreak, in 1980, was similar to the first in the number of people affected. AIDS patients accounted for nearly 50% of culture-proven cases during the third outbreak, in 1988.[14]

Water sprays or other dust suppression techniques should be used to reduce the amount of dust aerosolized during construction, excavation, or demolition in regions where *H. capsulatum* is endemic. During windy periods or other times when typical dust suppression techniques are ineffective, earthmoving activities should be interrupted. All earthmoving equipment (e.g., bulldozers, trucks, and front-end loaders) should have cabs with air-conditioning (if available) to protect their operators. Air filters on air-conditioners should be inspected on a regular schedule and cleaned or replaced as needed.

During filter cleaning or replacement of exceptionally dusty air filters, respiratory protection should be worn by the maintenance person if there is a potential for the dust to be aerosolized. Beds of all trucks carrying dirt or debris from a work site should be covered, and all trucks should pass through a wash station before leaving the site. When at a dump site, a truck operator should ensure that all individuals in the vicinity are in an area where they will not be exposed to dust aerosolized while the truck is emptied.

Water sprays and other suppression techniques may not be enough to control dust aerosolized during demolition of a building or other structure. Consequently, removal of accumulations of bird or bat manure before demolition may be necessary in some situations. Factors affecting decisions about pre-demolition removal of such accumulations include the quantity and locations of the material, the structural integrity or soundness of the building, weather conditions, proximity of the building to other buildings and structures, and whether nearby buildings are occupied by persons who may be at increased risk for developing symptomatic histoplasmosis (e.g., schools, day-care facilities, hospitals, clinics, jails, and prisons.)

City or county governments in regions where *H. capsulatum* is endemic should establish and enforce regulations concerning work practices that will control dust aerosolization at construction, excavation, and demolition sites. However, even in regions where *H. capsulatum* is not considered endemic, dust aerosolized during work activities in bird roosts has also resulted in outbreaks of histoplasmosis.[26,31] Consequently, regardless of whether a work site is in an endemic region, precautions should be taken at active and inactive bird roosts to prevent dust aerosolization.

Wearing Personal Protective Equipment

Because work practices and dust control measures to reduce worker exposures to *H. capsulatum* have not been fully evaluated, using personal protective equipment is still necessary during some activities. During removal of an accumulation of bat or bird manure from an enclosed area such as an attic, dust control measures should be used, but wearing a NIOSH-approved respirator and other items of personal protective equipment is also recommended to reduce further the risk of *H. capsulatum* exposure.

For some jobs involving exposures to airborne dusts, working conditions have changed little over the years despite improvements in other aspects of the industry. For example, inhalation of dust aerosolized from the dirt floors of chicken coops that contained *H. capsulatum* spores was reported more than 30 years ago as the cause of clinical cases of histoplasmosis in workers.[57-61] As the poultry industry has grown (there are now approximately 120,000 poultry farms in the United States[79]), the old-style chicken coop has been replaced by larger housing facilities. However, the floors of poultry houses are still dirt covered and provide an excellent medium for the growth of *H. capsulatum*. Ventilation systems in poultry houses are not primarily intended to reduce poultry workers' exposures to aerosolized dust, and dust measurements made during growing and catching chickens show that inhalation exposures of poultry workers to dust can be excessive.[80] Since ventilation systems designed especially to reduce airborne dust to "safe" levels in poultry houses would likely be economically and mechanically impractical, wearing a respirator is probably the most feasible method for protecting poultry workers.

Recommendations for selecting respirators to protect workers against inhalation exposures to airborne dust and *H. capsulatum* are described next. Following that, recommendations for personal protective equipment other than respirators are provided.

What Are the Advantages and Disadvantages of Various Kinds of Respirators for Protecting Workers Against Exposure to H. capsulatum?

Assigned Protection Factors

Respirators provide varying levels of protection, and people have developed histoplasmosis after disturbing material contaminated with *H. capsulatum* despite wearing respirators that they assumed would protect them.[55,81] Such unfortunate events demonstrate that when a respirator is needed, it must be carefully selected with an understanding of the circumstances associated with exposure to an airborne contaminant and the capabilities and limitations of the various kinds of respirators.

Because respirators provide different levels of protection, they are divided into classes, and each respirator class has been assigned a protection factor to help compare its protective capabilities with other respirator classes. An assigned protection factor is a unitless number determined statistically from a set of experimental or workplace data. This factor is the minimum level of protection expected for a substantial proportion (usually 95%) of properly fitted and trained respirator users.[82] When the effectiveness of a respirator is evaluated in a workplace, a protection factor is calculated for each respirator wearer and respirator combination by dividing the air concentration of a challenge agent by the air concentration of that agent inside the respirator wearer's face piece, hood, or helmet. For example, if air sampling measurements show equal concentrations of a contaminant inside and outside a respirator wearer's face piece, then the respirator provided no protection, and a protection factor of 1 would be calculated. Likewise, a protection factor of 5 means that a respirator wearer was exposed to one-fifth (20%) of the air concentration to which he or she would have been exposed if a respirator had not been used, a reduction of 80%. Similarly, a protection factor of 10 represents a one-tenth (10%) exposure (a 90% reduction), 50 represents a one-fiftieth (2%) exposure (a 98% reduction), and so on.

The assigned protection factors of respirators available for protecting workers against exposures to airborne materials contaminated with *H. capsulatum* range from 5 to 10,000.[83] Most disposable respirators represent the low end of the protection-factor scale. Self-contained breathing apparatuses operated in the pressure-demand mode, like those worn by firefighters, represent the high end. Within this range is a variety of negative-pressure, powered air-purifying, and supplied-air respirators that are available with half-face piece, full face piece, loose-fitting face piece, hood, or helmet.

References

1. Benenson AS, ed. [1995]. *Control of communicable diseases manual*. 16th ed. Washington, DC: American Public Health Association, pp. 237-240.

2. Johnson PC, Sarosi GA [1987]. Histoplasmosis. *Semin. Respir. Med.* 9 (2):145-151.

3. Larsh HW [1983]. Histoplasmosis. In: DiSalvo AF, ed. *Occupational mycoses*. Philadelphia, PA: Lea and Febiger, pp. 29-41.

4. Mitchell TG [1992]. Systemic mycoses. In: Joklik WK, Willett HP, Amos DB, Wifert CM, eds. *Zinsser microbiology*. 20th ed. Norwalk, CT: Appleton and Lange, pp. 1091-1112.

5. Wheat LJ, Connolly-Stringfield PA, Baker RL, Curfman MF, Eads ME, Israel KS, Norris SA, Webb DH, Zeckel ML [1990]. Disseminated histoplasmosis in the acquired immune deficiency syndrome: clinical findings, diagnosis and treatment, and review of the literature. *Med.* 69 (6):361-374.

6. Deepe GS [1994]. The immune response to Histoplasma capsulatum: unearthing its secrets. *J. Lab. Clin.* Med. 123:201-205.

7. Davies SF [1990]. Histoplasmosis: update 1989. *Semin. Respir. Infections* 5 (2):93-104.

8. Hajjeh RA [1995]. Disseminated histoplasmosis in persons infected with human immunodeficiency virus. *Clin. Infectious Dis.* 21 (Suppl 1):S108-S110.

9. Wheat LJ, Slama TG, Zeckel ML [1985]. Histoplasmosis in the acquired immune deficiency syndrome. *Am. J. Med.* 78:203-210.

10. Greenfield RA [1989]. Pulmonary infections due to higher bacteria and fungi in the immunocompromised host. *Semin. Respir. Med.* 10:68-77.

11. Selik RM, Karon JM, Ward [1997]. Effect of the human immunodeficiency virus epidemic on mortality from opportunistic infections in the United States in 1993. *J. Infect. Dis.* 176:632-636.

12. Schwarz J [1981]. Histoplasmosis of the eye. In: *Histoplasmosis. New York, NY*: Praeger Publishers, pp. 317-350.

13. Newell FW [1992]. Ophthalmology principles and concepts. 7th ed. St. Louis, MO: *Mosby Year Book*, p. 439.

14. Wheat LJ [1992]. Histoplasmosis in Indianapolis. *Clin. Infectious Dis.* 14 (Suppl 1):S91-S99.

15. Wheat J, French MLV, Kohler RB, Zimmerman SE, Smith CD, Slama TG [1982]. The diagnostic laboratory tests for histoplasmosis. *Ann. Int. Med.* 97 (5):680-685.

16. George RB, Penn RL [1986]. Histoplasmosis. In: Sarosi GA, Davies SF, eds. *Fungal diseases of the lung*. Orlando, FL: Harcourt Brace Jovanovich, pp. 69-85.

17. Bowman BH [1992]. Designing a PCR/probe detection system for pathogenic fungi. *Clin. Immunol. Newsletter* 12:65-69.

18. Check WA [1994]. Molecular techniques shed light on fungal genetics. *Am. Soc. Microbiol. News* 60:593-596.

19. Rippon JW [1988]. Chapter 15: Histoplasmosis (histoplasmosis capsulati and histoplasmosis farciminosum). In: *Medical mycology: the pathogenic fungi and the pathogenic actinomycetes*. 3rd ed. Philadelphia, PA: W.B. Saunders Company, pp. 381-423.

20. Wheat LJ, Kohler RB, Tewari RP:[1986]. Diagnosis of disseminated histoplasmosis by detection of Histoplasma capsulatum antigen in serum and urine specimens. *N. Engl. J. Med.* 314:83-88.

21. Wheat LJ, Connolly-Stringfield P, Kohler RB, Frame PT, Gupta MR [1989]. Histoplasma capsulatum polysaccharide antigen detection in diagnosis and management of disseminated histoplasmosis in patients with acquired immunodeficiency syndrome. *Am. J. Med.* 87:396-400.

22. Walsh TJ, Mitchell TG, Larone DH [1995]. Histoplasma, Blastomyces, Coccidioides, and other dimorphic fungi causing systemic mycoses. In: Murray PR, ed-in-chief. *Manual of clinical microbiology*. 6th ed. Washington, DC: American Society for Microbiology Press, pp. 749-764.

23. Edwards LB, Acquaviva FA, Livesay VT [1973]. Further observations on histoplasmin sensitivity in the United States. *Am. J. Epidemiol.* 98 (5):315-325.

24. Ajello L, Weeks RJ [1983]. Soil decontamination and other control measures. In: DiSalvo AF, ed. *Occupational mycoses*. Philadelphia, PA: Lea and Febiger, pp. 229-238.

25. Stobierski MG, Hospedales CJ, Hall WN, Robinson-Dunn B, Hoch D, Sheill DA [1996]. Outbreak of histoplasmosis among employees in a paper factory-Michigan, 1993. *J. Clin. Microbiol.* 34 (5):1220-1223.

26. Morse DL, Gordon MA, Matte T, Eadie G [1985]. An outbreak of histoplasmosis in a prison. *Am. J. Epidemiol.* 122 (2):253-261.

27. Bartlett PC, Weeks RJ, Ajello L [1982]. Decontamination of Histoplasma capsulatum-infested bird roost in Illinois. *Arch. Environ. Health* 37:221-223.

28. Gustafson TL, Kaufman L, Weeks R, Ajello L, Hutcheson RH, Wiener SL, et al. [1981]. Outbreak of acute pulmonary histoplasmosis in members of a wagon train. *Am. J. Med.* 71:759-765.

29. Chick EW, Compton SB, Pass III T, Mackey B, Hernandez C, Austin Jr E, et al. [1981]. Hitchcock's birds, or the increased rate of exposure to Histoplasma from blackbird roost sites. *Chest* 80 (4):434-438.

30. Storch G, Burford JG, George RB, Kaufman L, Ajello L [1980]. Acute histoplasmosis. Description of an outbreak in northern Louisiana. *Chest* 77:38-42.

31. DiSalvo AF, Johnson WM [1979]. Histoplasmosis in South Carolina: support for the microfocus concept. *Am. J. Epidemiol.* 109 (4):480-492.

32. Latham RH, Kaiser AB, Dupont WD, Dan BB [1980]. Chronic pulmonary histoplasmosis following the excavation of a bird roost. *Am. J. Med.* 68:504-508.

33. Sarosi GA, Parker JD, Tosh FE [1971]. Histoplasmosis outbreaks: their patterns. In: Ajello L, Chick EW, Furcolow ML, eds. Histoplasmosis: proceedings of the second national conference. Springfield, IL: Charles C. Thomas, pp. 123-128.

34. Tosh FE, Weeks RJ, Pfeiffer FR, Hendricks SL, Greer DL, Chin TDY [1967]. The use of formalin to kill Histoplasma capsulatum at an epidemic site. *Am. J. Epidemiol.* 85:259-265.

35. Tosh FE, Weeks RJ, Pfeiffer FR, Hendricks SL, Chin TDY [1966]. Chemical decontamination of soil containing Histoplasma capsulatum. *Am. J. Epidemiol.* 83:262-270.

36. Tosh FE, Doto IL, D'Alessio DJ, Medeiros AA, Hendricks SL, Chin TDY [1966]. The second of two epidemics of histoplasmosis resulting from work on the same starling roost. *Am. Rev. Respir. Dis.* 94:406-413.

37. Weeks RJ [1984]. Histoplasmosis sources of infection and methods of control. Atlanta, GA: Centers for Disease Control and Prevention.

38. Dean AG, Bates JH, Sorrels C, Sorrels T, Germany W, Ajello L, Kaufman L, McGrew C, Fitts A [1978]. An outbreak of histoplasmosis at an Arkansas courthouse, with five cases of probable reinfection. *Am. J. Epidemiol.* 108:36-46.

39. Raphael SS, Schwarz J [1953]. Occupational hazards from fungi causing deep mycoses. Arch. Ind. *Hyg. Occup. Med.* 8:154-165.

40. Felson B, Jones GF, Ulrich RP [1950]. Roentgenologic aspects of diffuse miliary granulomatous pneumonitis of unknown etiology: report of twelve cases with eighteen months' follow-up. *Am. J. Roentgenol. Radium Ther.* 64 (5):740-746.

41. Leslie L, Arnette C, Sikder A, Adams J, Holbrook C, Bond J, King B, Roberts K, Patrick MS, Palmer C, Finger R, Tomford JW, Rushton T [1995]. *Histoplasmosis-Kentucky*, 1995. MMWR 44 (38):701-703.

42. Lenhart, SW [1994]. Recommendations for protecting workers from Histoplasma capsulatum exposure during bat guano removal from a church's attic. *Appl. Occup. Environ. Hyg.* 9:230-236.

43. Gordon SM, Reines SS, Alvarado CS, Nolte F, Keyserling HL, Bryan J [1993]. Disseminated histoplasmosis caused by Histoplasma capsulatum in an immunocompromised adolescent after exploration of a bat cave. *Pediatric Infect. Dis. J.* 12 (1):102-104.

44. Sacks JJ, Ajello L, Crockett LK [1986]. An outbreak and review of cave-associated Histoplasma capsulati. *J. Med. Vet. Mycol.* 24:313-327.

45. Bartlett PC, Vonbehren LA, Tewari RP, Martin RJ, Eagleton L, Isaac MJ, Kulkarni PS [1982]. Bats in the belfry: an outbreak of histoplasmosis. *Am. J. Public Health* 72:1369-1372.

46. Schwarz J [1981]. Bats and soil. In: *Histoplasmosis. New York*, NY: Praeger Publishers, pp. 179-186.

47. Sorley DL, Levin ML, Warren JW, Flynn JPG, Gerstenblith J [1979]. Bat-associated histoplasmosis in Maryland bridge workers. *Am. J. Med.* 67:623-626.

48. Chick EW, Bauman DS, Lapp NL, Morgan WKC [1972]. A combined field and laboratory epidemic of histoplasmosis. *Am. Rev. Respir. Dis.* 105:968-971.

49. DiSalvo AF [1971]. The role of bats in the ecology of Histoplasma capsulatum. In: Ajello L, Chick EW, Furcolow ML,

eds. Histoplasmosis: proceedings of the second national conference. Springfield, IL: Charles C. Thomas, pp. 149-161.

50. Gordon MA, Ziment I [1967]. Epidemic of acute histoplasmosis in western New York State. *N.Y. State J. Med.* 67:235-243.

51. Ajello L, Hosty TS, Palmer J [1967]. Bat histoplasmosis in Alabama. *Am. J. Trop. Med. Hyg.* 16:329-331.

52. Hasenclever HF, Shacklette MH, Young RV, Gelderman GA [1967]. The natural occurrence of Histoplasma capsulatum in a cave—1. Epidemiologic aspects. *Am. J. Epidemiol.* 86 (1):238-245.

53. Shacklette MH, Hasenclever HF, Miranda EA [1967]. The natural occurrence of Histoplasma capsulatum in a cave—2. Ecologic aspects. *Am. J. Epidemiol.* 86 (1):246-252.

54. Shacklette MH, Hasenclever HF [1967]. The natural occurrence of Histoplasma capsulatum in a cave—3. Effect of flooding. *Am. J. Epidemiol.* 88 (2):210-252.

55. Campins H, Zubillaga C, Lopez LG, Dorante M [1956]. An epidemic of histoplasmosis in Venezuela. *Am. J. Trop. Med.* 5:690-695.

56. Englert E, Phillips AW [1953]. Acute diffuse pulmonary granulomatosis in bridge workers. *Am. J. Med.* 15:733-740.

57. Scalia SP [1961]. An outbreak of histoplasmosis in Baltimore County. *Maryland State Med. J.* 10:614-619.

58. Lehan PH, Furcolow ML [1957]. Epidemic histoplasmosis. *J. Chron. Dis.* 5 (4):489-503.

59. Furcolow ML, Menges RW, Larsh HW [1955]. An epidemic of histoplasmosis involving man and animals. *Ann. Int. Med.* 43:173-181.

60. Imbach MJ, Larsh HW, Furcolow ML [1954]. Epidemic histoplasmosis and airborne Histoplasma capsulatum. *Proc. Soc. Exper. Biol. and Med.* 85:72-74.

61. Zeidberg LD, Ajello L [1954]. Environmental factors influencing the occurrence of histoplasma capsulatum and Microsporum gypseum in soil. *J. Bacteriol.* 68:156-159.

62. Kier JH, Campbell CC, Ajello L, Sutliff WD [1954]. Acute bronchopneumonic histoplasmosis following exposure to infected garden soil. *J. Am. Med. Assoc.* 155:1230-1232.

63. Schwarz J [1981]. Global epidemiology and distribution of histoplasmosis. In: *Histoplasmosis. New York*, NY: Praeger Publishers, p. 87.

64. Hasenclever HF [1979]. Impact of airborne pathogens in outdoor systems: histoplasmosis. In: Edmonds RL, ed. *Aerobiology: the ecological systems approach*. Stroudsburg, PA: Dowden, Hutchinson and Ross, Inc., pp. 199-208.

65. Ward JI, Weeks M, Allen M, Hutcheson RH Jr., Anderson R, Fraser DW et al. [1979]. Acute histoplasmosis: clinical, epidemiologic and serologic findings of an outbreak associated with exposure to a fallen tree. *Am. J. Med.* 66:587-595.

66. Schlech WF, Wheat LJ, Ho JL, French MLV, Weeks RJ, Kohler RB, Deane CE, Eitzen HE, Band JD [1983]. Recurrent urban histoplasmosis, Indianapolis, Indiana, 1980-1981. *Am. J. Epidemiol.* 118:301-312.

67. Schwarz J, Kauffman CA [1977]. Occupational hazards from deep mycoses. *Arch. Dermatol.* 113:1270-1275.

68. Wheat LJ, Slama TG, Norton JA, Kohler RB, Eitzen HE, French MLV, Sathapatayavongs B [1982]. Risk factors for disseminated or fatal histoplasmosis, analysis of a large urban outbreak. *Ann. Intern. Med.* 96:159-163.

69. Kaplan JE, Masur H, Holmes KK, McNeil MM, Schonberger LB, Navin TR, et al. [1995]. USPHS/IDSA guidelines for the prevention of opportunistic infections in persons infected with human immunodeficiency virus: introduction. *Clin. Infect. Dis.* 21 (suppl 1):S1-S11.

70. Centers for Disease Control and Prevention (CDC) [1997]. 1997 USPHS/IDSA guidelines for the prevention of opportunistic infections in persons infected with human immunodeficiency virus. *MMWR* 46 (No. RR-12):1-46.

71. Wilcox KR Jr., Waisbren BA, Martin J [1958]. The Walworth, Wisconsin, epidemic of histoplasmosis. *Ann. Intern. Med.* 49:388-418.

72. Byrd RB, Leavey R, Trunk G [1975]. The Chanute histoplasmosis epidemic. *Chest* 68 (6):791-795.

73. Dealing with unwanted guests! [1997]. Austin, TX: Bat Conservation International, Inc.

74. Tuttle MD [1988]. America's neighborhood bats. Austin, TX: *University of Texas Press.*

75. Bat Conservation International, Inc. [1996]. Exclusion experts promote pest control industry changes. *Bats* 14 (2):10-11.

76. Courtsal FR [Date unknown]. Pigeons (rock doves). West Lafayette, IN: Purdue University.

77. Smith CD, Furcolow ML, Tosh FE [1964]. Attempts to eliminate Histoplasma capsulatumfrom soil. *Am. J. Hyg.* 79 (2):170-180.

78. CDC [1977]. Histoplasmosis control: decontamination of bird roosts, chicken houses and other point sources. Atlanta, GA: Centers for Disease Control and Prevention.

79. Olson DK, Bark SM [1996]. Health hazards affecting the animal confinement farm worker. *Am. Assoc. Occup. Health Nurses J.* 44 (4):198-204.

80. Lenhart SW, Morris PD, Akin RE, Olenchock SA, Service WS, Boone WP [1990]. Organic dust, endotoxin, and ammonia exposures in the North Carolina poultry processing industry. *Appl. Occup. Environ. Hyg.* 5 (9):611-618.

81. Furcolow ML [1965]. Environmental aspects of histoplasmosis. *Arch. Environ. Health* 10:4-10.

82. Myers WR, Lenhart SW, Campbell D, Provost G [1983]. Letter to the editor; topic: respirator performance terminology. *Am. Ind. Hyg. Assoc. J.* 44 (3):B25-B26.

83. NIOSH [1987]. NIOSH respirator decision logic. Cincinnati, OH: U.S. Department of Health and Human Services, Public Health Service, Centers for Disease Control, National Institute for Occupational Safety and Health, DHHS (NIOSH) Pub. No. 87-108.

Chapter 21

Idiopathic Pulmonary Fibrosis (IPF)

What Is Idiopathic Pulmonary Fibrosis (IPF)?

Idiopathic Pulmonary Fibrosis (IPF) is a disease of inflammation that results in scarring or fibrosis, of the lungs. In time, this fibrosis can build up to the point where the lungs are unable to provide oxygen to the tissues of the body.

Doctors use the word "idiopathic" (from the Greek "idio" meaning "peculiar" or "unusual" and "pathy" meaning "illness") to describe the disease, because the cause of IPF is unknown. Currently, researchers believe that IPF may result from either an autoimmune disorder, a condition in which the body's immune system attacks its own tissues, or the aftereffects of an infection, most likely a virus.

Whatever the trigger is for IPF, it appears to set off a series of events in which the inflammation and immune activity in the lungs—and, eventually, the fibrosis processes, too—become uncontrollable. In a few cases, heredity appears to play a part, possibly making some individuals more likely than others to get IPF.

In studies of patients with IPF, the average survival rate has been found to be 4 to 6 years after diagnosis. Those who develop idiopathic pulmonary fibrosis at a young age seem to have a longer survival.

National Heart, Lung, and Blood Institute (NHLBI), NIH Publication Number 93-2997, 1993. Text available on line at www.nhlbi.nih.gov/health/public.lung/other/idiopath.txt; cited April 2000.

How Common Is IPF?

The exact number of people who develop idiopathic pulmonary fibrosis each year is not known. It is known, however, that equal numbers of men and women get the illness and that most cases of IPF are diagnosed when the patients are between the ages of 40 and 70.

What Are the Symptoms of IPF?

Early symptoms of idiopathic pulmonary fibrosis are usually similar to those of other lung diseases. Very often, for example, patients suffer from a dry cough and dyspnea (shortness of breath). As the disease progresses, dyspnea becomes the major problem. Day-to-day activities such as climbing stairs, walking short distances, dressing, and even talking on the phone and eating become more difficult and sometimes nearly impossible. Enlargement (clubbing) of the fingertips may develop. The patient may also become less able to fight infection. In advanced stages of the illness, the patient may need oxygen all the time.

IPF can lead to death. Often the immediate cause is respiratory failure due to hypoxemia, right-heart failure, a heart attack, blood clot (embolism) in the lungs, stroke, or lung infection brought on by the disease.

What Is the Course of IPF?

Although the course of idiopathic pulmonary fibrosis varies greatly from person to person, the disease usually develops slowly, sometimes over years.

The early stages are marked by alveolitis, an inflammation of the air sacs called alveoli, in the lungs. The job of the air sacs is to allow the transfer of oxygen from the lungs into the blood and the elimination of carbon dioxide from the lungs and out of the body.

As IPF progresses, the alveoli become damaged and scarred, thus stiffening the lungs. The stiffening makes breathing difficult and brings on a feeling of breathlessness (dyspnea), especially during activities that require extra effort.

In addition, scarring of the alveoli reduces the ability of the lungs to transfer oxygen. The resulting lack of oxygen in the blood (hypoxemia) may cause increases in the pressure inside the blood vessels of the lungs, a situation known as pulmonary hypertension. The high blood pressure in the lungs then puts a strain on the right ventricle, the lower right side of the heart, which pumps the oxygen-poor blood into the lungs.

How Is IPF Diagnosed?

The first suspicion that a person may have idiopathic pulmonary fibrosis is usually based on the patient's symptoms and medical history. The doctor will try to confirm or rule out any suspicion by ordering one or more of the following tests.

Chest X-ray

A simple chest x-ray is a picture of the lungs and surrounding tissues, most often taken while the patient is standing up. In an IPF patient, the x-ray usually reveals shadows, mostly in the lower part of the lungs. In addition, lung size tends to appear smaller than normal.

Computed Tomography (CT)

A computed tomography scan of the chest is a series of x-rays that provide a view of the lungs that looks almost as if a slice had been made through the chest. During a CT scan, the patient lies inside a long, oval-shaped machine that permits x-ray beams to pass through the top, sides, and back of the body. A computer is used to combine all the pictures taken from these positions and thus gives the doctor a good look at what's going on inside the lungs and chest.

Blood Tests

When IPF is suspected, the doctor will analyze the patient's blood. A low level of oxygen in the arterial blood may reveal that the alveoli are not taking up enough oxygen.

Pulmonary Function Tests

Pulmonary function tests (PFTs) require the patient to breathe into a mouthpiece. The mouthpiece, in turn, is connected to a machine that measures the amount of air the patient breathes in and out over a specific period of time. The results tell the doctor how well the air passages in the lungs are functioning and how well the lungs are expanding.

Bronchoalveolar Lavage

Lung washings (bronchoalveolar lavage) are also helpful in arriving at a diagnosis of IPF. In this procedure, the doctor inserts a long,

narrow, flexible, lighted tube called a bronchoscope down the windpipe and into the lungs to remove fluid (lavage) and other materials from inside the lungs. The amounts of certain cells and proteins
found in the materials are measured to determine the stage of the
lung disease.

Even is some or all of the results from such tests are abnormal,
they are rarely sufficient to make a specific diagnosis of IPF. The only
way the doctor can confirm a diagnosis of IPF is by examining the
lung tissue; such tissue is usually obtained by an open lung biopsy.

Open Lung Biopsy

In an open lung biopsy, a chest surgeon makes cuts between the
ribs in the chest and removes small pieces of tissue from several places
in the lungs. The material is examined in the laboratory to determine
how much inflammation and fibrosis are in the lungs. It is the only
way to confirm whether the patient has IPF. If IPF is present, the
biopsy results are also the best way to find out how far the disease
has progressed and what the outlook is.

In a patient with no other significant illness, recovery from an open
lung biopsy is relatively quick. The hospital stay is usually 4 to 7 days;
some newer procedures require less surgery, bringing hospital stays
to 1 to 3 days.

Can IPF Be Treated?

The best chance of slowing the progress of IPF is by treatment as
soon as possible. Most IPF patients require treatment throughout life,
usually under the guidance of a lung specialist. Some major medical
centers and large teaching hospitals do research on the disease and
provide consultation and treatment to patients.

Treatment for idiopathic pulmonary fibrosis may vary a great deal.
It depends on many things, including the age of the patient and
stage of the disease. The aim of treatment is to reduce the inflammation of the alveoli and stop the abnormal process that ends in
fibrosis. Once scar tissue has formed in the lung, it cannot be returned to normal.

How Is IPF Treated?

Drugs are the primary way that IPF is treated. They are usually
prescribed for at least 3 to 6 months. This gives the doctor time to

see if a particular treatment is effective. A combination of tests is used to monitor how well a particular drug is working. The dose may have to be adjusted so that the medicine gives the best possible results with the least side effects. Most side effects are reduced when the dose is made smaller or the drug is stopped. Commonly used drugs are prednisone and cytoxan. Oxygen administration and, in special cases, transplantation of the lung are other choices.

Prednisone

A corticosteroid, prednisone, is the most common drug given to patients with idiopathic pulmonary fibrosis. About 25 to 35 percent of all patients respond favorably to this medicine. No one knows exactly how corticosteroids work or why some patients do well on prednisone while others do not. Patients take prednisone by mouth every morning, starting with a high dose for the first 4 to 8 weeks. As they improve, they gradually take smaller amounts. Changes in mood are one of the more common side effects of prednisone; most patients, however, can handle the mood changes—anxiety, depression, or sleeplessness—once they know what is causing the problem. A less common side effect is a rise in blood-sugar levels.

Cytoxan

Cyclophosphamide, also referred to as cytoxan, may be taken together with prednisone, or instead of it. Like prednisone, cytoxan is swallowed each day.

One of the more serious side effects of cyclophosphamide is leukopenia, a condition in which the number of white blood cells drops to a dangerously low level. Leukopenia can be controlled by regularly checking the blood count and adjusting the dose of cytoxan if necessary.

Other Medicines

Azathioprine, penicillamine, chlorambucil, vincristine sulfate, and colchicine have been used in a few patients with idiopathic pulmonary fibrosis. Their effectiveness in treating IPF, however, has not been adequately tested.

Oxygen

In addition to treatment with medicine, some patients may need oxygen, especially when blood oxygen becomes low. This treatment helps resupply the blood with oxygen. As a result, breathlessness is reduced, the patient can be more active, and the severity of pulmonary hypertension decreases.

Exercise

Regular exercise may be useful for patients with IPF. A daily walk or regular use of a stationary bicycle or treadmill can improve muscle strength and breathing ability and also increase overall strength. If needed, supplemental oxygen should be used; sometimes it is the only way a patient is able to do a reasonable amount of activity.

Lung Transplantation

Lung transplantation, either of both lungs or only one, is an alternative to drug treatment for patients in the severe, final stages of IPF. It is most often performed in patients under 60 years of age who do not respond to any form of treatment. The 1-year survival rate is approximately 60 percent.

How Will IPF Affect a Patient's Lifestyle?

Many IPF patients, particularly those in the early stages of the disease, respond to drug treatment and can continue to go about most of their normal activities, including working. Some patients with advanced IPF need to carry oxygen with them.

In addition to getting proper treatment, IPF patients can help themselves by following the same sensible health measures that everyone should observe. These include eating a healthy diet, maintaining proper weight, exercising regularly, and getting enough rest. Above all, IPF patients should not smoke. Pregnancy is not advisable because the illness puts an extra load on the heart and lungs.

As with many chronic illnesses, emotional support and psychological counseling can be of much help to the patient. Most doctors and patients agree that it is important for both patient and family to be as informed as possible about IPF. In this way, everyone involved can understand the illness and apply that information to what is happening in his or her own life.

Chapter 22

Legionnaires Disease

Legionnaires disease, which is also known as Legionellosis, is a form of pneumonia. It is often called Legionnaires disease because the first known outbreak occurred in the Bellevue Stratford Hotel that was hosting a convention of the Pennsylvania Department of the American Legion. In that outbreak, approximately 221 people contracted this previously unknown type of bacterial pneumonia, and 34 people died. The source of the bacterium was found to be contaminated water used to cool the air in the hotel's air conditioning system.

Legionnaires disease is most often contracted by inhaling mist from water sources such as whirlpool baths, showers, and cooling towers that are contaminated with Legionella bacteria. There is no evidence for person-to-person spread of the disease.

Symptoms

Symptoms of Legionnaires disease include fever, chills, and a cough that may or may not produce sputum. Other symptoms include abdominal pain, diarrhea, and confusion. This list of symptoms, however, does not readily distinguish Legionnaires disease from other types of pneumonia. Legionnaires disease is confirmed by laboratory

Text in this chapter is from "Legionnaires Disease," National Institute of Environmental Health Sciences (NIEHS), 1998, and "Legionellosis: Legionnaires Disease and Pontiac Fever," National Center for Infectious Diseases, Centers for Disease Control and Prevention (CDC), 2000.

tests that detect the presence of the bacterium, *Legionella pnuemophila*, or the presence of other bacteria in the family *Legionellaceae*. It is the most often treated with the antibiotic drug Erythromycin.

Although Legionnaires disease has a mortality rate of 5 to 15 percent, many people may be infected with the bacterium that causes the disease, yet not develop any symptoms. It is likely that many cases of Legionnaires disease go undiagnosed.

Legionnaires disease can be viewed as an example of how our physical environment affects our health. Relative humidity, temperature, and other environmental factors can alter the incidence and the fatality rates of infectious diseases, including Legionnaires disease. For example, cooling towers and evaporative condensers of large air conditioning systems have been associated with outbreaks of the disease, and the highest incidence of Legionnaires disease occurs in the warmest months of the year, the time when air conditioning systems are used the most.

Legionellosis

Legionellosis is an infection caused by the bacterium *Legionella pneumophila*. The disease has two distinct forms:

- Legionnaires disease, the more severe form of infection which includes pneumonia, and

- Pontiac fever, a milder illness.

Legionnaires disease acquired its name in 1976 when an outbreak of pneumonia occurred among persons attending a convention of the American Legion in Philadelphia. Later, the bacterium causing the illness was named Legionella.

How common is legionellosis in the United States?

An estimated 8,000 to 18,000 people get Legionnaires disease in the United States each year. Some people can be infected with the Legionella bacterium and have mild symptoms or no illness at all.

Outbreaks of Legionnaires disease receive significant media attention. However, this disease usually occurs as a single, isolated case not associated with any recognized outbreak. When outbreaks do occur, they are usually recognized in the summer and early fall, but cases may occur year-round. About 5% to 30% of people who have Legionnaires disease die.

What are the usual symptoms of legionellosis?

Patients with Legionnaires disease usually have fever, chills, and a cough, which may be dry or may produce sputum. Some patients also have muscle aches, headache, tiredness, loss of appetite, and, occasionally, diarrhea. Laboratory tests may show that these patients' kidneys are not functioning properly. Chest X-rays often show pneumonia. It is difficult to distinguish Legionnaires disease from other types of pneumonia by symptoms alone; other tests are required for diagnosis.

Persons with Pontiac fever experience fever and muscle aches and do not have pneumonia. They generally recover in 2 to 5 days without treatment.

The time between the patient's exposure to the bacterium and the onset of illness for Legionnaires disease is 2 to 10 days; for Pontiac fever, it is shorter, generally a few hours to 2 days.

How is legionellosis diagnosed?

The diagnosis of legionellosis requires special tests not routinely performed on persons with fever or pneumonia. Therefore, a physician must consider the possibility of legionellosis in order to obtain the right tests.

Several types of tests are available. The most useful tests detect the bacteria in sputum, find Legionella antigens in urine samples, or compare antibody levels to Legionella in two blood samples obtained 3 to 6 weeks apart.

Who gets legionellosis?

People of any age may get Legionnaires disease, but the illness most often affects middle-aged and older persons, particularly those who smoke cigarettes or have chronic lung disease. Also at increased risk are persons whose immune system is suppressed by diseases such as cancer, kidney failure requiring dialysis, diabetes, or AIDS. Those that take drugs that suppress the immune system are also at higher risk.

Pontiac fever most commonly occurs in persons who are otherwise healthy.

What is the treatment for legionellosis?

Erythromycin is the antibiotic currently recommended for treating persons with Legionnaires disease. In severe cases, a second drug, rifampin, may be used in addition. Other drugs are available for patients unable to tolerate erythromycin.

Pontiac fever requires no specific treatment.

How is legionellosis spread?

Outbreaks of legionellosis have occurred after persons have breathed mists that come from a water source (e.g., air conditioning cooling towers, whirlpool spas, showers) contaminated with Legionella bacteria. Persons may be exposed to these mists in homes, workplaces, hospitals, or public places. Legionellosis is not passed from person to person, and there is no evidence of persons becoming infected from auto air conditioners or household window air-conditioning units.

Where is the Legionella bacterium found?

Legionella organisms can be found in many types of water systems. However, the bacteria reproduce to high numbers in warm, stagnant water (90°-105° F), such as that found in certain plumbing systems and hot water tanks, cooling towers and evaporative condensers of large air-conditioning systems, and whirlpool spas. Cases of legionellosis have been identified throughout the United States and in several foreign countries. It is believed to occur worldwide.

What is being done to prevent legionellosis?

Improved design and maintenance of cooling towers and plumbing systems to limit the growth and spread of Legionella organisms are the foundations of legionellosis prevention.

During outbreaks, CDC and health department investigators seek to identify the source of disease transmission and recommend appropriate prevention and control measures, such as decontamination of the water source. Current research will likely identify additional prevention strategies.

Chapter 23

Lymphangioleiomyomatosis (LAM)

Lymphangioleiomyomatosis (LAM) is a rare lung disease that was first described in the medical literature by von Stossel in 1937. The disease is characterized by an unusual type of muscle cell that invades the tissue of the lungs, including the airways, and blood and lymph vessels. Over time, these muscle cells form into bundles and grow into the walls of the airways, and blood and lymph vessels, causing them to become obstructed.

Although these cells are not considered cancerous, they act somewhat like cancer cells in that they grow uncontrollably throughout the lung. Over time, the muscle cells block the flow of air, blood, and lymph to and from the lungs, preventing the lungs from providing oxygen to the rest of the body.

Kidney tumors that are often asymptomatic may also be found in patients with LAM.

Lymph and angio refer to the lymph and blood vessels. Leiomyomatosis refers to the formation of the bundles of the unusual muscle cells.

The cause of LAM is not known.

How Common Is LAM?

LAM affects almost exclusively women of childbearing age, although several cases have been reported in which the disease was

National Heart, Lung, and Blood Institute (NHLBI), 1995. Text available online at http://www.nhlbi.nih.gov/health/public/lung/other/lam.txt; cited April 2000.

thought to have developed after menopause. The international literature also includes reports of a few cases in men.

The precise number of people who have LAM is not known. It has been estimated that there may be up to several hundred women in the United States with the disease.

It also has been suggested that LAM has become more common during the past 5 to 10 years, although it may be that doctors are doing a better job of diagnosing it.

What Are the Symptoms of Lymphangioleiomyomatosis?

A common symptom of LAM is shortness of breath (dyspnea) with physical activity. In the early stages of disease, the person with LAM may experience shortness of breath only during strenuous exercise, but as the disease advances, there may be shortness of breath even at rest. Another common symptom is chest pain, and occasionally patients cough up small amounts of blood.

The symptoms associated with LAM are caused by the excessive growth of the muscle cells around the airways, and blood and lymph vessels. The excess muscle cells can block the airways, trapping air in the smallest air compartments in the lung (alveoli) and causing the person with LAM to have difficulty moving air out of the lungs. This results in a breakdown of the lung tissue and the formation of small cysts (air filled cavities).

Cysts near or on the surface of the lung (blebs) can rupture and, as air leaks from the lung into the chest cavity (pneumothorax), the lung or a part of the lung can collapse, causing pain. If the amount of air that leaks out is small, the lung may seal over the space and re-expand itself. If air continues to leak into the chest cavity, however, it may be necessary to re-expand the collapsed portion of the lung by removing the air that has leaked into the chest cavity. This is an in-patient procedure, done using a tube inserted through the chest wall into the chest cavity.

The excessive muscle growth may also block blood vessels in the lung, causing them to become distended with blood and even to rupture. This can result in the patient coughing up blood-stained sputum or blood (hemoptysis).

Obstruction of the lymphatic vessels by the excess muscle growth can lead to leakage of fluid into the chest cavity (pleural effusion). The fluid may be straw-colored (lymph), or fat-containing, milky white (chyle), or pinkish-red if it contains blood. A physician can remove some of this fluid with a needle and syringe to determine its composition and origin. If large amounts of this fluid accumulate in the chest cavity, it may have to be removed through a tube surgically inserted into the chest.

It is estimated that 30 to 50 percent of LAM patients will develop leakage of air into the chest cavity (pneumothorax), and up to 80 percent will have leakage of fluid into the chest cavity (pleural effusions). Coughing up blood-stained sputum or blood (hemoptysis) occurs less frequently.

What Is the Course of Lymphangioleiomyomatosis?

LAM is generally progressive, leading to increasingly impaired lung function. The rate of development can vary considerably among patients. As the disease advances, there is more extensive growth of muscle cells throughout the lung and repeated leakage of fluid into the chest cavity (pleural effusions). As an increasing number of cysts are formed, the lung takes on a honeycomb appearance.

The survival time following the diagnosis of LAM is uncertain. It has been reported to be less than 10 years, but new reports show patients living more than 20 years after diagnosis. The reason for the apparently increased survival time is unknown.

How Is Lymphangioleiomyomatosis Diagnosed?

The diagnosis of LAM can be difficult because many of the early symptoms are similar to those of other lung diseases, such as asthma, emphysema, or bronchitis. Often the person with LAM first goes to the physician complaining of chest pain and shortness of breath that was caused by a pneumothorax.

There are a number of tests the physician can do to confirm or rule out the existence of LAM.

Chest X-ray

This is a simple procedure that provides a picture of the lungs and other tissue in the chest. The chest x-ray is used to diagnose a pneumothorax or the presence of fluid in the chest cavity (pleural effusion).

Pulmonary Function Tests

The patient breathes through a mouthpiece into a machine (spirometer) that measures the volume of air in the lungs, the movement of air into and out of the lungs, and the movement of oxygen from the lungs into the blood.

Blood Tests

The patient's blood is analyzed to determine whether the lungs are providing an adequate supply of oxygen to the blood.

Computed Tomography (CT)

Computed tomography (CT) is the most definitive imaging test for diagnosing LAM.

The patient lies inside a long, cylindrical structure, and x-ray beams pass through the body from different angles, producing multiple images. A computer combines all of these images and provides a 3-dimensional picture of the inside of the lungs and chest. This is called a CT scan.

On a CT scan, the presence of thin-walled cysts spread relatively uniformly throughout the lungs usually means LAM.

Lung Biopsy

Although it is sometimes possible to diagnose LAM based on the above tests, the most definitive test for the diagnosis of LAM is an open lung biopsy. In this procedure, a few small pieces of lung tissue are removed through an incision made in the chest wall between the ribs.

Another procedure, thoracoscopy, is also being used in some patients to obtain lung tissue. In this procedure, tiny incisions are made in the chest wall, and a small lighted tube (endoscope) is inserted so that the interior of the lung can be viewed, and small pieces of tissue are removed.

Both procedures must be done in the hospital under general anesthesia. Another technique, called transbronchial biopsy, may also be used to obtain a small amount of lung tissue. A long, narrow, flexible, lighted tube (bronchoscope) is inserted down the windpipe (trachea), and into the lungs.

Bits of lung tissue are sampled, using a tiny forceps. This procedure is usually done in a hospital on an outpatient basis under local anesthesia. It is less reliable than an open lung biopsy because the amount of tissue that can be sampled is sometimes inadequate for diagnostic studies.

After the lung tissue is removed, it is examined in a pathology laboratory for the presence of the abnormal muscle cells and cystic changes characteristic of LAM.

How Is LAM Treated?

Because LAM affects almost exclusively women of childbearing age, physicians have thought that the hormone estrogen might be involved in the abnormal muscle cell growth that characterizes the disease, just as it is in the growth of smooth muscle in the uterus in a woman's childbearing years.

Although there is no evidence that there is a relationship between estrogen and LAM, the treatment of LAM has focused on reducing the production or effects of estrogen. Two treatments used are administration of medroxy-progesterone, a drug containing the hormone progesterone, or removal of the ovaries (oophorectomy). The response to treatment has been highly individual, and no therapy has been found to be effective for all LAM patients.

Oxygen therapy may be necessary if the disease continues to worsen and lung function is impaired.

For LAM patients with severe disease, lung transplantation is an established therapy. One year survival following transplant is approximately 70 percent, and 3-year survival is approximately 50 percent.

What Is the Effect Of LAM On the Patient's Lifestyle?

In the early stages of the disease, most patients can go about their daily activities, including attending school, going to work, and performing common physical activities, such as walking up a hill. In more advanced stages, the patient may have very limited ability to move around and may require oxygen full-time.

Patients with LAM should follow the same healthy lifestyle recommended for the general population, including eating a healthy diet, getting as much exercise as they can, as well as plenty of rest, and, of course, not smoking. Traveling to remote areas where medical attention is not readily available or to high altitudes where the blebs can expand and rupture should be considered carefully before undertaken.

In patients with normal lung function, there is probably no increased risk associated with pregnancy. However, in patients with compromised lung function, pregnancy is not advised.

There do not appear to be complications associated with oral contraceptives, but this issue should be discussed with the patient's pulmonologist and gynecologist.

Can a Patient Participate in LAM Research Programs at the National Heart, Lung, and Blood Institute?

Some LAM patients may be eligible to participate in clinical studies at the Warren Grant Magnuson Clinical Center of the National Institutes of Health in Bethesda, Maryland. Participants must meet the specific study requirements.

Glossary

Alveoli: Tiny sac-like air spaces in the lungs where transfer of carbon dioxide from blood into the lungs and oxygen from air into blood takes place.

Blebs: Cysts on or near the surface of the lungs.

Chest Cavity: Space in body surrounding the lungs.

Chyle: A milky fluid consisting of lymph and droplets of triglyceride fat that becomes mixed with the blood.

Dyspnea: Shortness of breath; difficult or labored breathing.

Hemoptysis: Coughing up blood or blood-stained sputum.

Lymph: A transparent, slightly yellow liquid found in the lymphatic vessels. Lymph is collected from tissue fluids throughout the body and returned to the blood via the lymphatic system.

Pleural effusion: Leakage of fluid into the chest cavity.

For Additional Information

The LAM Foundation
10105 Beacon Hills Drive
Cincinnati, OH 45241
Tel: 513-777-6889
Fax: 513-777-4109
Internet: http://lam.uc.edu
E-Mail: lam@one.net

Chapter 24

Lung Cancer

What Is Lung Cancer?

Lung cancer is cancer that usually starts in the lining of the bronchi, but can also begin in other areas of the respiratory system, including the trachea, bronchioles, or alveoli. Lung cancers are believed to develop over a period of many years.

Nearly all lung cancers are carcinomas, a cancer that begins in the lining or covering tissues of an organ. The tumor cells of each type of lung cancer grow and spread differently, and each type requires different treatment. More than 95 percent of lung cancers belong to the group called bronchogenic carcinoma.

Lung cancers are generally divided into two types:

- *Nonsmall cell lung cancer* is more common than small cell lung cancer. The three main kinds of non-small cell lung cancer are named for the type of cells in the tumor:

  Squamous cell carcinoma, also called epidermoid carcinoma, is the most common type of lung cancer in men. It often begins in the bronchi, and usually does not spread as quickly as other types of lung cancer.

  Adenocarcinoma usually begins along the outer edges of the lungs and under the lining of the bronchi. It is the most common type of lung cancer in women and in people who have never smoked.

Large cell carcinomas are a group of cancers with large, abnormal-looking cells. These tumors usually begin along the outer edges of the lungs.

- *Small cell lung cancer*, sometimes called oat cell cancer because the cancer cells may look like oats when viewed under a microscope, grows rapidly and quickly spreads to other organs.

It is important to find out what kind of lung cancer a person has. The different types of carcinomas, involving different regions of the lung, may cause different symptoms and are treated differently.

What Are the Symptoms of Lung Cancer?

The following are the most common symptoms for lung cancer, however, each individual may experience symptoms differently.

Lung cancer usually does not cause symptoms when it first develops, but they often become present after the tumor begins growing. A cough is the most common symptom of lung cancer.

Other symptoms include:

- constant chest pain
- shortness of breath
- wheezing
- recurring lung infections, such as pneumonia or bronchitis
- bloody or rust colored sputum
- hoarseness
- a tumor that presses on large blood vessels near the lung can cause swelling of the neck and face
- a tumor that presses on certain nerves near the lung causing pain and weakness in the shoulder, arm, or hand
- fever for unknown reason

Like all cancers, lung cancer can cause:

- fatigue
- loss of appetite

- loss of weight
- headache
- pain in other parts of the body not affected by the cancer
- bone fractures

Other symptoms can be caused by substances made by lung cancer cells—referred to as a paraneoplastic syndrome. Certain lung cancer cells produce a substance that causes a sharp drop in the level of sodium in the blood, which can cause many symptoms, including confusion and sometimes even coma.

None of these symptoms is a sure sign of lung cancer. Only a physician can tell whether a patient's symptoms are caused by cancer or by another problem. Consult your physician for a diagnosis.

What Are the Risk Factors for Lung Cancer?

A risk factor is anything that increases a person's chance of getting a disease such as cancer. Different cancers have different risk factors. Several risk factors make a person more likely to develop lung cancer:

- Smoking is the leading cause of lung cancer, with more than 90 percent of lung cancers thought to be a result of smoking.

Additional risk factors include:

- second-hand smoke—breathing in the smoke of others
- smoking marijuana cigarettes, which:

    contain more tar than tobacco cigarettes.

    are inhaled very deeply.

    are smoked all the way to the end where tar content is the highest.

    Because marijuana is an illegal substance, it is not possible to control whether it contains fungi, pesticides, and other additives.

- recurring inflammation, such as from tuberculosis and some types of pneumonia
- asbestos exposure

- talcum powder—While no increased risk of lung cancer has been found from the use of cosmetic talcum powder, some studies of talc miners and millers suggest a higher risk of lung cancer and other respiratory diseases from their exposure to industrial grade talc. Talcum powder is made from talc, a mineral which in its natural form may contain asbestos, although by law, all home-use talcum products (baby, body, and facial powders) have been asbestos-free.

- cancer-causing agents in the workplace, including:
    radioactive ores such as uranium
    arsenic
    vinyl chloride
    nickel chromates
    coal products
    mustard gas
    chloromethyl ethers

- radon—a radioactive gas that cannot been seen, tasted or smelled. It is produced by the natural breakdown of uranium

- family history

- personal history of lung cancer

- vitamin A deficiency—People who do not get enough vitamin A are at increased risk of lung cancer. Taking too much vitamin A may also increase lung cancer risk.

- air pollution—In some cities, air pollution may slightly increase the risk of lung cancer.

How Is Lung Cancer Diagnosed?

In addition to a complete medical history to check for risk factors and symptoms, and a physical examination to provide other information about signs of lung cancer and other health problems, procedures used to diagnose lung cancer include:

- chest x-ray—to look for any mass or spot on the lungs.

- other special x-rays and scans (such as the CT (computed tomography) scan)—can provide more precise information about the size, shape, and position of a tumor.

- sputum cytology—a study of phlegm (spit) cells under a microscope.

- needle biopsy—a needle is guided into the mass while the lungs are being viewed on a CT scan and a sample of the mass is removed and evaluated in the pathology laboratory under a microscope.

- bronchoscopy—a fiberoptic flexible, lighted tube is passed through the mouth into the bronchi to help find centrally located tumors or blockages, and gather samples of tissue or fluids to be examined under a microscope.

- mediastinoscopy—a process in which a small cut is made in the neck so that a tissue sample can be taken from the lymph nodes (mediastinal nodes) along the windpipe and the major bronchial tube areas to evaluate under a microscope.

- x-rays and scans of the brain, liver, bone, and adrenal glands— to determine if the cancer has spread from where it started into other areas of the body.

Other tests and procedures may be used as well.

Treatment for Lung Cancer

Specific treatment will be determined by your physician(s) based on:

- your age, overall health, and medical history
- extent of the disease
- your tolerance for specific medications, procedures, or therapies
- expectations for the course of the disease
- your opinion or preference

Surgery, radiation therapy, and chemotherapy may be used in the treatment of lung cancer.

Three main types of surgery are most often used in lung cancer treatment. The choice depends on the size and location of the tumor, the extent of the cancer, the general health of the patient, and other factors.

- Surgery

  segmental or wedge resection—to remove only a small part of the lung

  lobectomy—removal of an entire lobe of the lung

  pneumonectomy—removal of an entire lung

- radiation therapy (also called radiotherapy)—the use of high-energy rays to damage cancer cells and stop them from growing and dividing.

- chemotherapy—the use of drugs to kill cancer cells.

Chapter 25

Pneumonia

What Is Pneumonia?

Pneumonia is a serious infection or inflammation of your lungs. The air sacs in the lungs fill with pus and other liquid. Oxygen has trouble reaching your blood. If there is too little oxygen in your blood, your body cells can't work properly. Because of this and spreading infection through the body pneumonia can cause death.

Until 1936, pneumonia was the No.1 cause of death in the U.S. Since then, the use of antibiotics brought it under control. In 1996, pneumonia and influenza combined ranks as the fifth leading cause of death since 1979.

Pneumonia affects your lungs in two ways. Lobar pneumonia affects a section (lobe) of a lung. Bronchial pneumonia (or bronchopneumonia) affects patches throughout both lungs.

Causes of Pneumonia

Pneumonia is not a single disease. It can have over 30 different causes. There are five main causes of pneumonia:

- Bacteria
- Mycoplasmas
- Other agents, such as pneumocystis
- Viruses
- Various chemicals

Bacterial Pneumonia

Bacterial pneumonia can attack anyone from infants through the very old. Alcoholics, the debilitated, post-operative patients, people with respiratory diseases or viral infections and people who have weakened immune systems are at greater risk.

Pneumonia bacteria are present in some healthy throats. When body defenses are weakened in some way, by illness, old age, malnutrition, general debility or impaired immunity, the bacteria can multiply and cause serious damage. Usually, when a person's resistance is lowered, bacteria work their way into the lungs and inflame the air sacs.

The tissue of part of a lobe of the lung, an entire lobe, or even most of the lung's five lobes becomes completely filled with liquid (this is called "consolidation"). The infection quickly spreads through the bloodstream and the whole body is invaded.

The *streptococcus pneumoniae* is the most common cause of bacterial pneumonia. It is one form of pneumonia for which a vaccine is available.

Symptoms

The onset of bacterial pneumonia can vary from gradual to sudden. In the most severe cases, the patient may experience shaking chills, chattering teeth, severe chest pain, and a cough that produces rust-colored or greenish mucus.

A person's temperature often rises as high as 105° F. The patient sweats profusely, and breathing and pulse rate increase rapidly. Lips and nailbeds may have a bluish color due to lack of oxygen in the blood. A patient's mental state may be confused or delirious.

Viral Pneumonia

Half of all pneumonias are believed to be caused by viruses. More and more viruses are being identified as the cause of respiratory infection, and though most attack the upper respiratory tract, some produce pneumonia, especially in children. Most of these pneumonias are not serious and last a short time.

Influenza virus may be severe and occasionally fatal. The virus invades the lungs and multiplies, but there are almost no physical signs of lung tissue becoming filled with fluid. It finds many of its victims among those who have pre-existing heart or lung disease or are pregnant.

Symptoms

The initial symptoms of viral pneumonia are the same as influenza symptoms: fever, a dry cough, headache, muscle pain, and weakness. Within 12 to 36 hours, there is increasing breathlessness; the cough becomes worse and produces a small amount of mucus. There is a high fever and there may be blueness of the lips.

In extreme cases, the patient has a desperate need for air and extreme breathlessness. Viral pneumonias may be complicated by an invasion of bacteria, with all the typical symptoms of bacterial pneumonia.

Mycoplasma Pneumonia

Because of its somewhat different symptoms and physical signs, and because the course of the illness differed from classical pneumococcal pneumonia, mycoplasma pneumonia was once believed to be caused by one or more undiscovered viruses and was called "primary atypical pneumonia."

Identified during World War II, mycoplasmas are the smallest free-living agents of disease in humankind, unclassified as to whether bacteria or viruses, but having characteristics of both. They generally cause a mild and widespread pneumonia. They affect all age groups, occurring most frequently in older children and young adults. The death rate is low, even in untreated cases.

Symptoms

The most prominent symptom of mycoplasma pneumonia is a cough that tends to come in violent attacks, but produces only sparse whitish mucus. Chills and fever are early symptoms, and some patients experience nausea or vomiting. Patients may experience profound weakness which lasts for a long time.

Other Kinds of Pneumonia

Pneumocystis carinii pneumonia (PCP) is caused by an organism believed to be a fungus. PCP is the first sign of illness in many persons with AIDS, and perhaps 80 percent of AIDS patients (four out of five) will develop it sooner or later.

PCP can be successfully treated in many cases. It may recur a few months later, but treatment can help to prevent or delay its recurrence.

Other less common pneumonias may be quite serious and are occurring more often. Various special pneumonias are caused by the inhalation of food, liquid, gases or dust, and by fungi. Foreign bodies or a bronchial obstruction such as a tumor may promote the occurrence of pneumonia, although they are not causes of pneumonia.

Rickettsia (also considered an organism somewhere between viruses and bacteria) cause Rocky Mountain spotted fever, Q fever, typhus and psittacosis, diseases that may have mild or severe effects on the lungs. Tuberculosis pneumonia is a very serious lung infection and extremely dangerous unless treated early.

Treating Pneumonia

If you develop pneumonia, your chances of a fast recovery are greatest under certain conditions: if you're young, if your pneumonia is caught early, if your defenses against disease are working well, if the infection hasn't spread, and if you're not suffering from other illnesses.

In the young and healthy, early treatment with antibiotics can cure bacterial pneumonia and speed recovery from mycoplasma pneumonia, and a certain percentage of rickettsia cases. There is no clearly effective treatment yet for viral pneumonia, which usually heals on its own. Most people can be treated at home.

The drugs used to fight pneumonia are determined by the germ causing the pneumonia and the judgment of the doctor. After a patient's temperature returns to normal, medication must be continued according to the doctor's instructions, otherwise the pneumonia may recur. Relapses can be far more serious than the first attack.

Besides antibiotics, patients are given supportive treatment: proper diet and oxygen to increase oxygen in the blood when needed. In some patients, medication to ease chest pain and to provide relief from violent cough may be necessary.

The vigorous young person may lead a normal life within a week of recovery from pneumonia. For the middle-aged, however, weeks may elapse before they regain their accustomed strength, vigor, and feeling of well-being. A person recovering from mycoplasma pneumonia may be weak for an extended period of time.

In general, a person should not be discouraged from returning to work or carrying out usual activities but must be warned to expect some difficulties. Adequate rest is important to maintain progress toward full recovery and to avoid relapse. Remember, don't rush recovery!

Preventing Pneumonia Is Possible

Because pneumonia is a common complication of influenza (flu), getting a flu shot every fall is good pneumonia prevention.

Vaccine is also available to help fight pneumococcal pneumonia, one type of bacterial pneumonia. Your doctor can help you decide if you, or a member of your family, needs the vaccine against pneumococcal pneumonia. It is usually given only to people at high risk of getting the disease and its life-threatening complications.

The greatest risk of pneumococcal pneumonia is usually among people who:

- Have chronic illnesses such as lung disease, heart disease, kidney disorders, sickle cell anemia, or diabetes.

- Are recovering from severe illness

- Are in nursing homes or other chronic care facilities

- Are age 65 or older

If you are at risk, ask your doctor for the vaccine.

The vaccine is generally given only once. Ask your doctor about any revaccination recommendations. The vaccine is not recommended for pregnant women or children under age two. Since pneumonia often follows ordinary respiratory infections, the most important preventive measure is to be alert to any symptoms of respiratory trouble that linger more than a few days. Good health habits, proper diet and hygiene, rest, regular exercise, etc., increase resistance to all respiratory illnesses. They also help promote fast recovery when illness does occur.

If You Have Symptoms of Pneumonia

- Call your doctor immediately. Even with the many effective antibiotics, early diagnosis and treatment are important.

- Follow your doctor's advice. In serious cases, your doctor may advise a hospital stay. Or recovery at home may be possible.

- Continue to take the medicine your doctor prescribes until told you may stop. This will help prevent recurrence of pneumonia and relapse.

- Remember, even though pneumonia can be treated, it is an extremely serious illness. Don't wait, get treatment early.

Chapter 26

Primary Pulmonary Hypertension (PPH)

Primary, or unexplained, pulmonary hypertension (PPH) is a rare lung disorder in which the blood pressure in the pulmonary artery rises far above normal levels for no apparent reason. The pulmonary artery is the blood vessel carrying oxygen-poor blood from the right ventricle, one of the pumping chambers of the heart, to the lungs. In the lungs, the blood picks up oxygen and then flows to the left side of the heart, where it is pumped by the left ventricle to the rest of the body through the aorta.

Hypertension is the medical term for an abnormally high blood pressure. Normal mean pulmonary-artery pressure is approximately 14 mmHg at rest. In the PPH patient, the mean blood pressure in the pulmonary artery is greater than 25 mmHg at rest and 30 mmHg during exercise. This abnormally high pressure (pulmonary hypertension) is associated with changes in the small blood vessels in the lungs, resulting in an increased resistance to blood flowing through the vessels.

This increased resistance, in turn, places a strain on the right ventricle, which now has to work harder than usual against the resistance to move adequate amounts of blood through the lungs.

Incidence

The true incidence of PPH is unknown. The first reported case occurred in 1891, when E. Romberg, a German doctor, published a

National Heart, Lung, and Blood Institute (NHLBI), NIH Publication Number 96-3291, 1996. Text available online at http://www.nhlbi.nih.gov/health/public/lung/other/pph.txt; cited April 2000.

description of a patient who, at autopsy, showed thickening of the pulmonary artery but no heart or lung disease that might have caused the condition. In 1951, when 39 cases were reported by Dr. D.T. Dresdale in the United States, the illness received its name.

Between 1967 and 1973, a 10-fold increase in unexplained pulmonary hypertension was reported in central Europe. The rise was subsequently traced to aminorex fumarate, an amphetamine-like drug introduced in Europe in 1965 to control appetite. Only about 1 in 1,000 people who took the drug developed PPH. When they stopped taking the drug, some improved considerably; in others, the disease kept getting worse. Once aminorex was removed from the market, the incidence of PPH went down to normal levels.

More recently, in the United States and France, several cases of PPH have been associated with the appetite suppressants, fenfluramine and dexfenfluramine.

In the United States it has been estimated that 300 new cases of PPH are diagnosed each year; the greatest number are reported in women between the ages of 21 and 40. Indeed, at one time the disease was thought to occur among young women almost exclusively; we now know, however, that men and women in all age ranges, from very young children to elderly people, can develop PPH. Apparently it also affects people of all racial and ethnic origins equally.

Cause

There may be one or more causes of PPH; however, all remain unknown. The low incidence makes learning more about the disease extremely difficult. Studies of PPH also have been difficult because a good animal model of the disease has not been available.

Researchers think that in most people who develop PPH the blood vessels are particularly sensitive to certain internal or external factors and constrict, or narrow, when exposed to these factors. For example, people with Raynaud's disease seem more likely than others to develop PPH; Raynaud's disease is a condition in which the fingers and toes turn blue when cold because the blood vessels in the fingers and toes are particularly sensitive to cold. Diet suppressants, cocaine, HIV, and pregnancy are some of the factors that are thought to trigger constriction, or narrowing, in the pulmonary artery.

In about 6 to 10 percent of cases, PPH is familial; that is, it is inherited from other family members. The familial form of PPH is similar to the more common form of the disease, sometimes referred to as "sporadic" PPH.

Course of the Disease

Researchers believe that one of the ways PPH starts is with injury to the layer of cells (the endothelial cells) that line the small blood vessels of the lungs. This injury, which occurs for unknown reasons, may bring about changes in the way the endothelial cells interact with smooth muscle cells in the vessel wall. As a result, the smooth muscle contracts more than normal and thereby narrows the vessel.

The process eventually results in the development of extra amounts of tissue in the walls of the pulmonary arteries. The amount of muscle increases in some arteries, and muscle appears in the walls of arteries that normally have no muscle. With time, scarring, or fibrosis, of the arteries takes place, and they become stiff as well as thickened. Some vessels may become completely blocked. There is also a tendency for blood clots to form within the smaller arteries.

In response to the extra demands placed on it by PPH, the heart muscle gets bigger, and the right ventricle expands in size. Overworked and enlarged, the right ventricle gradually becomes weak and loses its ability to pump enough blood to the lungs. Eventually, the right side of the heart may fail completely, resulting in death.

Symptoms

In general, researchers find there is no correlation between the time PPH is thought to have started, the age at which it is diagnosed, and the severity of symptoms. In some patients, especially children, the disease progresses fairly rapidly.

The first symptom is frequently tiredness, with many patients thinking they tire easily because they are simply out of shape. Difficulty in breathing (dyspnea), dizziness, and even fainting spells (syncope) are also typical early symptoms. Swelling in the ankles or legs (edema), bluish lips and skin (cyanosis), and chest pain (angina) are among other symptoms of the disease.

Patients with PPH may also complain of a racing pulse; many feel they have trouble getting enough air. Palpitations, a strong throbbing sensation brought on by the increased rate of the heartbeat, can also cause discomfort.

Some people with PPH do not seek medical advice until they can no longer go about their daily routine. The more severe the symptoms, the more advanced the disease. In these more advanced stages, the patient is able to perform only minimal activity and has symptoms even when resting. The disease may worsen to the point where the patient is completely bedridden.

Diagnosis

PPH is rarely picked up in a routine medical examination. Even in its later stages, the signs of the disease can be confused with other conditions affecting the heart and lungs. Thus, much time can pass between the time the symptoms of PPH appear and a definite diagnosis is made.

PPH remains a diagnosis of exclusion. This means that it is diagnosed only after the doctor finds pulmonary hypertension and excludes or cannot find other reasons for the hypertension, such as a chronic obstructive pulmonary disease (chronic bronchitis and emphysema), blood clots in the lung (pulmonary thromboemboli), or some forms of congenital heart disease.

The first tests for PPH help the doctor determine how well the heart and lungs are performing. If the results of these tests do not give the doctor enough information, the doctor must perform a cardiac catheterization. The procedure, discussed below, is the way the doctor can make certain that the patient's problems are due to PPH and not to some other condition.

Electrocardiogram

The electrocardiogram (ECG) is a record of the electrical activity produced by the heart. An abnormal ECG may indicate that the heart is undergoing unusual stress.

In addition to the usual ECG performed while the patient is at rest, the doctor may order an exercise ECG. This ECG helps the doctor evaluate the performance of the heart during exercise, for example, walking a treadmill in the doctor's office.

Echocardiogram

In an echocardiogram, the doctor uses sound waves to map the structure of the heart by placing a slim device that looks like a microphone on the patient's chest. The instrument sends sound waves into the heart, which then are reflected back to form a moving image of the beating heart's structure on a TV screen. A record is made on paper or videotape. The moving pictures show how well the heart is functioning. The still pictures permit the doctor to measure the size of the heart and the thickness of the heart muscle; in the patient with severe pulmonary hypertension, the still pictures will show that the right heart is enlarged, while the left heart is either normal or reduced in size. Echocardiograms are helpful in excluding some other causes of pulmonary hypertension and can be useful in monitoring the response to treatment.

Pulmonary Function Tests

A variety of tests called pulmonary function tests (PFTs) evaluate lung function. In these procedures, the patient, with a nose clip in place, breathes in and out through a mouthpiece. The patient's breathing displaces the air held in a container suspended in water. As the container rises and falls in response to the patient's breathing, the movements produce a record, or spirogram, that helps the doctor measure lung volume (how much air the lungs hold) and the air flow in and out of the lungs. Some devices measure air flow electronically.

A mild restriction in air movement is commonly seen in patients with PPH. This restriction is thought to be due, in part, to the increased stiffness of the lungs resulting from both the changes in the structure and the high blood pressure in the pulmonary arteries.

Perfusion Lung Scan

A perfusion lung scan shows the pattern of blood flow in the lungs; it can also tell the doctor whether a patient has large blood clots in the lungs. In the perfusion scan, the doctor injects a radioactive substance into a vein. Immediately after the injection, the chest is scanned for radioactivity. Areas in the lung where blood clots are blocking the flow of blood will show up as blank or clear areas.

Two patterns of pulmonary perfusion are seen in patients with PPH. One is a normal pattern of blood distribution; the other shows a scattering of patchy abnormalities in blood flow.

A major reason for doing a perfusion scan is to distinguish patients with PPH from those whose pulmonary hypertension is due to blood clots in the lungs.

Right-Heart Cardiac Catheterization

In right-heart cardiac catheterization, the doctor places a thin, flexible tube, or catheter, through an arm, leg, or neck vein in the patient, and then threads the catheter into the right ventricle and pulmonary artery. Most important in terms of PPH is the ability of the doctor to get a precise measure of the blood pressure in the right side of the heart and the pulmonary artery with this procedure. It is the only way to get this measure, and must be performed in the hospital by a specialist.

During catheterization, the doctor can also evaluate the right heart's pumping ability; this is done by measuring the amount of blood pumped out of the right side of the heart with each heartbeat.

Functional Classification

Once PPH is diagnosed, most doctors will classify the disease according to the functional classification system developed by the New York Heart Association. It is based on patient reports of how much activity they can comfortably undertake.

- *Class 1*—Patients with no symptoms of any kind, and for whom ordinary physical activity does not cause fatigue, palpitation, dyspnea, or anginal pain.

- *Class 2*—Patients who are comfortable at rest but have symptoms with ordinary physical activity.

- *Class 3*—Patients who are comfortable at rest but have symptoms with less-than-ordinary effort.

- *Class 4*—Patients who have symptoms at rest.

Treatment

Some patients do well by taking medicines that make the work of the right ventricle easier. Anticoagulants, for example, can decrease the tendency of the blood to clot, thereby permitting blood to flow more freely. Diuretics decrease the amount of fluid in the body, further reducing the amount of work the heart has to do.

Until recently, nothing more could be done for people who have PPH. However, today doctors can choose from a variety of drugs that help lower blood pressure in the lungs and improve the performance of the heart in many patients.

Some patients also require supplemental oxygen delivered through nasal prongs or a mask if breathing becomes difficult; some need oxygen around the clock. In severely affected cases, a heart-lung, single lung, or double lung transplantation may be appropriate.

Drugs

Doctors now know that PPH patients respond differently to the different medicines that dilate, or relax, blood vessels and that no one drug is consistently effective in all patients. Because individual reactions vary, different drugs have to be tried before chronic or long-term treatment begins. During the course of the disease, the amount and type of medicine may also have to be changed.

To find out which medicine works best for a particular patient, doctors evaluate the drugs during cardiac catheterization. This way they can see the effect of the medicine on the patient's heart and lungs. They can also adjust the dose to reduce the side effects that may occur— for example, systemic low blood pressure (hypotension); nausea; angina; headaches; or flushing.

To determine whether a drug is improving a patient's condition, both the pulmonary pressure and the amount of blood being pumped by the heart (the cardiac output) must be evaluated. A decrease in pulmonary pressure alone, for example, does not necessarily mean that the patient is recovering; cardiac output must either increase or remain unchanged. The most desirable response is a decrease in pressure and an increase in cardiac output. Once the patient has reached a stable condition, he or she can go home, returning every few weeks or months to the doctor for followup.

At present, approximately one-quarter to one-half of patients can be treated with calcium channel blocking drugs given by mouth. By relaxing the smooth muscle in the walls of the heart and blood vessels, these calcium channel blockers improve the ability of the heart to pump blood.

A vasodilator, prostacyclin, is helping some severely ill patients who are unresponsive to treatment with calcium channel blockers. The drug, which has been studied in clinical trials, imitates the natural prostacyclin that the body produces on its own to dilate blood vessels.

Prostacyclin also seems to help prevent blood clots from forming.

Prostacyclin is administered intravenously by a portable, battery-operated pump. The pump is worn attached to a belt around the waist or carried in a small shoulder pack. The medication is then slowly and continuously pumped into the body through a permanent catheter placed in a vein in the neck.

Protstacyclin seems to improve pulmonary hypertension and permit more physical activity. It is sometimes used as a bridge to help those patients waiting for a transplant, while in other cases it is used for long-term treatment.

Transplantation

The first heart-lung transplant was performed in this country in 1981. Many of these operations were performed for patients with PPH. The survival rate is the same as for other patients with heart-lung transplants, about 60 percent for 1 year, and 37 percent for 5 years.

The single lung transplant is the most common method of transplant used in cases of PPH. This procedure, in which one lung—either the left or right—is replaced, was first performed in 1983 in patients with pulmonary fibrosis. Double lung transplants are also done to treat PPH.

There are fewer complications with the single lung transplant than with the heart-lung transplant, and the survival rate is on the order of 70 percent for 1 year. A surprising finding is the remarkable ability of the right ventricle to heal itself. In patients with lung transplants, both the structure and function of the right ventricle markedly improve. Complications of transplantation include rejection by the body of the transplanted organ, and infection. Patients take medications for life to reduce their body's immune system's ability to reject "foreign" organs.

The Primary Pulmonary Hypertension Patient Registry

In 1981, the National Heart, Lung, and Blood Institute (NHLBI) established the first PPH-patient registry in the world. The registry followed 194 people with PPH over a period of at least 1 year and, in some cases, for as long as 7.5 years. Much of what we know about the illness today stems from this study.

At the time the patients enrolled in the registry, 75 percent were in functional classes 3 or 4. They had an average mean pulmonary artery pressure three times the normal, an abnormally high pressure in the right side of the heart, and a reduced cardiac output. In making the diagnosis of PPH, investigators found no complications arising from cardiac catheterization.

The study findings show that pulmonary artery pressure in patients who had symptoms for less than 1 year was similar to that in patients who had symptoms for more than 3 years. Researchers also found that patients whose only symptom was difficulty in breathing upon exercise already had very high pulmonary artery pressure. This suggests that the pulmonary artery pressure rises to high levels early in the course of the disease.

No correlations could be found between the cause of PPH and cigarette smoking, occupation, place of residence, pregnancy, use of appetite suppressants, or use of prescription drugs, including oral contraceptives. This study was designed to serve only as a registry, so it was not possible to evaluate the effectiveness of treatment.

Because we still do not understand the cause or have a cure for PPH, NHLBI remains committed to supporting basic and clinical studies of this illness. Basic research studies are focusing on the possible involvement of immunologic and genetic factors in the cause and progression of PPH, looking at agents that cause narrowing of the pulmonary blood vessels, and identifying factors that cause growth of smooth muscle and formation of scar tissue in the vessel walls. Most important is finding a reliable way to diagnose PPH early in the course of the disease that does not require cardiac catheterization.

Living with Primary Pulmonary Hypertension

With the cause of primary pulmonary hypertension still unknown, there is at present no known way to prevent or cure this disease. However, many patients report that by changing some parts of their lifestyle, they can go about many of their daily tasks. For example, they do relaxation exercises, try to reduce stress, and adopt a positive mental attitude.

People with PPH go to school, work at home or outside the home part-time or full-time, and raise their children. Indeed, many patients with PPH do not look sick, and some feel perfectly well much of the time as long as they do not strain themselves physically.

Walking is good exercise for many patients. Some patients with advanced PPH carry portable oxygen when they go out; patients who find walking too exhausting may use a wheelchair or motorized scooter. Others stay busy with activities that are not of a physical nature.

For the patient who lives at a high altitude, a move to a lower altitude—where the air is not so thin, and thus the amount of oxygen is higher—can be helpful. Medical care is important, preferably by a doctor who is a pulmonary vascular specialist. These specialists are usually located at major research centers.

PPH patients can also help themselves by following the same sensible health measures that everyone should observe. These include eating a healthy diet, not smoking, and getting plenty of rest. Pregnancy is not advised because it puts an extra load on the heart. Oral contraceptives are not recommended, and other methods of birth control should be used.

Most doctors and patients agree that it is important for both patient and family to be as informed as possible about PPH. In this way everyone can understand the illness and apply that information to what is happening. In addition to family and close friends, support groups can help the PPH patient.

Glossary of Terms for This Chapter

Angina: Chest pain that originates in the heart.

Aorta: Blood vessel that delivers oxygen-rich blood from the left ventricle to the body; it is the largest blood vessel in the body.

Atrium: One of the two receiving chambers of the heart. The right atrium receives oxygen-poor blood from the body. The left atrium receives oxygen-rich blood from the lungs. The plural of atrium is atria.

Blood pressure: The pressure of blood against the walls of a blood vessel or heart chamber. Unless there is reference to another location, such as the pulmonary artery or one of the heart chambers, it refers to the pressure in the systemic arteries, as measured, for example, in the forearm.

Cardiac output: Total amount of blood being pumped by the heart over a particular period of time.

Catheter: Thin, flexible medical tube; one use is to insert it into a blood vessel to measure blood pressure.

Clinical trials: Medical studies of patients that evaluate the effectiveness of treatment.

Constrict: Tighten; narrow.

Cyanosis: A bluish color in the skin because of insufficient oxygen.

Diastolic pressure: The lowest pressure to which blood pressure falls between contractions of the ventricles.

Dilate: Relax; expand.

Dyspnea: A sensation of difficulty in breathing.

Edema: Swelling due to the buildup of fluid.

Endothelial cells: The delicate lining, only one cell thick, of the organs of circulation.

Fibrosis: Process by which inflamed tissue becomes scarred.

Heartbeat: One complete contraction of the heart.

Hyperreactive: Describes a situation in which a body tissue is especially likely to have an exaggerated reaction to a particular situation.

Hypertension: Abnormally high blood pressure.

Hypotension: Abnormally low blood pressure.

Lung volume: The amount of air the lungs hold.

Mean blood pressure: The average blood pressure, taking account of the rise and fall that occurs with each heartbeat. It is often estimated by multiplying the diastolic pressure by two, adding the systolic pressure, and then dividing this sum by three.

Palpitation: The sensation of rapid heartbeats.

Perfusion: Flow.

Pulmonary artery: Blood vessel delivering oxygen-poor blood from the right ventricle to the lungs.

Pulmonary hypertension: Abnormally high blood pressure in the arteries of the lungs.

Smooth muscle: Muscle that performs automatic tasks, such as constricting blood vessels.

Spirogram: A record of the amounts of air being moved in and out of the lungs.

Syncope: Fainting; temporary loss of consciousness.

Systemic: Relating to a process that affects the body generally; in this instance, the way in which blood is supplied through the aorta to all body organs except the lungs.

Systolic pressure: The highest pressure to which blood pressure rises with the contraction of the ventricles.

Vasodilator: An agent that widens blood vessels.

Ventricle: One of the two pumping chambers of the heart. The right ventricle receives oxygen-poor blood from the right atrium and pumps it to the lungs through the pulmonary artery. The left ventricle receives oxygen-rich blood from the left atrium and pumps it to the body through the aorta.

For More Information

Pulmonary Hypertension Association (PHA)
817 Silver Spring Ave.
Suite No. 303
Silver Spring, MD 20910
Toll Free: 800-748-7274

Chapter 27

Psittacosis

Many species of birds can carry a form of the organism Chlamydia that can cause the disease psittacosis (sit-ah-COH-sis). The name is derived from a group of birds called psittacine, which includes parrots and parakeets. But the disease also may occur in pigeons, ducks and chickens. Infected birds may not appear ill but can still transmit the germs to humans.

People exposed to infected birds acquire the disease by inhaling airborne organisms from bird droppings. The illness causes fever, cough (usually without sputum), aching muscles and headache. The incubation period is about 1 to 2 weeks. Physical examination and a chest X-ray usually reveal signs of pneumonia similar to that due to many other causes.

Fortunately, psittacosis infection almost always responds well to treatment with one of the tetracycline antibiotics if given for a sufficient period of time. In some instances, the pneumonia may be extensive and severe, requiring treatment in an intensive care unit. In other instances, it may be so mild that it goes undiagnosed and resolves over a period of weeks or months.

Chapter 28

Pulmonary Embolism

What Is Pulmonary Embolism?

Pulmonary embolism, a severe and life-threatening condition, is the blocking of the pulmonary artery by foreign matter such as:

- a blood clot (thrombus) or pieces of it
- fat
- air
- tumor tissue

Conditions that may contribute to pulmonary embolism include:

- heart disease
- chronic obstructive pulmonary diseases
- extended bed rest
- surgery
- cancer
- paralysis
- aging
- sickle cell disease

What Are the Symptoms of Pulmonary Embolism?

The following are the most common symptoms for pulmonary embolism, however, each individual may experience symptoms differently.

Signs and symptoms of pulmonary embolism may be similar to those of a heart attack or a lung disorder such as pneumonia. They include:

- sudden chest pain
- chronic cough, sometimes mixed with blood-streaked sputum
- severe dyspnea (difficulty in breathing)
- excessive perspiring
- shock
- cyanosis (bluish skin color)
- anxiety
- loss of consciousness

The symptoms of pulmonary embolism may resemble other conditions or medical problems. Consult your physician for a diagnosis.

How Is Pulmonary Embolism Diagnosed?

Pulmonary embolism is difficult to diagnose. Non-invasive tests cannot be used in the diagnosis of pulmonary embolism. Often, the physician must eliminate the possibility of other lung diseases, before determining that the condition is pulmonary embolism. A test called V/Q scan, a nuclear ventilation-perfusion study of the lungs, may be used, as well as a pulmonary angiography. New diagnostic methods are under investigation.

Treatment for Pulmonary Embolism

Specific treatment will be determined by your physician(s) based on:

- your age, overall health, and medical history
- extent of the disease
- your tolerance for specific medications, procedures, or therapies
- expectations for the course of the disease
- your opinion or preference

The immediate treatment for pulmonary embolism is anticoagulant therapy to dissolve the clot and return blood flow. Oxygen and sedatives also be used to make the patient comfortable. Surgery to remove the embolism may also be performed.

Chapter 29

Respiratory Distress Syndrome (RDS)

Why Is RDS an Important Concern?

Three thousand newborn babies die each year of respiratory distress syndrome (RDS). In addition, about 30,000 babies in the United States have RDS each year.

What Is RDS?

Also called hyaline membrane disease, RDS is a lung disorder, found mainly in newborn babies who are born prematurely. The disease causes difficulty in breathing because the lungs are immature and lack enough surfactant, a detergent-like substance that keeps the lungs' air spaces open. RDS leads to the gradual collapse of the lungs, which results in harm to other organs. The babies who recover are also at greater risk of other problems such as heart failure, kidney failure, intestinal disease, bleeding into the brain, chronic lung disease, cerebral palsy, and, later in life, learning disorders.

Treatment

RDS is expensive, with the special medical care alone costing this nation more than $100 million each year. Prevention or improved treatment would not only save this expense, but would also reduce the suffering of the baby and family, and improve the quality of life for these babies.

Who Is Affected?

Nearly all babies born before 32 weeks of pregnancy will have RDS, and about 25 percent of these very premature babies will die of RDS and associated problems.

How Is RDS Treated?

The usual treatment is to give the baby oxygen and assisted breathing with a mechanical respirator. Recently, treatment has included giving babies replacement surfactant.

What Is the Role of Endocrinology?

Endocrine research has contributed to both preventing and treating RDS more effectively.

Animal studies have shown that hormone treatment can accelerate lung development before birth and improve the lungs' functioning after birth. These studies have led to a safe and effective new treatment for women who are about to give birth prematurely. These women now receive betamethasone, a synthetic adrenal hormone, which cuts the RDS rate in half and prevents other health problems as well. This treatment also increases the effectiveness of the artificial surfactant that is given to newborns with RDS.

Because some treated babies still develop RDS, further research is needed to clarify how hormones regulate lung development and to discover other methods of preventing or treating RDS. Recent basic and clinical studies suggest that babies treated with the combination of two hormones given to the mother—adrenal and thyroid hormones—have less RDS and less long-term lung disease than those with mothers receiving only one hormone.

Further studies have discovered that other types of hormones can also stimulate lung development, suggesting that more advances in treatment may be forthcoming. Continued basic and clinical endocrine research is needed to determine the safety and effectiveness of current treatments and to develop new and more effective approaches.

Basic studies on how hormones affect lung development led directly to clinical studies on how to prevent RDS. Similarly, current basic endocrine research on hormone effects has led to the recent clinical trials of combined hormonal therapy.

Chapter 30

Respiratory Sleep Disorders

Sleep disorders run the gamut from inability to sleep (insomnia) to sleeping too much (hyper-somnolence) and also include parasomnias (such as sleepwalking and movement disorders).

The most sleep disorder associated with respiratory problems is sleep apnea (cessation of breathing). Discrete apneas (cessation of ventilation for more than 10 seconds) are frequent occurrences in otherwise normal individuals (without underlying lung disease) and may have an important impact on their general health and well-being. However, this condition often goes unrecognized or misdiagnosed.

Apneas generally are classified into three types: obstructive, mixed and central.

Obstructive apneas are the most common and are caused by a sleep-induced collapse of the pharyngeal airway. Although the explanation for this phenomenon is subject to debate, the obstruction probably results from sleep-induced decrease in upper airway muscle tone in an individual with a small pharyngea airway. This condition afflicts men much more frequently than it does women, which some believe may be due to hormonal influences.

Central apneas are far less common and are characterized by simultaneous cessation of respiratory effort and airflow. These usually result from an instability in the mechanisms controlling ventilation The two most frequent causes of this kind of ventilatory instability are a variety of neurologic disorders and congestive heart failure.

Mixed apneas, as the name indicates, are a combination of obstructive and central apnea phenomena. They begin as a central pause and are followed by inspiratory effort against an occluded airway.

Consequences

Two apnea-related events produce the consequences of sleep-disordered breathing. First, the afflicted individual generally has to wakeup up to resume breathing at the end of an apnea. If apneas occur regularly, the sleep pattern can be disrupted, causing chronic sleep deprivation and hypersomnolence during the day. The latter is the most common complaint of patients with sleep apnea. (Hypersomnolence also can result from not spending enough time in bed, disrupted sleep due to periodic movements, narcolepsy—recurrent, uncontrollable episodes of sleep—and a variety of other causes.)

Hypersomnolence can be mild and manifested only by falling asleep while watching television or reading. However, it can be severe and cause a person to fall asleep during activities such as driving, eating, working, talking, etc, These consequences can range from annoying to life-threatening.

Sleep apnea patients frequently experience intellectual deterioration (impaired memory and concentration), personality changes (somatic-depressive patterns) and sexual dysfunction (impotence) that is most likely explained by the sleep disruption described above.

The second group of consequences results from recurrent hypoxemia and hypercapnia caused by sleep-induced apnea. These blood gas abnormalities can result in serious effects, including arrhythmia, systemic and pulmonary hypertension, cor pulmonale and even modest lung disease.

Recognition and Diagnosis

The most common respiratory sleep disorder by far is obstructive sleep apnea (OSA). OSA affects between 2% and 5% of adult male population (a figure seven times the incidence in women). The physician therefore must have a high clinical suspicion and carefully question the patient to recognize this disorder, as most suffers breath quite normally when awake.

The onset of sleep apnea is often subtle and gradual, such that many patients fail to recognize the symptoms. People with this disorder often think they're just tired from overwork and stress or that it's just a function of getting older. Most patients with OSA are not aware that they stop breathing hundreds of times during the night and rarely recognize the brief arousal that occurs at the end of apnea.

Warning signs include:

1. reports by a bed partner that the patient stopped breathing (apnea)

2. loud, frequent snoring of long duration, and

3. hypersomnolence or irresistible sleepiness during the day.

Other indications include male gender, obesity, systemic hypertension and increasing age. To summarize, the typical sufferer of sleep apnea is an obese male, about 45 years of age, with high blood pressure who snores loudly at night and is sleepy during the day.

A single one of these variables should not strongly suggest the presence of this disorder. However, the presence of several of these signs or symptoms indicates the need for further evaluation.

Patients with central sleep apnea can differ from those described above. These individuals rarely snore and often complain of insomnia, with frequent arousals during the night.

It's important for the physician to distinguish between a patient who is always sleepy and one who complains of excessive fatigue, lack of energy and low motivation. Chronic fatigue can originate from a host of other conditions, including depression, cardiovascular disease, etc.

Sleep Evaluation

A full polysomnographic evaluation is probably indicated if the presence of several of the above signs and symptoms create a reasonable clinical suspicion that sleep apnea is present. Less expensive screening procedures are actively investigated, but currently are not generally accepted in diagnosing sleep apnea syndromes.

A formal sleep study consists of an all-night sleep evaluation that monitors sleep stages, nasal and oral airflow, chest-abdominal wall motion and arterial oxygen saturation, as well as cardiac electrical activity. Sleep is staged, apneas and hypopneas (reduction in ventilation for more than 10 seconds) quantitated, the severity of associated arterial oxygen desaturation recorded and any arrythmias noted.

Treatment

Therapy should be initiated if the polysomnogram demonstrates frequent apneas (probably greater than 15 or 20 events per hour of sleep) and the patient is clearly symptomatic. In the absence of clear symptoms when fewer apneas are observed, the decision is less clear-cut. Unfortunately, the upper limit of normal apneic frequency is poorly defined. There no absolute "cutoffs" in apnea frequency or severity of arterial oxygen desaturation that indicate a need for treatment. Therefore, treatment is usually aimed at symptoms (primarily hypersomnolence) and the physiologic sequelae of recurrent hypoxia and hypercapnia. Each patient's therapy must be individualized based on symptoms, polysomnographic information and the risk or discomfort of the contemplated treatment.

Patients with minimal disease can benefit from simple therapies, while more severely afflicted individuals may require more drastic approaches. It is also frequently appropriate to simply follow patients with relatively mild disease and few symptoms.

The first step in treatment should be to seek reversible causes of nocturnal pharyngeal collapse. Surgically remediable abnormalities of the upper airway, such as tonsillar hypertrophy, severe nasal obstruction or a pharyngeal tumor fall into this group. Such pathology is rare, but it should be carefully excluded. Hyperthyroidism should also be considered.

Once these possibilities are eliminated, simple forms of therapy can be instituted when applicable. One step is to discontinue alcohol or sedative use near bedtime. Avoiding sleeping on back also can help. Another effective way to reduce or eliminate obstructive apnea is weight reduction if the patient is obese. Substantial weight loss is often required, but moderate weight reduction may be helpful in some patients.

Aggressive Therapy

If these initial remedies are inapplicable or ineffective, more aggressive therapy may be indicated.

Medications for OSA (protriptyline or progesterone) has generally proved unsatisfactory. The most widely used form of therapy for OSA is nasal continuous positive airway pressure (CPAP). Currently in widespread use, nasal CPAP utilizes a sealed nasal mask combined with a high-flow blower. The mechanism is believed to work by pneumatically splinting the airway open during sleep. Although this treatment works very well, some patients consider the CPAP equipment too cumbersome and inconvenient to wear to bed each night. However, as technology steadily improves, so does patient compliance and satisfaction.

Signs and Symptoms of Obstructive Sleep Apnea

- Reported respiratory cessation by bed partner
- Snoring (loud, longstanding and frequent)
- Hypersomnolence or irresistible sleepiness
- Male gender
- Obesity
- Systemic hypertension
- Increasing age

Another option for OSA therapy is uvulopalatopharyngoplasty (UPPP).

UPPP is a procedure designed to increase airway size by removing the uvula, a portion of the soft palate and other redundant tissue in the pharyngeal airway. A success rate of only about 50% and inability to predict who will respond successfully has recently made this alternative less popular.

Tracheostomy also remains a viable and definitive form of therapy for OSA and should be considered in extreme cases. However, many patients prefer less invasive approaches.

Treatment of central sleep apnea has been less satisfactory than that of OSA. The most commonly used modalities include acetazolamide, low flow oxygen administration and nasal CPAP.

Recognition of the signs that characterize an apneic sufferer can help the office practitioner focus on the problem, make necessary distinctions and recommend appropriate evaluation and treatment. By reducing or eliminating symptoms, the physician can improve the quality of life for many patients and possibly prolong life for some.

Bibliography

Connaughton JJ, Catterall JR, Elton RA, Stradling JR, Douglas NJ. "Do sleep studies contribute to the management of patients with severe chronic obstructive pulmonary disease?" *Am Rev Respir Dis* 1988;138:341-344.

Fletcher Ec, Schaof JW, Miller J, Fletcher JG, "Long-term cardiopulmonary sequelae in patients with sleep apnea and chronic lung disease," *Am Rev Respir Dis* 1987; 135: 525-533.

He J, Kyger MH, Zorick FJ, Conway W, Roth T. "Mortality and apnea index in obstructive sleep apnea." *Chest* 1988; 94:9-14.

Roehrs T, Zorick F, Wittig R, Conway W, Roth T. "Predictors of objective daytime sleepiness in patients with sleep-related breathing disorders." *Chest* 1989; 95:1202-1206.

Sanders MH, Gruendl CA, Rogers RM. "Patient compliance with nasal CPAP therapy for sleep apnea." *Chest* 1986; 90:330-333.

Strohl KP, Chemiack NS, Gothe B. "Physiologic basis of therapy for sleep apnea." *Am Rev Respir Dis* 1986; 134:791-802.

Chapter 31

Respiratory Syncytial Virus (RSV)

Clinical Features

Respiratory syncytial virus (RSV) is the most common cause of bronchiolitis and pneumonia among infants and children under 1 year of age. Illness begins most frequently with fever, runny nose, cough, and sometimes wheezing. During their first RSV infection, between 25% and 40% of infants and young children have signs or symptoms of bronchiolitis or pneumonia, and 0.5% to 2% require hospitalization. Most children recover from illness in 8 to 15 days. The majority of children hospitalized for RSV infection are under 6 months of age. RSV also causes repeated infections throughout life, usually associated with moderate-to-severe cold-like symptoms; however, severe lower respiratory tract disease may occur at any age, especially among the elderly or among those with compromised cardiac, pulmonary, or immune systems.

The Virus

RSV is a negative-sense, enveloped RNA virus. The virion is variable in shape and size (average diameter of between 120 and 300 nm), is unstable in the environment (surviving only a few hours on environmental surfaces), and is readily inactivated with soap and water and disinfectants.

Centers for Disease Control and Prevention (CDC), 1999.

Epidemiologic Features

RSV is spread from respiratory secretions through close contact with infected persons or contact with contaminated surfaces or objects. Infection can occur when infectious material contacts mucous membranes of the eyes, mouth, or nose, and possibly through the inhalation of droplets generated by a sneeze or cough. In temperate climates, RSV infections usually occur during annual community outbreaks, often lasting 4 to 6 months, during the late fall, winter, or early spring months. The timing and severity of outbreaks in a community vary from year to year. RSV spreads efficiently among children during the annual outbreaks, and most children will have serologoic evidence of RSV infection by 2 years of age.

Diagnosis

Diagnosis of RSV infection can be made by virus isolation, detection of viral antigens, detection of viral RNA, demonstration of a rise in serum antibodies, or a combination of these approaches. Most clinical laboratories use antigen detection assays to diagnose infection.

Treatment

For children with mild disease, no specific treatment is necessary other than the treatment of symptoms (e.g., acetaminophen to reduce fever). Children with severe disease may require oxygen therapy and sometimes mechanical ventilation. Ribavirin aerosol may be used in the treatment of some patients with severe disease. Some investigators have used a combination of immune globulin intravenous (IGIV) with high titers of neutralizing RSV antibody (RSV-IGIV) and ribavirin to treat patients with compromised immune systems.

Prevention

Development of an RSV vaccine is a high research priority, but none is yet available. Current prevention options include good infection-control practices, RSV-IGIV, and an anti-RSV humanized murine monoclonal antibody. RSV-IGIV or the anti-RSV humanized murine monoclonal antibody can be given during the RSV outbreak season to prevent serious complications of infection in some infants and children at high risk for serious RSV disease (e.g., those with chronic lung disease and prematurely born infants with or without chronic lung disease).

Frequent hand washing and not sharing items such as cups, glasses, and utensils with persons who have RSV illness should decrease the spread of virus to others. Excluding children with colds or other respiratory illnesses (without fever) who are well enough to attend child care or school settings will probably not decrease the transmission of RSV, since it is often spread in the early stages of illness. In a hospital setting, RSV transmission can and should be prevented by strict attention to contact precautions, such as hand washing and wearing gowns and gloves.

Respiratory Syncytial Virus (RSV) in the Child Care Setting

RSV causes infections of the upper respiratory tract (like a cold) and the lower respiratory tract (like pneumonia). It is the most frequent cause of lower respiratory infections, including pneumonia, in infants and children under 2 years of age. Almost 100 percent of children in child care get RSV in the first year of their life, usually during outbreaks during the winter months. In most children, symptoms appear similar to a mild cold. About half of the infections result in lower respiratory tract infections and otitis media. An RSV infection can range from very mild to life-threatening or even fatal. Children with heart or lung disease and weak immune systems are at increased risk of developing severe infection and complications. RSV causes repeated symptomatic infections throughout life.

RSV is spread through direct contact with infectious secretions such as by breathing them in after an infected person has coughed or by touching a surface an infected person has contaminated by touching it or coughing on it. A young child with RSV may be infectious for 1 to 3 weeks after symptoms subside.

The most effective preventive measure against the spread of RSV and other respiratory viral infections is careful and frequent hand washing. Once one child in a group is infected with RSV, spread to others is rapid. Frequently, a child is infectious before symptoms appear. Therefore, an infected child does not need to be excluded from child care unless he or she is not well enough to participate in usual activities.

If a child or adult in the child care facility develops an illness caused by RSV infection make sure that procedures regarding hand washing, hygiene, disposal of tissues used to clean nasal secretions, and cleaning and disinfection of toys are followed. If multiple cases occur, cohorting or separating ill children from well/recovered children may help to reduce the spread of RSV. Do not exclude ill children unless they are unable to participate comfortably in activities or require a level of care that would jeopardize the health and safety of the other children in your care.

Chapter 32

Sudden Infant Death Syndrome (SIDS)

Sudden Infant Death Syndrome (SIDS) is the diagnosis given for the sudden death of an infant under one year of age that remains unexplained after a complete investigation, which includes an autopsy, examination of the death scene, and review of the symptoms or illnesses the infant had prior to dying and any other pertinent medical history. Because most cases of SIDS occur when a baby is sleeping in a crib, SIDS is also commonly known as crib death.

SIDS is the leading cause of death in infants between 1 month and 1 year of age. Most SIDS deaths occur when a baby is between 1 and 4 months of age. African American children are two to three times more likely than white babies to die of SIDS, and Native American babies are about three times more susceptible. Also, more boys are SIDS victims than girls.

What Are the Risk Factors for SIDS?

A number of factors seem to put a baby at higher risk of dying from SIDS. Babies who sleep on their stomachs are more likely to die of SIDS than those who sleep on their backs. Mothers who smoke during pregnancy are three times more likely to have a SIDS baby, and exposure to passive smoke from smoking by mothers, fathers, and others in the household doubles a baby's risk of SIDS. Other risk factors include mothers who are less than 20 years old at the time of their

National Institute of Child Health and Human Development (NICHD), April 1997, modified April 2000.

first pregnancy, babies born to mothers who had no or late prenatal care, and premature or low birth weight babies.

What Causes SIDS?

Mounting evidence suggests that some SIDS babies are born with brain abnormalities that make them vulnerable to sudden death during infancy. Studies of SIDS victims reveal that many SIDS infants have abnormalities in the "arcuate nucleus," a portion of the brain that is likely to be involved in controlling breathing and waking during sleep. Babies born with defects in other portions of the brain or body may also be more prone to a sudden death. These abnormalities may stem from prenatal exposure to a toxic substance, or lack of a vital compound in the prenatal environment, such as sufficient oxygen. Cigarette smoking during pregnancy, for example, can reduce the amount of oxygen the fetus receives.

Scientists believe that the abnormalities that are present at birth may not be sufficient to cause death. Other possibly important events occur after birth such as lack of oxygen, excessive carbon dioxide intake, overheating or an infection. For example, many babies experience a lack of oxygen and excessive carbon dioxide levels when they have respiratory infections that hamper breathing, or they rebreathe exhaled air trapped in underlying bedding when they sleep on their stomachs.

Normally, infants sense such inadequate air intake, and the brain triggers the babies to wake from sleep and cry, and changes their heartbeat or breathing patterns to compensate for the insufficient oxygen and excess carbon dioxide. A baby with a flawed arcuate nucleus, however, might lack this protective mechanism and succumb to SIDS. Such a scenario might explain why babies who sleep on their stomachs are more susceptible to SIDS, and why a disproportionately large number of SIDS babies have been reported to have respiratory infections prior to their deaths. Infections as a trigger for sudden infant death may explain why more SIDS cases occur during the colder months of the year, when respiratory and intestinal infections are more common.

The numbers of cells and proteins generated by the immune system of some SIDS babies have been reported to be higher than normal. Some of these proteins can interact with the brain to alter heart rate and breathing during sleep, or can put the baby into a deep sleep. Such effects might be strong enough to cause the baby's death, particularly if the baby has an underlying brain defect.

Some babies who die suddenly may be born with a metabolic disorder. One such disorder is medium chain acylCoA dehydrogenase deficiency, which prevents the infant from properly processing fatty acids. A build-up of these acid metabolites could eventually lead to a rapid and fatal disruption in breathing and heart functioning. If there is a family history of this disorder or childhood death of unknown cause, genetic screening of the parents by a blood test can determine if they are carriers of this disorder. If one or both parents is found to be a carrier, the baby can be tested soon after birth.

What Might Help Lower the Risk of SIDS?

There currently is no way of predicting which newborns will succumb to SIDS; however, there are a few measures parents can take to lower the risk of their child dying from SIDS.

Good prenatal care, which includes proper nutrition, no smoking or drug or alcohol use by the mother, and frequent medical check-ups beginning early in pregnancy, might help prevent a baby from developing an abnormality that could put him or her at risk for sudden death. These measures may also reduce the chance of having a premature or low birth weight baby, which also increases the risk for SIDS. Once the baby is born, parents should keep the baby in a smoke-free environment.

Parents and other caregivers should put babies to sleep on their backs as opposed to on their stomachs. Studies have shown that placing babies on their backs to sleep has reduced the number of SIDS cases by as much as a half in countries where infants had traditionally slept on their stomachs. Although babies placed on their sides to sleep have a lower risk of SIDS than those placed on their stomachs, the back sleep position is the best position for infants from 1 month to 1 year. Babies positioned on their sides to sleep should be placed with their lower arm forward to help prevent them from rolling onto their stomachs.

Many parents place babies on their stomachs to sleep because they think it prevents them from choking on spit-up or vomit during sleep. But studies in countries where there has been a switch from babies sleeping predominantly on their stomachs to sleeping mainly on their backs have not found any evidence of increased risk of choking or other problems.

In some instances, doctors may recommend that babies be placed on their stomachs to sleep if they have disorders such as gastroesophageal reflux or certain upper airway disorders which predispose them to choking or breathing problems while lying on their backs. If a parent is unsure about the best sleep position for their baby, it is always a good idea to talk to the baby's doctor or other health care provider.

A certain amount of tummy time while the infant is awake and being observed is recommended for motor development of the shoulder. In addition, awake time on the stomach may help prevent flat spots from developing on the back of the baby's head. Such physical signs are almost always temporary and will disappear soon after the baby begins to sit up.

Parents should make sure their baby sleeps on a firm mattress or other firm surface. They should avoid using fluffy blankets or covering as well as pillows, sheepskins, blankets, or comforters under the baby. Infants should not be placed to sleep on a waterbed or with soft stuffed toys.

Recently, scientific studies have demonstrated that bed sharing, between mother and baby, can alter sleep patterns of the mother and baby. These studies have led to speculation that bed sharing, sometimes referred to as co-sleeping, may also reduce the risk of SIDS. While bed sharing may have certain benefits (such as encouraging breast feeding), there are not scientific studies demonstrating that bed sharing reduces SIDS. Some studies actually suggest that bed sharing, under certain conditions, may increase the risk of SIDS. If mothers choose to sleep in the same beds with their babies, care should be taken to avoid using soft sleep surfaces. Quilts, blankets, pillows, comforters, or other similar soft materials should not be placed under the baby. The bed sharer should not smoke or use substances such as alcohol or drugs which may impair arousal. It is also important to be aware that unlike cribs, which are designed to meet safety standards for infants, adult beds are not so designed and may carry a risk of accidental entrapment and suffocation.

Babies should be kept warm, but they should not be allowed to get too warm because an overheated baby is more likely to go into a deep sleep from which it is difficult to arouse. The temperature in the baby's room should feel comfortable to an adult and overdressing the baby should be avoided.

There is some evidence to suggest that breast feeding might reduce the risk of SIDS. A few studies have found SIDS to be less common in infants who have been breastfed. This may be because breast milk can provide protection from some infections that can trigger sudden death in infants.

Parents should take their babies to their health care provider for regular well baby check-ups and routine immunizations. Claims that immunizations increase the risk of SIDS are not supported by data, and babies who receive their scheduled immunizations are less likely to die of SIDS. If an infant ever has an incident where he or she stops breathing and turns blue or limp, the baby should be medically evaluated for the cause of such an incident.

Although some electronic home monitors can detect and sound an alarm when a baby stops breathing, there is no evidence that such monitors can prevent SIDS. A panel of experts convened by the National Institutes of Health in 1986 recommended that home monitors not be used for babies who do not have an increased risk of sudden unexpected death. The monitors are recommended, however, for infants who have experienced one or more severe episodes during which they stopped breathing and required resuscitation or stimulation, premature infants with apnea, and siblings of two or more SIDS infants. If an incident has occurred or if an infant is on a monitor, parents need to know how to properly use and maintain the device, as well as how to resuscitate their baby if the alarm sounds.

How Does a SIDS Baby Affect the Family?

A SIDS death is a tragedy that can prompt intense emotional reactions among surviving family members. After the initial disbelief, denial, or numbness begins to wear off, parents often fall into a prolonged depression. This depression can affect their sleeping, eating, ability to concentrate, and general energy level. Crying, weeping, incessant talking, and strong feelings of guilt or anger are all normal reactions. Many parents experience unreasonable fears that they, or someone in their family, may be in danger. Over-protection of surviving children and fears for future children is a common reaction.

As the finality of the child's death becomes a reality for the parents, recovery occurs. Parents begin to take a more active part in their own lives, which begin to have meaning once again. The pain of their child's death becomes less intense but not forgotten. Birthdays, holidays, and the anniversary of the child's death can trigger periods of intense pain and suffering.

Children will also be affected by the baby's death. They may fear that other members of the family, including themselves, will also suddenly die. Children often also feel guilty about the death of a sibling and may feel that they had something to do with the death. Children may not show their feelings in obvious ways. Although they may deny being upset and seem unconcerned, signs that they are disturbed include intensified clinging to parents, misbehaving, bed wetting, difficulties in school, and nightmares. It is important to talk to children about the death and explain to them that the baby died because of a medical problem that occurs only in infants in rare instances and cannot occur in them. The National Institute of Child Health and Human Development (NICHD) continues to support research aimed at uncovering what causes SIDS, who is at risk for the disorder, and ways to lower the risk of sudden infant death. Inquiries regarding research programs should be directed to Dr. Marian Willinger, 301-496-5575.

Families with a baby who has died from SIDS may be aided by counseling and support groups. Examples of these groups include the following:

Association of SIDS and Infant Mortality Programs
c/o Minnesota SIDS Center
2525 Chicago Ave. South
Minneapolis, MN 55404
Tel: 612-813-6285
Fax: 612-813-7344
Internet: http://www.asip1.org

National SIDS Resource Center
2070 Chain Bridge Road
Suite 450
Vienna, VA 22182
Tel: 703-821-8955
Fax: 703-821-2098
Internet: http://www.sidscenter.org
E-Mail: sids@circlesolutions.com

SIDS Alliance
(a national network of SIDS support groups)
1314 Bedford Avenue
Suite 210
Baltimore, MD 21208
Toll Free: 800-221-7437
Tel: 410-653-8226
Fax: 410-653-8709
Internet: http://www.sidsalliance.org
E-Mail: info@sidsalliance.org

Chapter 33

Sleep Apnea

What Is Sleep Apnea?

Sleep apnea is a serious, potentially life-threatening condition that is far more common than generally understood. First described in 1965, sleep apnea is a breathing disorder characterized by brief interruptions of breathing during sleep. It owes its name to a Greek word, apnea, meaning "want of breath." There are two types of sleep apnea: central and obstructive. Central sleep apnea, which is less common, occurs when the brain fails to send the appropriate signals to the breathing muscles to initiate respirations.

Obstructive sleep apnea is far more common and occurs when air cannot flow into or out of the person's nose or mouth although efforts to breathe continue.

In a given night, the number of involuntary breathing pauses or "apneic events" may be as high as 20 to 30 or more per hour. These breathing pauses are almost always accompanied by snoring between apnea episodes, although not everyone who snores has this condition. Sleep apnea can also be characterized by choking sensations. The frequent interruptions of deep, restorative sleep often lead to early morning headaches and excessive daytime sleepiness.

Early recognition and treatment of sleep apnea is important because it may be associated with irregular heartbeat, high blood pressure, heart attack, and stroke.

National Heart, Lung, and Blood Institute (NHLBI), NIH Publication Number 95-3798, 1995. Text available online at http://www.nhlbi.nih.gov/health/public/sleep/sleepapn.txt; cited April 2000.

Who Gets Sleep Apnea?

Sleep apnea occurs in all age groups and both sexes but is more common in men (it may be underdiagnosed in women) and possibly young African Americans. It has been estimated that as many as 18 million Americans have sleep apnea. Four percent of middle-aged men and 2 percent of middle-aged women have sleep apnea along with excessive daytime sleepiness. People most likely to have or develop sleep apnea include those who snore loudly and also are overweight, or have high blood pressure, or have some physical abnormality in the nose, throat, or other parts of the upper airway. Sleep apnea seems to run in some families, suggesting a possible genetic basis.

What Causes Sleep Apnea?

Certain mechanical and structural problems in the airway cause the interruptions in breathing during sleep. In some people, apnea occurs when the throat muscles and tongue relax during sleep and partially block the opening of the airway. When the muscles of the soft palate at the base of the tongue and the uvula (the small fleshy tissue hanging from the center of the back of the throat) relax and sag, the airway becomes blocked, making breathing labored and noisy and even stopping it altogether. Sleep apnea also can occur in obese people when an excess amount of tissue in the airway causes it to be narrowed. With a narrowed airway, the person continues his or her efforts to breathe, but air cannot easily flow into or out of the nose or mouth. Unknown to the person, this results in heavy snoring, periods of no breathing, and frequent arousals (causing abrupt changes from deep sleep to light sleep). Ingestion of alcohol and sleeping pills increases the frequency and duration of breathing pauses in people with sleep apnea.

How Is Normal Breathing Restored During Sleep?

During the apneic event, the person is unable to breathe in oxygen and to exhale carbon dioxide, resulting in low levels of oxygen and increased levels of carbon dioxide in the blood. The reduction in oxygen and increase in carbon dioxide alert the brain to resume breathing and cause an arousal. With each arousal, a signal is sent from the brain to the upper airway muscles to open the airway; breathing is resumed, often with a loud snort or gasp. Frequent arousals, although necessary for breathing to restart, prevent the patient from getting enough restorative, deep sleep.

What Are the Effects of Sleep Apnea?

Because of the serious disturbances in their normal sleep patterns, people with sleep apnea often feel very sleepy during the day and their concentration and daytime performance suffer. The consequences of sleep apnea range from annoying to life-threatening. They include depression, irritability, sexual dysfunction, learning and memory difficulties, and falling asleep while at work, on the phone, or driving. It has been estimated that up to 50 percent of sleep apnea patients have high blood pressure.

Although it is not known with certainty if there is a cause and effect relationship, it appears that sleep apnea contributes to high blood pressure. Risk for heart attack and stroke may also increase in those with sleep apnea. In addition, sleep apnea is sometimes implicated in sudden infant death syndrome.

When Should Sleep Apnea Be Suspected?

For many sleep apnea patients, their spouses are the first ones to suspect that something is wrong, usually from their heavy snoring and apparent struggle to breathe. Coworkers or friends of the sleep apnea victim may notice that the individual falls asleep during the day at inappropriate times (such as while driving a car, working, or talking). The patient often does not know he or she has a problem and may not believe it when told. It is important that the person see a doctor for evaluation of the sleep problem.

How Is Sleep Apnea Diagnosed?

In addition to the primary care physician, pulmonologists, neurologists, or other physicians with specialty training in sleep disorders may be involved in making a definitive diagnosis and initiating treatment. Diagnosis of sleep apnea is not simple because there can be many different reasons for disturbed sleep. Several tests are available for evaluating a person for sleep apnea.

Polysomnography is a test that records a variety of body functions during sleep, such as the electrical activity of the brain, eye movement, muscle activity, heart rate, respiratory effort, air flow, and blood oxygen levels. These tests are used both to diagnose sleep apnea and to determine its severity.

The Multiple Sleep Latency Test (MSLT) measures the speed of falling asleep. In this test, patients are given several opportunities to fall asleep during the course of a day when they would normally be awake. For each opportunity, time to fall asleep is measured. People without sleep problems usually take an average of 10 to 20 minutes to fall asleep. Individuals who fall asleep in less than 5 minutes are likely to require some treatment for sleep disorders. The MSLT may be useful to measure the degree of excessive daytime sleepiness and to rule out other types of sleep disorders.

Diagnostic tests usually are performed in a sleep center, but new technology may allow some sleep studies to be conducted in the patient's home.

How Is Sleep Apnea Treated?

The specific therapy for sleep apnea is tailored to the individual patient based on medical history, physical examination, and the results of polysomnography.

Medications are generally not effective in the treatment of sleep apnea. Oxygen administration may safely benefit certain patients but does not eliminate sleep apnea or prevent daytime sleepiness. Thus, the role of oxygen in the treatment of sleep apnea is controversial, and it is difficult to predict which patients will respond well. It is important that the effectiveness of the selected treatment be verified; this is usually accomplished by polysomnography.

Behavioral Therapy

Behavioral changes are an important part of the treatment program, and in mild cases behavioral therapy may be all that is needed. The individual should avoid the use of alcohol, tobacco, and sleeping pills, which make the airway more likely to collapse during sleep and prolong the apneic periods. Overweight persons can benefit from losing weight.

Even a 10 percent weight loss can reduce the number of apneic events for most patients. In some patients with mild sleep apnea, breathing pauses occur only when they sleep on their backs. In such cases, using pillows and other devices that help them sleep in a side position is often helpful.

Physical or Mechanical Therapy

Nasal continuous positive airway pressure (CPAP) is the most common effective treatment for sleep apnea. In this procedure, the patient wears a mask over the nose during sleep, and pressure from an air blower forces air through the nasal passages. The air pressure is adjusted so that it is just enough to prevent the throat from collapsing during sleep. The pressure is constant and continuous. Nasal CPAP prevents airway closure while in use, but apnea episodes return when CPAP is stopped or used improperly.

Variations of the CPAP device attempt to minimize side effects that sometimes occur, such as nasal irritation and drying, facial skin irritation, abdominal bloating, mask leaks, sore eyes, and headaches. Some versions of CPAP vary the pressure to coincide with the person's breathing pattern, and others start with low pressure, slowly increasing it to allow the person to fall asleep before the full prescribed pressure is applied.

Dental appliances that reposition the lower jaw and the tongue have been helpful to some patients with mild sleep apnea or who snore but do not have apnea. Possible side effects include damage to teeth, soft tissues, and the jaw joint. A dentist or orthodontist is often the one to fit the patient with such a device.

Surgery

Some patients with sleep apnea may need surgery. Although several surgical procedures are used to increase the size of the airway, none of them is completely successful or without risks. More than one procedure may need to be tried before the patient realizes any benefits.

Some of the more common procedures include removal of adenoids and tonsils (especially in children), nasal polyps or other growths, or other tissue in the airway and correction of structural deformities. Younger patients seem to benefit from these surgical procedures more than older patients.

Uvulopalatopharyngoplasty (UPPP) is a procedure used to remove excess tissue at the back of the throat (tonsils, uvula, and part of the soft palate). The success of this technique may range from 30 to 50 percent. The long-term side effects and benefits are not known, and it is difficult to predict which patients will do well with this procedure.

Laser-assisted uvulopalatoplasty (LAUP) is done to eliminate snoring but has not been shown to be effective in treating sleep apnea. This procedure involves using a laser device to eliminate tissue in the back of the throat. Like UPPP, LAUP may decrease or eliminate snoring but not sleep apnea itself. Elimination of snoring, the primary symptom of sleep apnea, without influencing the condition may carry the risk of delaying the diagnosis and possible treatment of sleep apnea in patients who elect LAUP. To identify possible underlying sleep apnea, sleep studies are usually required before LAUP is performed.

Tracheostomy is used in persons with severe, life-threatening sleep apnea. In this procedure, a small hole is made in the windpipe and a tube is inserted into the opening. This tube stays closed during waking hours, and the person breathes and speaks normally. It is opened for sleep so that air flows directly into the lungs, bypassing any upper airway obstruction. Although this procedure is highly effective, it is an extreme measure that is poorly tolerated by patients and rarely used.

Other Procedures

Patients in whom sleep apnea is due to deformities of the lower jaw may benefit from surgical reconstruction. Finally, surgical procedures to treat obesity are sometimes recommended for sleep apnea patients who are morbidly obese.

National Center on Sleep Disorders Research (NCSDR)

The mission of the NCSDR is to support research, training, and education about sleep disorders. The center is located within the National Heart, Lung, and Blood Institute (NHLBI) of the National Institutes of Health. The NHLBI supports a variety of research and training programs focusing on cardiopulmonary disorders in sleep, designed to fill critical gaps in the understanding of the causes, diagnosis, treatment, and prevention of sleep-disordered breathing.

For More Information

Information about sleep disorders research can be obtained from the NCSDR. In addition, the NHLBI Information Center can provide you with sleep education materials as well as other publications relating to heart, lung, and blood diseases.

National Center on Sleep Disorders Research
Two Rockledge Centre
Suite 10038
6701 Rockledge Drive MSC 7920
Bethesda, MD 20892-7920
Tel: 301-435-0199
Fax: 301-480-3451
Internet: http://www.nhlbi.nih.gov/about/ncsdr
E-Mail: ncsdr@nih.gov

Chapter 34

Sarcoidosis

Sarcoidosis is a disease due to inflammation. It can appear in almost any body organ, but most often starts in the lungs or lymph nodes.

No one yet knows what causes sarcoidosis. The disease can appear suddenly and disappear. Or it can develop gradually and go on to produce symptoms that come and go, sometimes for a lifetime.

As sarcoidosis progresses, small lumps, or granulomas, appear in the affected tissues. In the majority of cases, these granulomas clear up, either with or without treatment. In the few cases where the granulomas do not heal and disappear, the tissues tend to remain inflamed and become scarred (fibrotic).

Sarcoidosis was first identified over 100 years ago by two dermatologists working independently, Dr. Jonathan Hutchinson in England and Dr. Caesar Boeck in Norway. Sarcoidosis was originally called Hutchinson's disease or Boeck's disease. Dr. Boeck went on to fashion today's name for the disease from the Greek words "sark" and "oid," meaning flesh-like. The term describes the skin eruptions that are frequently caused by the illness.

Usual Symptoms

Shortness of breath (dyspnea) and a cough that won't go away can be among the first symptoms of sarcoidosis. But sarcoidosis can also

National Heart, Lung, and Blood Institute (NHLBI), NIH Publication Number 95-3093, 1995. Available online at http://www.nhlbi.nih.gov/health/public/lung/other/sarcoidosis/index.htm; cited April 2000.

show up suddenly with the appearance of skin rashes. Red bumps (erythema nodosum) on the face, arms, or shins, and inflammation of the eyes are also common symptoms. It is not unusual, however, for sarcoidosis symptoms to be more general. Weight loss, fatigue, night sweats, fever, or just an overall feeling of ill health can also be clues to the disease.

Who Gets Sarcoidosis?

Sarcoidosis was once considered a rare disease. We now know that it is a common chronic illness that appears all over the world. Indeed, it is the most common of the fibrotic lung disorders, and occurs often enough in the United States for Congress to have declared a national Sarcoidosis Awareness Day in 1990.

Anyone can get sarcoidosis. It occurs in all races and in both sexes. Nevertheless, the risk is greater if you are a young black adult, especially a black woman, or of Scandinavian, German, Irish, or Puerto Rican origin. No one knows why.

Because sarcoidosis can escape diagnosis or be mistaken for several other diseases, we can only guess at how many people are affected. The best estimate today is that about 5 in 100,000 white people in the United States have sarcoidosis. Among black people, it occurs more frequently, in probably 40 out of 100,000 people.

Overall, there appear to be 20 cases per 100,000 in cities on the east coast and somewhat fewer in rural locations. Some scientists, however, believe that these figures greatly underestimated the percentage of the U.S. population with sarcoidosis. Sarcoidosis mainly affects people between 20 to 40 years of age. White women are just as likely as white men to get sarcoidosis, but the black female gets sarcoidosis two times as often as the black male.

Sarcoidosis also appears to be more common and more severe in certain geographic areas. It has long been recognized as a common disease in Scandinavian countries, where it is estimated to affect 64 out of 100,000 people. But it was not until the mid-1940s—when a large number of cases were identified during mass chest x-ray screening for the Armed Forces—that its high prevalence was recognized in North America.

What Sarcoidosis Is Not

Much about sarcoidosis remains unknown. Nevertheless, if you have the disease, you can be reassured about several things.

Sarcoidosis is usually not crippling. It often goes away by itself, with most cases healing in 24 to 36 months. Even when sarcoidosis lasts longer, most patients can go about their lives as usual. Sarcoidosis is not a cancer. It is not contagious, and your friends and family will not catch it from you. Although it can occur in families, there is no evidence that sarcoidosis is passed from parents to children.

Inflammatory phases in lung sarcoidosis. Magnified views show how illness may affect the normal lung, going from alveolitis, to granuloma formation, to fibrosis.

Some Things We Don't Know about Sarcoidosis

Sarcoidosis is currently thought to be associated with an abnormal immune response. Whether a foreign substance is the trigger; whether that trigger is a chemical, drug, virus, or some other substance; and how exactly the immune disturbance is caused are not known.

Researchers supported by the National Heart, Lung, and Blood Institute are trying to solve some of these mysteries. Among the research questions they are trying to answer are:

- Does sarcoidosis have many causes, or is it produced by a single agent?

- In which body organ does sarcoidosis actually start?

- How does sarcoidosis spread from one part of the body to another?

- Do heredity, environment, and lifestyle play any role in the appearance, severity, or length of the disease?

- Is the abnormal immune response seen in patients a cause or an effect of the disease?

- How can sarcoidosis be prevented?

Course of the Disease

In general, sarcoidosis appears briefly and heals naturally in 60 to 70 percent of the cases, often without the patient knowing or doing anything about it. From 20 to 30 percent of sarcoidosis patients are left with some permanent lung damage. In 10 to 15 percent of the patients, sarcoidosis can become chronic.

When either the granulomas or fibrosis seriously affect the function of a vital organ—the lungs, heart, nervous system, liver, or kidneys, for example—sarcoidosis can be fatal. This occurs 5 to 10 percent of the time.

Some people are more at risk than others; no one knows why.

No one can predict how sarcoidosis will progress in an individual patient. But the symptoms the patient experiences, the doctor's findings, and the patient's race can give some clues. For example, a sudden onset of general symptoms such as weight loss of feeling poorly are usually taken to mean that the course of sarcoidosis will be relatively short and mild. Dyspnea and possibly skin sarcoidosis often indicate that the sarcoidosis will be more chronic and severe.

White patients are more likely to develop the milder form of the disease. Black people tend to develop the more chronic and severe form.

Sarcoidosis rarely develops before the age of 10 or after the age of 60. However, the illness—with or without symptoms—has been reported in younger as well as in older people. When symptoms do appear in these age groups, the symptoms are those that are more general in nature, for example, tiredness, sluggishness, coughing and a general feeling of ill health.

Diagnosis

Preliminary diagnosis of sarcoidosis is based on the patient's medical history, routine tests, a physical examination, and a chest x-ray.

The doctor confirms the diagnosis of sarcoidosis by eliminating other diseases with similar features. These include such granulomatous diseases as berylliosis (a disease resulting from exposure to beryllium metal), tuberculosis, farmer's lung disease (hypersensitivity pneumonitis), fungal infections, rheumatoid arthritis, rheumatic fever, and cancer of the lymph nodes (lymphoma).

Signs and Symptoms

In addition to the lungs and lymph nodes, the body organs more likely than others to be affected by sarcoidosis are the liver, skin, heart, nervous system, and kidneys, in that order of frequency. Patients can have symptoms related to the specific organ affected, they can have only general symptoms, or they can be without any symptoms whatsoever. Symptoms also can vary according to how long the illness has been under way, where the granulomas are forming, how much tissue has become affected, and whether the granulomatous process is still active.

Even when there are no symptoms, a doctor can sometimes pick up signs of sarcoidosis during a routine examination, usually a chest x-ray, or when checking out another complaint. The patient's age and race or ethnic group can raise an additional red flag that a sign or symptom of illness could be related to sarcoidosis. Enlargement of the salivary or tear glands and cysts in bone tissue are also among sarcoidosis signals.

Some Sarcoidosis Sites

Lungs

The lungs are usually the first site involved in sarcoidosis. Indeed, about 9 out of 10 sarcoidosis patients have some type of lung problem, with nearly one-third of these patients showing some respiratory symptoms—usually coughing, either dry or with phlegm, and dyspnea. Occasionally, patients have chest pain and a feeling of tightness in the chest.

It is thought that sarcoidosis of the lungs begins with alveolitis (inflammation of the alveoli), the tiny sac like air spaces in the lungs where carbon dioxide and oxygen are exchanged. Alveolitis either clears up spontaneously or leads to granuloma formation. Eventually fibrosis can form, causing the lung to stiffen and making breathing even more difficult.

Eyes

Eye disease occurs in about 20 to 30 percent of patients with sarcoidosis, particularly in children who get the disease. Almost any part of the eye can be affected—the membranes of the eyelids, cornea, outer coat of the eyeball (sclera), retina, and lens. The eye involvement can start with no symptoms at all or with reddening or watery eyes. In a few cases, cataracts, glaucoma, and blindness can result.

Skin

The skin is affected in about 20 percent of sarcoidosis patients. Skin sarcoidosis is usually marked by small, raised patches on the face. Occasionally the patches are purplish in color and larger. Patches can also appear on limbs, face, and buttocks.

Other symptoms include erythema nodosum, mostly on the legs and often accompanied by arthritis in the ankles, elbows, wrists, and hands. Erythema nodosum usually goes away, but other skin problems can persist.

Nervous System

In an occasional case (1 to 5 percent), sarcoidosis can lead to neurological problems. For example, sarcoid granulomas can appear in the brain, spinal cord, and facial and optic nerves. Facial paralysis and other symptoms of nerve damage call for prompt treatment.

Laboratory Tests

No single test can be relied on for a correct diagnosis of sarcoidosis. X-rays and blood tests are usually the first procedures the doctor will order. Pulmonary function tests often provide clues to diagnosis. Other tests may also be used, some more often than others.

Many of the tests that the doctor calls on to help diagnose sarcoidosis can also help the doctor follow the progress of the disease and determine whether the sarcoidosis is getting better or worse.

Chest X-ray

A picture of the lungs, heart, as well as the surrounding tissues containing lymph nodes, where infection-fighting white blood cells form, can give the first indication of sarcoidosis. For example, a swelling of the lymph glands between the two lungs can show up on an x-ray. An x-ray can also show which areas of the lung are affected.

Pulmonary Function Tests

By performing a variety of tests called pulmonary function tests (PFT), the doctor can find out how well the lungs are doing their job of expanding and exchanging oxygen and carbon dioxide with the blood. The lungs of sarcoidosis patients cannot handle these tasks as well as they should; this is because granulomas and fibrosis of lung tissue decrease lung capacity and disturb the normal flow of gases between the lungs and the blood.

One PFT procedure calls for the patient to breathe into a machine, called a spirometer. It is a mechanical device that records changes in the lung size as air is inhaled and exhaled, as well as the time it takes the patient to do this.

Blood Tests

Blood analyses can evaluate the number and types of blood cells in the body and how well the cells are functioning. They can also measure the levels of various blood proteins known to be involved in immunological activities, and they can show increases in serum calcium levels and abnormal liver function that often accompany sarcoidosis.

Blood tests can measure a blood substance called angiotensin-converting enzyme (ACE). Because the cells that make up granulomas secrete large amounts of ACE, the enzyme levels are often high in patients with sarcoidosis. ACE levels, however, are not always high in sarcoidosis patients, and increased ACE levels can also show up in other illnesses.

Bronchoalveolar Lavage

This test uses an instrument called a bronchoscope—a long, narrow tube with a light at the end—to wash out, or lavage, cells and other materials from inside the lungs. This wash fluid is then examined for the amount of various cells and other substances that reflect inflammation and immune activity in the lungs. A high number of white blood cells in this fluid usually indicates an inflammation in the lungs.

Biopsy

Microscopic examination of specimens of lung tissue obtained with a bronchoscope, or of specimens of other tissues, can tell a doctor where granulomas have formed in the body.

Gallium Scanning

In this procedure, the doctor injects the radioactive chemical element gallium-67 into the patient's vein. The gallium collects at places in the body affected by sarcoidosis and other inflammatory conditions. Two days after the injection, the body is scanned for radioactivity. Increases in gallium uptake at any site in the body indicate that inflammatory activity has developed at the site and also give an idea of which tissue, and how much tissue, has been affected. However, since any type of inflammation causes gallium uptake, a positive gallium scan does not necessarily mean that the patient has sarcoidosis.

Kveim Test

This test involves injecting a standardized preparation of sarcoid tissue material into the skin. On the one hand, a unique lump formed at the point of injection is considered positive for sarcoidosis. On the other hand, the test result is not always positive even if the patient has sarcoidosis.

The Kveim test is not used often in the United States because no test material has been approved for sale by the U.S. Food and Drug Administration. However, a few hospitals and clinics may have some standardized test preparation prepared privately for their own use.

Slit-Lamp Examination

An instrument called a slit lamp, which permits examination of the inside of the eye, can be used to detect silent damage from sarcoidosis.

Management

Fortunately, many patients with sarcoidosis require no treatment. Symptoms, after all, are usually not disabling and do tend to disappear spontaneously.

When therapy is recommended, the main goal is to keep the lungs and other affected body organs working and to relieve symptoms. The disease is considered inactive once the symptoms fade. After many years of experience with treating the disease, corticosteroids remain the primary treatment for inflammation and granuloma formation. Prednisone is probably the corticosteroid most often prescribed today. There is no treatment at present to reverse the fibrosis that might be present in advanced sarcoidosis.

Occasionally, a blood test will show a high blood level of calcium accompanying sarcoidosis. The reasons for this are not clear. Some scientists believe that this condition is not common. When it does occur, the patient may be advised to avoid calcium-rich foods, vitamin D, or sunlight, or to take prednisone; this corticosteroid quickly reverses the condition.

Because sarcoidosis can disappear even without therapy, doctors sometimes disagree on when to start the treatment, what dose to prescribe, and how long to continue the medicine. The doctor's decision depends on the organ system involved and how far the inflammation has progressed. If the disease appears to be severe-especially in the lungs, eyes, heart, nervous system, spleen, or kidneys—the doctor may prescribe corticosteroids.

Corticosteroid treatment usually results in improvement. Symptoms often start up again, however, when it is stopped. Treatment, therefore, may be necessary for several years, sometimes for as long as the disease remains active or to prevent relapse.

Frequent checkups are important so that the doctor can monitor the illness and, if necessary, adjust the treatment. Corticosteroids, for example, can have side effects—mood swings, swelling, and weight gain because the treatment tends to make the body hold on to water; high blood pressure; high blood sugar; and craving for food. Long-term use can affect the stomach, skin, and bones. This situation can bring on stomach pain, an ulcer, or acne, or cause the loss of calcium from bones. However, if the corticosteroid is taken in carefully prescribed, low doses, the benefits from the treatment are usually far greater than the problems.

Most people with sarcoidosis lead a normal life.

Besides corticosteroids, various other drugs have been tried, but their effectiveness has not been established in controlled studies. These drugs include chloroquine and D-penicillamine. Several drugs such as chlorambucil, azathioprine, methotrexate, and cyclophosphamide, which might suppress alveolitis by killing the cells that produce granulomas, have also been used. None has been evaluated in controlled clinical trials, and the risk of using these drugs is high, especially in pregnant women.

Cyclosporine, a drug used widely in organ transplants to suppress immune reaction, has been evaluated in one controlled trial. It was found to be unsuccessful.

Research Status in Sarcoidosis

Goals of the National Heart, Lung, and Blood Institute

There are many unanswered questions about sarcoidosis. Identifying the agent that causes the illness, along with the inflammatory mechanisms that set the stage for the alveolitis, granuloma formation, and fibrosis that characterize the disease, is the major aim of the National Heart, Lung, and Blood Institute's program on sarcoidosis. Development of reliable methods of diagnosis, treatment, and eventually, the prevention of sarcoidosis is the ultimate goal.

Originally, scientists thought that sarcoidosis was caused by an acquired state of immunological inertness (anergy). This notion was revised a few years ago, when the technique of bronchoalveolar lavage provided access to a vast array of cells and cell-derived mediators operating in the lungs of sarcoidosis patients. Sarcoidosis is now believed to be associated with a complex mix of immunological disturbances involving simultaneous activation, as well as depression, of certain immunological functions.

Immunological studies on sarcoidosis patients show that many of the immune functions associated with thymus-derived white blood cells, called T-lymphocytes or T-cells, are depressed. The depression of this cellular component of systemic immune response is expressed in the inability of the patients to evoke a delayed hypersensitivity skin reaction (a positive skin test), when tested by the appropriate foreign substance, or antigen, underneath the skin.

In addition, the blood of sarcoidosis patients contains a reduced number of T-cells. These T-cells do not seem capable of responding normally when treated with substances known to stimulate the growth of laboratory-cultured T-cells. Neither do they produce their normal complement of immunological mediators, cytokines, through which the cells modify the behavior of other cells.

In contrast to the depression of the cellular immune response, humoral immune response of sarcoidosis patients is elevated. The humoral immune response is reflected by the production of circulating antibodies against a variety of exogenous antigens, including common viruses. This humoral component of systemic immune response is mediated by another class of lymphocytes known as B-lymphocytes, or B-cells, because they originate in the bone marrow.

In another indication of heightened humoral response, sarcoidosis patients seem prone to develop autoantibodies (antibodies against endogenous antigens) similar to rheumatoid factors. With access to the cells and cell products in the lung tissue compartments through the bronchoalveolar technique, it also has become possible for researchers to complement the above investigations at the blood level with analysis of local inflammatory and immune events in the lungs.

In contrast to what is seen at the systemic level, the cellular immune response in the lungs seems to be heightened rather than depressed. The heightened cellular immune response in the diseased tissue is characterized by significant increases in activated T-lymphocytes with certain characteristic cell-surface antigens, as well as in activated alveolar macrophages.

This pronounced, localized cellular response is also accompanied by the appearance in the lung of an array of mediators that are thought to contribute to the disease process; these include interleukin-1, interleukin-2, B-cell growth factor, B-cell differentiation factor, fibroblast growth factor and fibronectin.

Because a number of lung diseases follow respiratory tract infections, ascertaining whether a virus can be implicated in the events leading to sarcoidosis remains an important area of research. Some recent observations seem to provide suggestive leads on this question. In these studies, the genes of cytomegalovirus (CMV), a common disease-causing virus, were introduced into lymphocytes, and the expression of the viral genes was studied. It was found that the viral genes were expressed both during acute infection of the cells and when the virus was not replicating in the cells. However, this expression seemed to take place only when the T-cells were activated by some injurious event.

In addition, the product of a CMV gene was found capable of activating the gene in alveolar macrophage responsible for the production of interleukin-1. Since interleukin-1 levels are found to increase in alveolar macrophage from patients with sarcoidosis, this suggests that certain viral genes can enhance the production of inflammatory components associated with sarcoidosis.

Whether these findings implicate viral infections in the disease process in sarcoidosis is unclear. Future research with viral models may provide clues to the molecular mechanisms that trigger alterations in lymphocyte and macrophage regulation leading to sarcoidosis.

In 1995, the National Heart, Lung, and Blood Institute started a multicenter case control study of the etiology of sarcoidosis. The investigation is planned to last six years and will collect information and specimens for use in investigation of environmental, occupational, lifestyle, and genetic risk factors for sarcoidosis. Examination of the natural history of sarcoidosis is planned in patients at early and late stages of the disease. Such information should improve our understanding of the cause(s) of sarcoidosis and provide insight into how to better prevent and treat the disease.

Living with Sarcoidosis

The cause of sarcoidosis still remains unknown, so there is at present no known way to prevent or cure this disease. However, doctors have had a great deal of experience in management of the illness.

If you have sarcoidosis, you can help yourself by following sensible health measures. You should not smoke. You should also avoid exposure to other substances such as dusts and chemicals that can harm your lungs.

Patients with sarcoidosis are best treated by a lung specialist or a doctor who has a special interest in sarcoidosis. Sarcoidosis specialists are usually located at major research centers. If you have any symptoms of sarcoidosis, see your doctor regularly so that the illness can be watched and, if necessary, treated. If it heals naturally, sarcoidosis is unlikely to recur. Nevertheless, if you have had sarcoidosis, or are suspected of having the illness but have no symptoms now, be sure to have physical checkups every year, including an eye examination.

Although severe sarcoidosis can reduce the chances of becoming pregnant, particularly for older women, many young women with sarcoidosis have given birth to healthy babies while on treatment. Patients planning to have a baby should discuss the matter with their doctor. Medical checkups all through pregnancy and immediately thereafter are especially important for sarcoidosis patients. In some cases, bed rest is necessary during the last 3 months of pregnancy.

In addition to family and close friends, a number of local lung organizations, other nonprofit health organizations, and self-help groups are available to help patients cope with sarcoidosis. By keeping in touch with them, you can share personal feelings and experiences. Members also share specific information on the latest scientific advances, where to find sarcoidosis specialists, and how to improve one's self-image.

For More Information

Additional information on sarcoidosis is available from a number of sources. For the names of U.S. scientists working on sarcoidosis or physicians specializing in the disease, write to:

National Heart, Lung, and Blood Institute
Division of Lung Diseases
2 Rockledge Center
6701 Rockledge Drive
MSC 7952
Suite 10018
Bethesda, MD 20892-7952
Tel: 301-496-4236
Internet: http://www.nhlbi.nih.gov
E-Mail: nhlbiingo@rover.nhlbi.nih.gov

Other Sources

Information and publications for sarcoidosis patients and their families are available from:

National Institute of Allergy and Infectious Diseases
9000 Rockville Pike
Building 31
Room 7A32
Bethesda, MD 20892
Internet: http://www.niaid.nih.gov

Sarcoidosis Family Aid and Research Foundation
460A Central Avenue
East Orange, NJ 07018
Toll Free: 800-223-6429

Help from the American Lung Association

Many local chapters of the American Lung Association host support groups for sarcoidosis patients. The address and telephone number of the chapter nearest to you should be in your local telephone directory. Or you can write or call the association's national headquarters:

American Lung Association
1740 Broadway
New York, NY 10019-4374
Tel: 212-315-8700
Internet: http://www.lungusa.org
E-Mail: info@lungsusa.org

Patient Support Groups

Following are addresses of organizations that provide additional information and patient support groups on sarcoidosis:

Sarcoidosis Networking
13925 80th Street East
Puyallup, WA 98372
Tel: 206-845-3108

National Sarcoidosis Resources Center
P.O. Box 1593
Piscataway, NJ 08855-1593
Tel: 908-699-0733

Sarcoidosis Research Institute

3475 Central Avenue
Memphis, TN 38111
Tel: 901-327-5454
Internet: http://www.sarcoidcenter.com/sriccontents.htm
E-Mail: sarcoid@sarcoidcenter.com

Chapter 35

Silicosis

What Is Silicosis?

Silicosis is a disabling, nonreversible and sometimes fatal lung disease caused by overexposure to respirable crystalline silica. Silica is the second most common mineral in the earth's crust and is a major component of sand, rock, and mineral ores. Overexposure to dust that contains microscopic particles of crystalline silica can cause scar tissue to form in the lungs, which reduces the lungs' ability to extract oxygen from the air we breathe. Typical sand found at the beach does not pose a silicosis threat.

More than 1 million U.S. workers are exposed to crystalline silica. Each year, more than 250 American workers die with silicosis. There is no cure for the disease, but it is 100 percent preventable if employers, workers, and health professionals work together to reduce exposures. In addition to silicosis, inhalation of crystalline silica particles has been associated with other diseases, such as bronchitis and tuberculosis. Some studies also indicate an association with lung cancer.

Who Is at Risk?

Working in any dusty environment where crystalline silica is present potentially can increase a person's chances of getting silicosis.

U.S. Department of Labor, 1996; text available on the National Institute for Occupational Safety and Health (NIOSH) website at http://www.cdc.gov.niosh/silfact1.html; cited April 2000.

239

If a number of workers are working in a dusty environment and one is diagnosed with the silicosis, the others should be examined to see if they might also be developing silicosis.

Some examples of the industries and activities that pose the greatest potential risk for worker exposure include:

- construction (sandblasting, rock drilling, masonry work, jack hammering, tunneling)
- stone cutting (sawing, abrasive blasting, chipping, grinding)
- glass manufacturing
- mining (cutting or drilling through sandstone and granite)
- agriculture (dusty conditions from disturbing the soil, such as plowing or harvesting)
- foundry work (grinding, moldings, shakeout, core room)
- shipbuilding (abrasive blasting)
- ceramics, clay, and pottery
- railroad (setting and laying track)
- manufacturing of soaps and detergents
- manufacturing and use of abrasives

More than 100,000 workers in the United States encounter high-risk, silica exposures through sandblasting, rock drilling, and mining. Workers who remove paint and rust from buildings, bridges, tanks, and other surfaces; clean foundry castings; work with stone or clay; etch or frost glass; and work in construction are at risk of overexposure to crystalline silica.

What Are the Types, Symptoms and Complications of Silicosis?

There are three types of silicosis, depending upon the airborne concentration of crystalline silica to which a worker has been exposed:

- *Chronic silicosis* usually occurs after 10 or more years of overexposure.

- *Accelerated silicosis* results from higher exposures and develops over 5-10 years.

- *Acute silicosis* occurs where exposures are the highest and can cause symptoms to develop within a few weeks or up to 5 years.

Chronic silicosis, the most common form of the disease, may go undetected for years in the early stages; in fact, a chest X-ray may not reveal an abnormality until after 15 or 20 years of exposure. The body's ability to fight infections may be overwhelmed by silica dust in the lungs, making workers more susceptible to certain illnesses, such as tuberculosis. As a result, workers may exhibit one or more of the following symptoms:

- shortness of breath following physical exertion
- severe cough
- fatigue
- loss of appetite
- chest pains
- fever

How Can Workers Determine If They Have Silicosis?

A medical examination that includes a complete work history and a chest X-ray and lung function test is the only sure way to determine if a person has silicosis. Workers who believe they are overexposed to silica dust should visit a doctor who knows about lung diseases. The National Institute for Occupational Safety and Health (NIOSH) recommends that medical examinations occur before job placement or upon entering a trade, and at least every 3 years thereafter.

Chapter 36

Tuberculosis (TB)

Tuberculosis (TB) is an infectious disease caused by a germ (bacterium) called *Mycobacterium tuberculosis*. This germ primarily affects the lungs and may infect anyone at any age.

In the United States, the number of TB cases steadily decreased until 1986 when an increase was noted; TB has continued to rise since. Today, ten million individuals are infected in the U.S., as evidenced by positive skin tests, with approximately 26,000 new cases of active disease each year. The increase in TB cases is related to HIV/AIDS, homelessness, drug abuse and immigration of persons with active infections.

How Is TB Contracted?

TB is a contagious or infectious disease that is spread from person-to-person. A person is usually infected by inhaling the germs which have been sprayed into the air by someone with the active disease who coughs.

However, inhaling the germ does not usually mean you will develop active disease. A person's natural body defenses are usually able to control the infection so that it does not cause disease. In this case, the person would be infected, but not have active disease. Only about 10% of those infected will actually develop TB in their lifetimes.

Active disease can occur in an infected person when the body's resistance is low or if there is a large or prolonged exposure to the germs that overcome the body's natural defenses. The body's response to active TB infection produces inflammation which can eventually damage the lungs.

The amount of damage may be quite extensive, yet the symptoms may be minimal. The usual symptoms of disease due to TB are:

- Fever
- Night sweats
- Cough
- Loss of appetite
- Weight Loss
- Blood in the sputum (phlegm)
- Loss of energy

Diagnosing TB

To diagnose TB, your clinician will gather five important pieces of information:

- Symptoms
- History of possible exposure and onset of symptoms
- Tuberculin skin test or PPD
- Chest X-ray
- Sputum test

Tuberculin Skin Test

The tuberculin skin test (or PPD) is performed with an extract of killed tuberculosis germs that is injected into the skin. If a person has been infected with tuberculosis, a lump will form at the site of the injection—this is a positive test. This generally means that TB germs have infected the body. It does not usually mean the person has active disease. People with positive skin tests but without active disease cannot transmit the infection to others.

Chest X-Ray

If a person has been infected with TB, but active disease has not developed, the chest X-ray usually will be normal. Most people with a positive PPD have normal chest X-rays and continue to be healthy. For such persons, preventive drug therapy may be recommended.

However, if the germ has attacked and caused inflammation in the lungs, an abnormal shadow is usually visible on the chest X-rays. For these persons, aggressive diagnostic studies (sputum tests) and treatment usually are appropriate.

Sputum Test

Samples of sputum coughed up from the lungs can be tested to see if TB germs are present. The sputum is examined under a microscope (a "sputum smear") to look for evidence of the presence of TB organisms. The organisms are then grown in the laboratory to identify them as TB germs and to determine what medications are effective in treating them. These studies are referred to as culture and susceptibility testing. State health department laboratories and reference laboratories can perform such testing.

Treatment of TB

Individuals with a positive tuberculin skin test may or may not receive preventive drug therapy depending on the exposure history, the timing of the skin test conversion (when the test changes from negative to positive) and other factors in the individual's medical history. When it is known that a person has recently been in close contact with an individual with active tuberculosis and has developed a positive tuberculin skin test, preventive treatment is advisable due to a relatively high risk of developing active disease. Isoniazid (INH) may be prescribed for six to nine months as preventive treatment and for twelve months in persons who are HIV positive.

Since the advent of anti-tuberculosis drugs in the 1940s, the treatment of drug-susceptible tuberculosis has become highly effective if administered and taken properly. Treatment no longer requires prolonged hospital stays. In many cases, a patient with a new case of TB can be treated at home. Others will enter the hospital to be placed on a medication program and to be isolated until the disease is controlled. When the person is no longer infectious, he or she can leave the hospital and continue on medication at home. Hospitalization in such cases may be a few weeks to several months depending on the severity of the disease and the effectiveness of the treatment program. In most cases, a treatment program for drug-susceptible TB involves taking two or four drugs for a period of time ranging from six to nine months. Medications may include isoniazid, rifampin, pyrazinamide, ethambutol or streptomycin. It is necessary to take multiple drugs and to take all of the doses prescribed, because all of the TB germs cannot be destroyed by one drug.

It is important to realize that hospitalization for a TB patient, when necessary, represents only the beginning of treatment. Since active TB is slow to respond completely to therapy, medications prescribed by a clinician must be taken faithfully for a long period of time (at least 6 months, in some cases for a year or more). If the TB medications are not taken regularly, serious complications may develop:

- the organisms may become resistant to one or more of the drugs,

- there may be an increased risk of toxic reactions from the drugs and

- there is a high risk of disease relapse or recurrence.

Given the many effective medications available today, the chances are excellent that tuberculosis in an individual can be cured. It is important, however, for the patient to understand the disease and to cooperate fully in the therapy program.

Drug-Resistant TB

In a small percentage of cases, the initial treatment does not go as planned. It may be that the patient is not taking the medications regularly, the medication program is not sufficient for a particular infection or the medications are not absorbed properly. In these patients, there is a tendency for the germs to become resistant to some or all of the drugs. Sometimes a person has initial drug-resistant disease. In other words, the TB germs they contracted were from a person with drug-resistant TB.

Drug-resistant TB is very difficult to treat and requires more and different medications for a longer period of treatment. Sometimes, surgery is needed to remove areas of destroyed lung that contain many millions of germs that are inaccessible to antibiotics. A person with drug-resistant TB should be treated by a specialist with considerable experience in managing the disease and this treatment should be initiated in a hospital setting.

Chapter 37

Drug-Resistant Tuberculosis

Multi-drug-resistant tuberculosis (MDR TB) is a form of tuberculosis that is resistant to two or more of the primary drugs used for the treatment of tuberculosis. Resistance to one or several forms of treatment occurs when the bacteria develops the ability to withstand antibiotic attack and relay that ability to their progeny. Since that entire strain of bacteria inherits this capacity to resist the effects of the various treatments, resistance can spread from one person to another. On an individual basis, however, inadequate treatment or improper use of the anti-tuberculosis medications remains an important cause of drug-resistant tuberculosis.

Even though throughout the late 1980s and early 1990s the incidence of tuberculosis was on the rise, recent trends indicate that the number of tuberculosis cases reported have been continuously declining. During the period of 1992 to 1997, the total number of tuberculosis cases reported decreased by 26 percent.

Several factors have been identified as contributing to this substantial decline, including demographic changes and increased federal and other resources for state and local tuberculosis control efforts.

In 1997, the CDC reported that 1.3 percent of tuberculosis cases (from states that reported drug susceptibility) were resistant to both isoniazid and rifampin. Certain areas, however, have been shown to have much higher rates. Forty-seven percent of all MDR TB cases were reported from New York and California.

247

A strain of MDR TB originally develops when a case of drug-susceptible tuberculosis is improperly or incompletely treated. This occurs when a physician does not prescribe proper treatment regimens or when a patient is unable to adhere to therapy. Improper treatment allows individual TB bacilli that have natural resistance to a drug to multiply. Eventually the majority of bacilli in the body are resistant.

Once a strain of MDR TB develops it can be transmitted to others just like a normal drug-susceptible strain. Airborne transmission has been the cause of several well-publicized cases of nosocomial (hospital-based) outbreaks of MDR TB in New York City and Florida. These outbreaks were responsible for the deaths of several patients and health care workers, a majority of whom were coinfected with HIV.

Persons at risk for MDR TB include:

- persons who have been exposed to someone with active MDR TB, especially if they are immunocompromised

- TB patients who have failed to take medications as prescribed

- TB patients who have been prescribed an ineffective treatment regimen

- persons who have been previously treated for TB and experience a recurrence

- persons from other countries and areas in the U.S. with a high incidence of MDR TB

As with drug susceptible tuberculosis, MDR TB has been a particular concern among HIV-infected persons. Some of the factors that have contributed to the number of cases of MDR TB, both in general and among HIV-infected individuals are:

- delayed diagnosis and delayed determination of drug susceptibility, which may take several weeks

- susceptibility of immunosuppressed individuals for not only acquiring MDR TB but for rapid disease progression, which may result in rapid transmission of the disease to other immunosuppressed patients

- inadequate respiratory isolation procedures and other environmental safety conditions, especially in confined areas such as prisons

- noncompliance or intermittent compliance with antituberculosis drug therapy.

MDR TB is more difficult to treat than drug-susceptible strains of TB. The success of treatment depends upon how quickly a case of TB is identified as drug resistant and whether an effective drug therapy is available. The second-line drugs used in cases of MDR TB are often less effective and more likely to cause side effects.

Tests to determine the resistance of a particular strain to various drugs usually take several weeks complete. During the delay the patient may be treated with a drug regimen that is ineffective.

Once a strain's drug resistance is known, an effective drug regimen must be identified and begun. Some strains of MDR TB are resistant to seven or more drugs, making the identification of effective drugs difficult. To deal with this problem, it is recommended that newly discovered cases of TB in populations at high risk for MDR TB be treated with four drugs rather than the standard three as part of initial treatment.

Treatment for MDR TB involves drug therapy over many months or years. Despite the longer course of treatment, the cure rate decreases from over 90 percent for nonresistant strains of TB to 50 percent or less for MDR TB.

Because it is difficult for some people to successfully complete their tuberculosis treatment, several innovations have been developed. One of these is the use of incentives and enablers, which may be transportation, tokens or food coupons that are given to patients each time they appear at the clinic or doctor's office for treatment. Incentives and enablers are combined with the use of directly observed therapy (DOT). DOT is a system of treatment in which the patient is administered his or her medication by a nurse or health worker and observed taking the medication.

One recent innovation in TB treatment is the recent FDA approval of Rifater. Rifater is a medication that combines the three main drugs (isoniazid, rifampin, and pyrazinamide) used to treat tuberculosis into one pill. This reduces the number of pills a patient has to take each day and makes it impossible for the patient to take only one of the three medications, a common path to the development of MDR TB.

In June 1998, the U.S. Food and Drug Administration approved the first new drug for pulmonary tuberculosis in 25 years. The drug, rifapentine (Priftin), has been approved for use with other drugs to fight TB. One potential advantage of rifapentine is that it can be taken less often in the final four months of treatment—once a week compared with twice a week for the standard regimen.

Chapter 38

Pediatric Tuberculosis

Since 1992, the trend has reversed, and the rate has begun to decline again. Between 1992 and 1997 the incidence of tuberculosis cases among children 14 and younger born in the United States decreased 25 percent, while the total number of cases in all ages decreased 38 percent.

Cases of active tuberculosis and asymptomatic TB infection in children are of great concern. They indicate that transmission of tuberculosis has occurred recently. Many adults who develop active tuberculosis were infected many years ago, when their immune systems were stronger and able to protect them. Children, particularly infants, could have been infected only recently because of their age. When a child is diagnosed with active tuberculosis, it means that someone close to them, almost always an adult, must have active tuberculosis and is possibly transmitting the disease to others as well.

Diagnosis of tuberculosis in children is difficult and poses problems that are not present in adults. Children are less likely to have obvious symptoms of tuberculosis. In addition, sputum samples are difficult to collect from children. Culture and drug susceptibility results from tests of the adult source case often have to be relied upon for diagnosing and properly treating tuberculosis in a child.

Tuberculosis in infants and children younger than 4 years of age is much more likely to spread throughout the body through the bloodstream. In addition, children are at much greater risk of developing tuberculous meningitis, a very dangerous form of the disease that affects the central nervous system. For these reasons, prompt diagnosis and immediate treatment of tuberculosis are critical in pediatric cases.

In general, the same methods are used in treating tuberculosis in children as are used in treating tuberculosis in adults. At least six months of treatment with three or four drugs is the recommended course of therapy for both adults and children. The primary difference between treatment for adults and children is the use of ethambutol. One of the side effects of ethambutol is impaired vision. Because this effect is difficult to monitor in young children, ethambutol is not routinely recommended for children under eight years old.

The best method to prevent cases of pediatric tuberculosis is to find, diagnose, and treat cases of active tuberculosis among adults. Children almost never contract tuberculosis from other children or transmit it themselves. Adults are usually the ones who pass tuberculosis on to children. Improved contact investigations and use of directly observed therapy should improve the success rate of finding and treating adult cases of tuberculosis and therefore reduce the number of cases of pediatric tuberculosis.

Some groups of children are at greater risk for tuberculosis than others. These include:

- children living in a household with an adult who has active tuberculosis

- children living in a household with an adult who is at high risk for contracting TB

- children infected with HIV or another immunocompromising condition

- children born in a country that has a high prevalence of tuberculosis

- children from communities that are medically underserved

Chapter 39

Upper Respiratory Infections

Children and Croup

Croup is a viral infection that usually affects children between the ages of three months to five years. In most cases, croup follows an upper respiratory infection. This illness is most often seen in the fall and winter during the cold season. Croup tends to reoccur during childhood, but attacks disappear as the child grows.

Common symptoms of croup include a low grade fever, a brassy, barking cough, a hoarse cry, inspiratory stridor (a harsh sound from the windpipe during inhalation) and difficulty breathing. These symptoms are caused by swelling and muscle spasm in the throat and windpipe. Symptoms usually appear in the evening and worsen at night. Croup may last from several days to several weeks. Parents should expect a complete recovery.

Treatment of Croup at Home

In most cases, croup can be treated effectively at home. Treatment with cool mist will relieve some of the distress of croup. Cool mist is effective in reducing fever, reducing the swelling in the airway and liquefying mucus secretions in the airway for easy expectoration. Cool mist therapy may be delivered by directing a vaporizer into the crib or playpen. The crib or playpen should be covered with a sheet to create a warm humid environment. Another option may be to run the shower or tub water in the bathroom with the door closed for fifteen minutes or so. This creates an environment high in humidity to relieve the coughing and other symptoms associated with croup.

In addition the cool mist therapy, the child should receive adequate rest and drink plenty of fluids. Because crying increases respiratory distress, care should be taken to comfort and soothe the child.

Finally, it is very important to closely monitor the child with croup. Parents should be aware of signs of increasing airway obstruction and seek medical care if the child is experiencing respiratory distress. If the child experiences continuous respiratory stridor, retractions around the neck or ribs (skin sinking in) or severe breathing difficulty, it is important to seek prompt medical care.

Medical Management of Croup

Treatment of croup in the doctor's office or hospital is similar to treatment at home. Cool mist therapy in a croup tent will help relieve some of the distress of croup symptoms. Inhaled medications and/or oral corticosteroids may be prescribed to decrease the swelling and spasm of the upper airways. Because croup is a viral infection, antibiotics are generally not used.

In addition to a croup tent and other medications, a doctor's office or hospital can provide constant monitoring of the child's breathing. Doctors and nurses can ensure the child is breathing and receiving enough oxygen. This is important in severe cases of croup.

Colds and Upper Respiratory Infections

Colds are typically viral infections of the upper respiratory tract. Symptoms can include:

- a scratchy, sore throat
- sneezing
- nasal discharge, which is watery at first, then thick
- extreme tiredness
- muscle aches
- low grade fever
- an overall sick feeling

Colds are highly contagious and are spread through touching contaminated surfaces, coughing and sneezing. Over 200 different viruses can cause a cold. Some of the common viruses include: rhino virus, respiratory syncytial virus (RSV), corona virus, para-influenza and influenza.

Some people are more prone to colds than others. A child in preschool may "catch" as many as four to eight colds per year. Generally, there is an increased frequency of colds during fall and winter months because of closer, indoor contact with other people.

A cold usually runs its course without complications in one to two weeks. If you have cold symptoms lasting longer than two weeks, report this to your doctor. Also, report symptoms of a nasal discharge which has an odor or is colored as this can indicate a sinus infection.

Treatment

Because there is no cure for the common cold, treatment is aimed at relieving symptoms. Saline (salt water) nose drops or sprays may be helpful in relieving nasal congestion, especially for infants. "Over-the-counter" decongestant sprays can relieve symptoms temporarily, but should not be used for more than three days. Longer use can lead to rebound congestion with more symptoms of congestion. Oral (tablet or syrup) decongestants may also relieve nasal symptoms.

Antihistamines in tablet or syrup form may be of some benefit in reducing mucus production. In general, aspirin is not recommended for children under 18 and for many persons with asthma. Ask your doctor about taking acetaminophen (Tylenol) for relieving pain and fever. Antibiotics and vitamin C are not helpful in relieving symptoms of the common cold.

Frequent hand washing and use of disposable tissues may help decrease the spread of cold germs. In fact, hand washing may be the single most effective way to reduce the spread of infections! Experimental vaccines have not proven successful because there are so many possible viruses that can cause a cold.

Acute Bronchitis

Acute bronchitis is an inflammation and irritation of the bronchial tubes (airways) in the lungs. It is usually caused by an infection or, more rarely, by an exposure to chemicals. Symptoms generally include cough with mucus, chest discomfort, fever and extreme tiredness.

Acute infectious bronchitis can be caused by many bacteria and viruses. In children, viruses are the most common infectious cause of bronchitis. It is important to note that severe cases of bronchitis may progress to pneumonia.

Treatment

A clinician can determine if a bronchial infection is due to a virus or bacteria. An antibiotic is prescribed if you have a bacterial bronchitis. If you have a viral bronchitis, however, an antibiotic may not be prescribed. This is because an antibiotic is not effective against a viral infection and unnecessary use of antibiotics can lead to "drug-resistant" bacteria. Your clinician may prescribe an antibiotic if you have developed a secondary bacterial infection on top of the pre-existing viral infection. It is important that the antibiotic is the correct one to kill the specific bacteria of your infection.

Additional medications may be prescribed to ease your breathing. Bronchodilator medications are given if you experience wheezing or shortness of breath. Corticosteroid medications may be used to decrease inflammation and irritation in your airways. These prescription medicines are available as tablets, syrups or inhalers (sprays).

How long the bronchitis lasts is affected by your general state of health, the virus or bacteria involved and how soon you get treatment. Avoiding smoke and other irritants, good nutrition with plenty of fluids, rest and medication are all important. Sometimes viral bronchitis can cause asthma-like symptoms. This is more common in persons with a history of asthma or allergy. This condition's main symptom is a dry, hacking cough that lasts four to eight weeks or longer after the initial infection is over. The cough may be triggered by cold, dry air, smoke or dust. Bronchodilator and corticosteroid medications may be prescribed for persistent or severe cases. Your doctor can discuss your medications, restrictions and anticipated recovery time.

Acute bronchitis is different from chronic bronchitis which develops from long-term irritation of the airways and is most often associated with smoking. Even persons who inhale second-hand smoke are at risk for developing chronic bronchitis!

Avoiding exposure to smoke, frequent hand washing and the use of disposable tissues can decrease the number of acute bronchitis infections. Also, ask your doctor about yearly flu (influenza) vaccines.

Chapter 40

Other Lung Disorders and Conditions

Actinomycosis

Actinomycosis is a long-lasting disease caused by a microorganism (*Actinomyces israelii*) that is normally present in the mouth and throat. Infection occurs most commonly in the jaw or neck, usually following dental trauma, and sometimes in the abdominal membrane or lungs. Hard, very slow-growing swellings form and eventually turn into abscesses. When the abscesses break down, pus is discharged through several openings in the skin. Treatment with penicillin is usually effective.

Atelectasis

Atelectasis is either complete or partial collapse of a lung. The term refers to two distinct conditions. The first is the failure of the lungs to expand at birth, and the second is the collapsed (airless) condition of a segment of a lung. This collapse is generally caused by an obstruction in the tube (bronchus) leading to the lung, or by excessive secretion of mucus in the airway. Such a condition can occur in several respiratory disorders, particularly in pneumonia but also in bronchitis. Pressure from outside the lungs from a tumor, for example, can also press on part of a lung and cause a collapse.

Treatment

If the cause of the collapse is a blocked bronchus, such an obstruction may be removed by using a special instrument called a bronchoscope. Atelectasis from other causes can often be corrected by breathing exercises and respiratory therapy treatments.

Complications

If excessive amounts of mucus are the cause of the collapse, the mucus build-up can become infected. Atelectasis following surgery may cause a fever.

Black Lung

Black lung is the common name for the lung disorder anthracosis. The normal pink color of the lungs is turned black by the inhalation of coal dust or smoke. Once a common disorder only among coal miners, anthracosis is now also found in city dwellers.

Symptoms

In the early stages the symptoms resemble those of bronchitis, with coughing and shortness of breath. If the cause is not removed, over a period of years the coughing gradually gets worse. Diagnosis is confirmed by an X-ray examination.

Treatment

The lung damage caused by the inhaled dust cannot be repaired, nor can it be treated directly. Breathing clean air halts the progress of the disease and may help reduce the severity of the symptoms. A victim should avoid further exposure to dust particles.

Fungal Infection

Fungal infection may be caused by microscopic fungi or their spores. Many antifungal drugs are available for the treatment of superficial (skin, hair, mouth, vagina) and systemic (deep) fungal infections. Since fungi are more resistant than bacteria to treatment, a longer duration of treatment is usually required to cure a fungal infection. Table 40.1 lists some of the common fungal disorders and their basic characteristics.

Histoplasmosis

Histoplasmosis is an infection caused by the fungus *Histoplasma capsulatum*, which grows in soil enriched with droppings from birds or bats. It is most common in the Mississippi, Missouri, and Ohio river areas. Histoplasmosis originates in the lungs when spores of the fungus are inhaled and may spread in the bloodstream to other parts of the body. Histoplasmosis may be mild or acute or, rarely, progressive and eventually fatal, if untreated. Mild histoplasmosis has no obvious symptoms. The only sign of infection is the presence of calcified spots on the lungs, which can be detected on a chest X ray. The primary acute form of severe histoplasmosis is characterized by a cough, breathlessness, hoarseness, coughing up of blood, and fever. There may also be chills, muscle pains, weight loss, and fatigue. Occasionally, the disease spreads to other parts of the body; this is called progressive disseminated histoplasmosis. Severe forms of the disease may be seen in people with impaired immune systems, such as those with AIDS. The infection can be treated with antifungal drugs.

Table 40.1. Common Fungal Disorders

Disorder	*Basic Characteristics*
Actinomycosis	Fibrous masses about the mouth or tongue, that burst and become sinuses or ulcers; also abscesses in the lungs
Aspergillosis	Lumps in the skin, ears, sinuses, and especially, the lungs
Athlete's Foot	Skin eruptions on the foot, usually between the toes
Blastomycosis	Lesions all over the body but, especially, infection of the lungs
Candidiasis	White patches inside the mouth that later become shallow ulcers; may also occur in the vagina
Histoplasmosis	Infection of the lungs, ulcers in the gastrointestinal tract, and possible skin lesions
Ringworm	Raised, round sores of the skin

Pneumoconiosis

Pneumoconiosis is a general term for any chronic lung disease caused by the inhalation of dust particles. It is usually caused by environmental or occupational factors, such as the inhalation of coal dust particles during coal mining. There are three main types of pneumoconiosis.

1. Simple pneumoconiosis results from the deposition of inert dust in the lungs and is apparently harmless. For example, iron, tin, and carbon dust do not seem to cause any adverse effects.

2. Irritant dusts, such as silica and asbestos, can cause silicosis or asbestosis. These diseases cause scarring and gradual destruction of the lung tissue.

3. Organic dusts may cause a form of allergic reaction. For example, byssinosis is caused by cotton fiber dust, and bagassosis is caused by sugar cane residue.

Symptoms

Simple pneumoconiosis seldom produces symptoms. Coal dust, however, may cause scarring and destruction of lung tissue similar to that caused by silica and asbestos. Pneumoconiosis that results from irritant dusts may cause increasing breathlessness, coughing, and spitting of blood. Asbestosis may develop into lung cancer.

The main symptom of pneumoconiosis that is caused by organic dusts is asthma. In some cases, this may be complicated with bronchitis.

Treatment

There is no cure for this condition. It is essential that a person change jobs or living environment at the first suspicion of pneumoconiosis. It is impossible to remove the dust particles once they have reached the lungs, and lung deterioration is likely to continue for some time after a person has stopped inhaling the dust. Dust suppression and regular medical examinations are essential. Proper use of respirators and masks in hazardous environments can decrease the risk of developing pneumoconiosis.

Bronchopneumonia

Bronchopneumonia, also called bronchial pneumonia, is a contagious infection of the lungs. This type of pneumonia is localized, mainly in the smaller branches of the bronchial tubes, called bronchioles.

Bronchopneumonia can be caused by pneumococci, certain other bacteria, or by viruses. The bronchioles become inflamed as they clog with pus and mucus, resulting in one or more of the following symptoms: coughing, chest pains, fever, blood-streaked sputum, chills, and difficulty in breathing.

Treatment is with antibiotic drugs and bed rest. Hospitalization for diagnostic tests and treatment may be necessary for some patients.

Pleurisy

Pleurisy is the inflammation of the pleura, a membrane that lines the inside of the chest and covers the lungs. Normally, the two surfaces of the membrane are moist and allow the lungs to move smoothly over the chest wall when a person breathes. When the pleura is inflamed, the surfaces become dry and rough and rub together. This condition, known as dry pleurisy, causes intense pain, which is made worse by coughing or deep breathing.

As the condition develops, the pain usually ceases because fluid forms in the pleural cavity and separates the inflamed surfaces of the pleura. If a large amount of fluid forms (wet pleurisy or pleural effusion), the underlying lung may collapse, causing breathlessness.

Causes

Usually, pleurisy is caused by an infection of the pleura or of the underlying lung, as may occur with pneumonia. Pleurisy may also be caused by a pulmonary infarction; the spread of disease from elsewhere in the body, such as cancer; or a generalized disease, such as kidney failure.

Treatment

Treatment is directed toward the underlying cause. Initially, painkillers and anti-inflammatory drugs may be given and, if the patient has a fever, antibiotics may be prescribed. When a specific diagnosis has been made, the appropriate treatment can be given, such as anticoagulants for a pulmonary infarction.

Complications

Injury to the pleura or lung cancer may cause bleeding into the pleural cavity (hemothorax). Pleurisy that is caused by infection may result in an accumulation of pus in the pleural cavity (empyema). This may require antibiotic treatment and surgical drainage. Pleural effusions that are caused by cancer tend to recur. They may need treatment with cytotoxic drugs.

Empyema

Empyema is the accumulation of pus in a body cavity. It generally occurs because of a secondary bacterial infection that accompanies a lung disorder, for example, pneumonia or pleurisy. Infection may also come from the outside, for example, as the result of a stab wound. The symptoms of empyema include fever and sweating, other serious illness, chest pain that is worse with inspiration, and cough.

Treatment

The pus must be removed. This can be done either by sucking it out through a hollow needle (aspiration) or by a surgical operation to remove part of a rib and drain the pus away through a tube. Antibiotic drugs are prescribed to combat the infection, and the underlying cause is treated at the same time.

Pneumothorax

Pneumothorax is the presence of air or gas in the pleural cavity, the space between the lungs and the chest wall. The condition prevents the normal expansion of the lungs, thereby impairing breathing. It may result in a collapsed lung.

Causes

The most common cause of a pneumothorax is a penetrating injury of the chest wall. This is known as a traumatic pneumothorax. Rarely, injury may cause a life-threatening form of traumatic pneumothorax in which a flap of tissue acts as a valve that allows air to be drawn into the chest, but not to be blown out again. The pressure within the chest rises rapidly and causes both lungs to collapse. With the accumulation of air on one side the mediastinum shifts, causing collapse of the other side. This condition is known as a tension pneumothorax.

A spontaneous pneumothorax is caused by air leaking from the lungs. This may be the result of an underlying disease, such as emphysema, or of a congenital weakness of the lungs.

Pneumothorax may also be produced artificially, as by the surgical introduction of a needle into the pleural cavity to collapse a lung in the treatment of pulmonary tuberculosis.

Symptoms

The symptoms of pneumothorax vary widely, depending on the cause of the disorder. The main symptoms of a traumatic pneumothorax are breathlessness and severe chest pains. A tension pneumothorax causes extreme breathing difficulty and may be rapidly fatal.

The symptoms of a spontaneous pneumothorax range from slight breathlessness on exertion to the sudden onset of severe chest pains and extreme breathing difficulty.

Treatment

A patient with a traumatic pneumothorax requires hospitalization so that the air in the pleural cavity can be removed by insertion of a tube into the chest wall. Then the injury is treated. A tension pneumothorax requires emergency medical treatment; the rapid removal of air from the pleural cavity may be lifesaving.

Most patients with a small, spontaneous pneumothorax do not require treatment because the air is gradually reabsorbed. Occasionally, the condition may recur, in which case surgery may be necessary.

Embolism

Embolism is an obstruction of an artery, or less commonly, a vein, by material that has been carried there in the bloodstream. This material is called an embolus and may be a blood clot (thrombus), a clump of cancer cells, fat globules from the site of a broken bone (fat embolus), infected tissue from an abscess, or an air bubble (air embolus).

Symptoms

If the embolus is small, there may be no immediate symptoms. A large embolus can totally obstruct a blood vessel, and the area of tissue supplied by it dies. If this occurs in the heart, the patient suffers myocardial infarction. An obstructed vessel in the brain causes a stroke. If an embolus blocks the femoral artery, the patient experiences acute cramp-like pain in the leg, which quickly becomes white and cold. An embolus in the lung (pulmonary embolism) produces symptoms similar to those of coronary thrombosis: severe pain, shock, collapse, and the coughing of bloodstained mucus. An embolus in the kidney causes hematuria (bloody urine).

Treatment

Treatment depends on the size, nature, and location of the embolus. Severe obstructions, such as those occurring with pulmonary embolism, require emergency hospital treatment. The patient is treated for shock and given oxygen and anticoagulant drugs. Sometimes, surgery (embolectomy) is performed, particularly if the embolus is in an artery of the arm or leg.

Part Three

Diagnosis

Chapter 41

Arterial Blood Gas Analysis (ABG)

How Your Doctor Diagnoses Lung Disease

If you have symptoms that suggest a respiratory disorder, your doctor will want to know about your medical history, especially any risk factors for lung disease, such as cigarette smoking, and about any family history of respiratory diseases, such as cystic fibrosis and emphysema. The doctor will ask about workplace or other exposure to materials (such as asbestos and coal) that can damage the lungs, any history of allergies, and any seasonal variation of symptoms. It will be important for you to inform your doctor of anything usual or unusual you believe may be related to your breathing.

During the physical exam, the doctor will check your blood pressure, examine your chest, listen to it with a stethoscope, and look for signs of respiratory disease. The doctor will also percuss your lungs by placing one hand on your chest and thumping it with the fingers of the other hand. The resultant vibration helps in evaluating the size and condition of the lungs.

In many cases, the doctor will also order a chest X-ray. If you have had a previous chest X-ray, the films will be compared to check for new abnormalities. Sometimes a diagnosis can be suggested at this stage or, depending on your symptoms and X-ray findings, more tests may be needed. In general, the more sophisticated and invasive tests are usually performed last.

Arterial Blood Gas Analysis (ABG)

Where It's Done: Doctor's office, commercial pulmonary function laboratory, or hospital.

Who Does It: Doctor, respiratory therapist, or pulmonary lab technician.

How Long It Takes: 5-10 minutes.

Discomfort/Pain: Puncture can be painful.

Results Ready When: Minutes.

Special Equipment: Blood gas syringe and needle, and blood gas analyzer.

Risks/Complications: Can cause injury to the artery (rarely).

Other Names: None.

Purpose: To evaluate the lungs' ability to provide blood with oxygen and remove carbon dioxide, and to measure the acidity of the blood.

How It Works

The blood's acidity and concentrations of various gases in the blood can be measured in the laboratory and compared with normal values to determine how well the lungs are working.

Preparation

The person performing the test may first check your circulation by pressing on the radial and ulnar arteries of your wrist. When the arteries are pressed, the palm will turn white; when they are released again, they will become pink and flush. Failure to flush within 5 seconds indicates decreased blood flow.

If this test indicates that the artery on the wrist cannot be used as a puncture site, blood may be drawn from an artery elsewhere in the body.

Test Procedure

The site to be punctured is scrubbed clean, and a blood sample is drawn from the artery in a needle puncture.

The blood sample is analyzed in a laboratory for the presence of oxygen and carbon dioxide and for pH.

After the Test

After the needle is removed from the artery, you are instructed to compress the puncture site with a sterile gauze for at least five minutes—or longer if you have clotting problems, are taking anticoagulant therapy, or are taking aspirin or an aspirin like medication.

A bandage is placed over the puncture site and should be kept in place for 30 to 60 minutes.

Factors Affecting Results

- Hyperventilation (from pain or anxiety).

- Cigarette smoking.

- Carbon monoxide inhalation.

Interpretation

Abnormal measurements may signal the presence of various disorders including lung disease.

Advantages

It provides immediate and accurate assessment of gases in the blood and blood acidity.

Disadvantages

It's invasive.

The Next Step

Your doctor will make an assessment of your lungs based on the ABG results. Treatment, including oxygen therapy, may be decided.

Chapter 42

Body Plethysmography

General Information

Where It's Done: Doctor's office, commercial pulmonary function laboratory, or hospital.

Who Does It: Doctor, respiratory therapist, or pulmonary lab technician.

How Long It Takes: 20 minutes.

Discomfort/Pain: Some people feel claustrophobic, and some are uncomfortable breathing against a closed shutter.

Results Ready When: Immediately to 1-2 days.

Special Equipment: Body plethysmograph, or "body box," pneumotachograph, shutter, transducers, mouthpiece, nose clip, and oscilloscope.

Risks/Complications: None.

Other Names: Airway Resistance or Thoracic Gas Volume.

Purpose

- To measure the volume of air in the lungs.

- To diagnose lung disease or assess its severity.

- To determine whether the airways are obstructed and to what extent.

How It Works

The test is conducted inside a tightly sealed box where changes in air pressure and volume as you inhale and exhale can be measured and compared to normal values for someone of your age, sex, height, and weight.

Preparation

- Avoid eating heavy meals for three hours before the test.

- Wear comfortable clothing that doesn't restrict breathing.

- Loose-fitting dentures may be removed.

- A clip is placed over your nose.

Test Procedure

You sit inside a plethysmograph, a glass-walled, airtight box about the size of a refrigerator, and insert the mouthpiece into your mouth with your lips sealed around it. The door of the plethysmograph is closed and tightly sealed. You breathe quietly through the mouthpiece, then are instructed to pant lightly. While you are panting, place your palms flat on your cheeks to make sure the air you exhale is leaving your mouth and not filling your cheeks instead.

As you perform various breathing exercises, the pressure in the breathing tube and in the box are recorded.

You will be talked through the test by a technician who is usually sitting right next to the plethysmograph.

After the Test

You remove the nose clip and exit the plethysmograph. You replace dentures if necessary, and are free to leave.

Factors Affecting Results

- Lack of a tight seal over the mouthpiece.

- Bulging of the cheeks during breathing out.

Interpretation

Pressure of the exhaled air against the shutter and changes in lung volume are used to evaluate the ability of your lungs to fill up with air, and to assess the flow of air through the airways.

Advantages

It's noninvasive.

Disadvantages

It detects a problem but doesn't identify its cause.

The Next Step

Test results should help your doctor more precisely understand your pulmonary physiology.

Chapter 43

Bronchial Challenge Test

General Information

Where It's Done: Doctor's office, commercial pulmonary function laboratory, or hospital.

Who Does It: Doctor, respiratory therapist, or pulmonary lab technician.

How Long It Takes: 60 minutes to 2 hours.

Discomfort/Pain: Test can be tiring and can cause shortness of breath or other symptoms of lung disease in people with abnormally sensitive airways.

Results Ready When: 1-2 days.

Special Equipment: Pulmonary function analyzer or spirometer, mouthpiece, nose clip, compressed gas nebulizers, compressed gas source, dosimeter, and various doses of methacholine solution.

Risks/Complications: Possible severe airway constriction. Should not be performed in people who have known severe asthma or whose pulmonary function measurements are significantly below normal.

Other Names: Bronchial provocation test, bronchial inhalation challenge, methacholine challenge, and histamine challenge.

Purpose

- To detect asthma when it is suspected despite normal pulmonary function.

- To identify substances or exposures that trigger asthma attacks, particularly in people with occupational asthma.

- To evaluate the effectiveness of drugs in preventing airway constriction.

How It Works

The test replicates in a controlled setting the conditions in the environment that may be causing your airways to constrict.

Preparation

Certain drugs, particularly bronchodilators, must be avoided prior to the test. Ask your doctor for instructions regarding specific medications. Do not smoke or take caffeine for six hours before the test.

Avoid exercise and exposure to cold air for two hours before the test.

Patient Tip

Caffeine is found not only in coffee and tea but also in chocolate, cola drinks, and in some asprin-combinaton analgesic products. These should all be avoided prior to the test because caffeine can affect test results.

Test Procedure

Baseline pulmonary function tests are performed using a spirometer. If it is necessary to test the effectiveness of a drug in preventing airway constriction, you will receive the drug before continuing the test. You breathe in aerosolized methacholine through a nebulizer for about two minutes. Then, after a 30-second wait, you exhale forcefully through the mouthpiece. Methacholine is a histamine, a substance released in an allergic response. In the test, it simulates the conditions in the airways after exposure to an allergy-causing substance.

Other substances suspected of causing airway constriction, such as chemicals in the workplace, may be used in subsequent tests. If your symptoms seem to worsen with cold air exposure, a controlled amount of cold air may be pumped into your mouthpiece instead. If exercise is suspected of triggering asthma, you will be instructed to exercise. Spirometry tests are repeated. The tests may be repeated with higher concentrations of methacholine, colder air, or after more strenuous exercise.

After the Test

You remove the nose clip, replace the dentures if necessary, and are free to resume normal activities. You may wheeze or cough for 30 to 60 minutes after the test, and may need a bronchodilator to decrease symptoms.

Factors Affecting Results

Failure to follow instructions, such as not holding your breath or exhaling with maximum force. Anxiety or fatigue. Recent or current chest infection, a cold, or other respiratory disease. Bronchodilators, sedatives, and other drugs that may affect breathing. Other procedures, such as positive-pressure-breathing therapy, performed a few hours before the test.

Interpretation

The results before and after the challenge (the tested exposure) are compared. If your lung function dropped 20% or more after exposure to cold, exercise, methacholine, or to whatever substance is used for the test, your airways are abnormally sensitive to these exposures. It is likely that in normal circumstances, that exposures or various substances that trigger allergic reactions may cause your airways to narrow and trigger asthma attacks. Diagnosis of asthma, however, can only be made after test results are correlated with your symptoms, because abnormal sensitivity of the airways may be present in various disorders, including, among others, chronic obstructive pulmonary disease, bronchiolitis, and cystic fibrosis.

Advantages

It's highly reliable.

Disadvantages

- There is a risk of causing severe airway constriction.

- Results can only be interpreted in the light of symptoms.

The Next Step

Based on the test results, your doctor may be better able to decide if treatment is needed or to adjust your treatment.

Chapter 44

Bronchoscopy

General Information

Where It's Done: Hospital or surgical center.

Who Does It: Doctor (pulmonary specialist or chest surgeon) and radiology technician or respiratory therapist.

How Long It Takes: 30 minutes to 2 hours.

Discomfort/Pain: Procedure may cause some irritation in the throat and/or coughing; slight discomfort when IV line is inserted.

Results Ready When: 2 days.

Special Equipment: Bronchoscope and bronchoscopy instruments.

Risks/Complications: Bleeding, fever, infection (uncommon), collapse of the lung (in 2-5% of cases), cessation of heartbeat or breathing (very rare).

Other Names: Flexible fiber-optic bronchoscopy or rigid bronchoscopy.

Purpose

- To detect or rule out structural and other abnormalities of the airways, bronchial tumors, or the presence of a foreign body.

- To obtain samples of lung secretions and tissues for analysis.

- To obtain samples of lung tissue for analysis.

How It Works

A thin fiber-optic tube with a light source is passed into the airways in the lungs (bronchi), allowing the doctor to see the tracheal and bronchial structures.

Preparation

- You must fast for eight to 12 hours prior to the procedure.

- You remove clothing above the waist and don a hospital gown.

- Atropine and codeine or other medication may be injected intramuscularly to dry up saliva and suppress coughing.

- A local anesthetic is sprayed into your mouth and/or nose, depending on which way the scope will be passed into your lungs (see Figure 44.1). Alternatively, anesthesia is injected under your chin on both sides of your neck to numb the voice box area.

- Electrocardiography electrodes are placed on your chest for monitoring your heartbeat, a blood pressure cuff is placed on your arm, and an oximeter is attached to your finger, earlobe, or toe to measure oxygen saturation in your blood.

- A soft tube that delivers oxygen is inserted into your nose or mouth, and an intravenous (IV) infusion is placed on your arm in order to administer medications.

Patient Tips

If you must take medication during the fast, you may take it with small sips of water. Up to a week before the test, you should stop taking any medication, such as aspirin or Coumarin (Coumadin), that may cause excess bleeding.

Test Procedure

The doctor inserts a long viewing tube, called a bronchoscope, through your nose or mouth. If it is introduced through your mouth, you are asked to hold a plastic mouthpiece called a bite block between your teeth, to prevent you from accidentally biting the tube.

The bronchoscope is usually a flexible fiber-optic tube about the width of a pen. If a large foreign body must be removed or a large biopsy sample is required, the doctor may use a rigid bronchoscope—a hollow metal tube with a light source and a viewing device—which requires general anesthesia.

Through the bronchoscope, the doctor inspects your voice box, windpipe, and the branches of the airways.

Secretions from the lungs may be removed through the bronchoscope to clear the airways; the washings can be cultured or examined under a microscope.

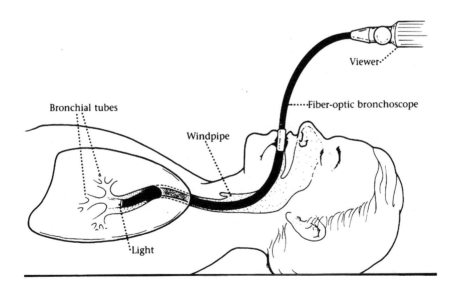

Figure 44.1. *This test entails inserting a viewing tube with magnifying and lighting devices through the mouth or nose and down the windpipe (trachea) and into the lung's bronchial tubes.*

Bronchoalveolar lavage, in which a sterile saline solution is introduced into the lung through the bronchoscope and sucked back out, may be performed to diagnose infection or other conditions. Usually, the lavage is performed in the portion of the lung that looks abnormal on the chest X-ray.

Bronchial brushing, in which a tiny brush on a long wire is introduced through the bronchoscope and rubbed against the airways or alveoli, may be used to obtain tissue samples from the lung. Samples are analyzed for the presence of fungi, bacteria, or other infectious agents, and for the presence of abnormal cells.

Tissue may also be removed (called endobronchial or transbronchial biopsy) with the help of tiny forceps. The lung has no pain sensation, but you may feel a tug when the tissue sample is removed. While the biopsy is performed, a fluoroscope, an X-ray device, may be used to visualize the lung. The picture, which is transmitted onto a TV monitor, helps the doctor guide the instruments.

A needle may be inserted through the bronchoscope to puncture a lymph node and aspirate (withdraw) cells.

Bronchoscopy may also be used to place radiation therapy catheters or stents.

After the Test

All monitoring equipment, the oxygen tube, and the IV infusion are removed. if the test included a biopsy, a chest X-ray is performed to make sure the lung has not been punctured and no air has entered the pleural cavity. If the test was performed under local anesthesia, you will be free to leave after sedation has worn off, which usually takes about two hours (you should have someone drive you home). If bronchoscopy was conducted under general anesthesia, you will be discharged to your hospital room or the recovery area. Avoid eating or drinking until the gag reflex returns, which may take two to four hours. You may experience hoarseness, mild fever, and coughing up small amounts of blood for about 24 hours. If you cough up large quantities of blood, have trouble breathing, have high fever, or experience pain, contact your doctor or go to a hospital emergency department immediately.

Factors Affecting Results

Excessive coughing or gagging can interfere with obtaining adequate results or even prevent the test from being completed.

Interpretation

Sometimes the doctor may establish or confirm the diagnosis simply by viewing the airways. In other cases, examinations of the tissue samples and secretions removed from the lung provide additional information.

Advantages

- The test is less invasive than surgical biopsy and can be performed on an outpatient basis.
- It requires only local anesthesia.
- It entails relatively low risk and little discomfort.
- It allows the doctor to view the airways directly.
- It produces reliable results.

Disadvantages

- It's more invasive than imaging techniques.
- The biopsy sample may be too small to diagnose some disorders, particularly noninfectious inflammatory lung diseases.
- The doctor can see only the airways, not the lung tissue itself.

The Next Step

If the bronchoscopy renders a diagnosis, no further testing may be needed, and treatment can be started. If the bronchoscopy does not yield a diagnosis, further testing may be required, including surgical biopsy, needle aspiration of the lung, or further radiographic evaluation.

Chapter 45

Chest Magnetic Resonance Imaging (MRI)

General Information

Where It's Done: Diagnostic clinic, radiology lab, or hospital.

Who Does It: Radiologist or qualified technician.

How Long It Takes: 30-90 minutes.

Discomfort/Pain: None, but some people find the noise and being in a confined space upsetting.

Results Ready When: Often within a few hours.

Special Equipment: MRI scanner, computer, and display screen or monitor; film or magnetic tape recorder.

Risks/Complications: None, unless the patient has an implanted pacemaker or other implanted metal devices.

Other Names: Nuclear magnetic resonance imaging.

Purpose: To obtain two-dimensional views of an internal organ or structure.

How It Works

MRI uses a powerful magnetic field and radio waves to alter the natural alignment of hydrogen atoms within the body.

Computers record the activity of the hydrogen atoms and translate that into images.

Preparation

- All jewelry, hair clips, and other metal objects must be removed.

- Some facilities ask patients to disrobe and put on a hospital gown; other allow patients to wear clothing so long as it doesn't have metal parts. (Watches should be removed, and pockets emptied of credit cards and other objects that will be damaged by exposure to the magnetic field or will interfere with the images.)

- A contrast medium may be injected before some studies (e.g. Gadolinium may be injected before an MRI study of the brain): people who are claustrophobic or have difficulty lying still may be given a sedative. Otherwise, no special preparation is required.

Test Procedure

- You will be instructed to lie as still as possible on a narrow table that slides into a tubelike structure that holds the magnet.

- A loud thumping or hammering noise will e heard during the test; you may request earplugs or listen to music with earphones to reduce the noise level.

- At certain points during the test, the noise will stop and you will be able to hear instructions from the doctor or technician administering the test.

Variations

Echoplanar MRI is a new technique that allows for rapid accumulation of data such as cardiac motion.

After the Test

You can resume your pretest activities immediately.

Factors Affecting Results

Movement, extreme obesity, and the presence of metal objects can all affect results.

Interpretation

A radiologist or other medical specialist interprets the results.

Advantages

- MRI offers increased-contrast resolution, enabling better visualization of soft tissues. Also, it allows for multiplanar imaging, as opposed to CT, which is usually only axial.

- It provides highly detailed information without exposing the body to radiation. In many instances, it provides more useful images than CT scanning and ultrasound.

Disadvantages

- It is expensive and not available in many small hospitals and rural areas.

- It also cannot be sued for patients with implanted pacemakers and certain other metal objects.

Chapter 46

Chest Radiography

General Information

Where It's Done: Hospital, commercial lab, or doctor's office.

Who Does It: X-ray technician.

How Long It Takes: 10-15 minutes.

Discomfort/Pain: None.

Results Ready When: Several minutes to 1-2 days.

Special Equipment: X-ray machine (portable or stationary).

Risks/Complications: Risks associated with radiation, particularly during pregnancy.

Other Names: Chest x-ray, chest roentgenography, and chest films.

Purpose

- To evaluate the lungs, as well as the chest cage, for the presence of abnormalities.

- To evaluate the size of the heart. To establish the size and location of an abnormality prior to performing other tests, such as a biopsy.

- To screen for lung disease in people who have occupational exposure to potentially toxic substances such as asbestos.

How It Works

X-rays (electromagnetic energy emitted by an X-ray tube) are absorbed by the body tissue. When the tissue is exposed to special photographic film, various types of tissue show up as shadows, dark gray areas, or white opaque areas.

Preparation

You remove clothing and jewelry above the waist and don a hospital gown. If your hair is long, you must pin it up on your head so that no locks hang over your chest or shoulders.

Test Procedure

The technician positions you against the X-ray machine. You are asked to take a deep breath and hold it without moving while an X-ray picture is taken. Pictures are usually taken from the front and the side. Depending on the suspected problem, additional X-rays may be taken at different angles.

After the Test

You dress and are free to leave. The film is processed in a developing machine, and X-ray pictures are produced.

Factors Affecting Results

- If you move during the test, the image may be distorted.

- Images obtained with portable X-ray machines tend to be of poorer quality than those taken with stationary X-ray equipment. Portable X-rays are usually done only if you are hospitalized and physically unable to go to the X-ray department.

Interpretation

The doctor studies the X-ray picture and determines whether all chest structures look normal.

Advantages

- It's relatively inexpensive and widely available.
- It's painless and fast.

Disadvantages

- It involves exposure, although minimal, to radiation.
- It may not provide adequate information about lungs and other soft tissues.

The Next Step

A normal X-ray usually requires no further testing.

An abnormal X-ray may require monitoring (observation), confirmation by another test such as a chest CT scan or MRI, or a biopsy of the abnormality.

Chapter 47

Chest Tomography

General Information

Where It's Done: Hospital radiology unit or outpatient diagnostic clinic.

Who Does It: Radiologist or technician.

How Long It Takes: 30-45 minutes.

Discomfort/Pain: None unless contrast medium is used; some people find it uncomfortable to remain still during the test.

Results Ready When: Often in a few hours; may take longer in some cases and other places.

Special Equipment: Revolving CT scanner (camera), X-ray and computer equipment, and monitor.

Other Names: Computed axial tomography (CAT) scan or computed transaxial tomography.

Purpose

- To obtain a better image of the lung and chest structures than with regular chest X-rays.

- To evaluate the potential spread of cancers, including lung tumors.

- To determine the anatomy of chest structures prior to surgery.

How It Works

- Multiple X-rays are taken as the CT X-ray penetration through the specific plane(s) of the body part(s) examined, and gives each a numeric value (density coefficient).

- A computer calculates the amount of X-ray penetration through the specific planes(s) of the body part(s) examined, and gives each a numeric value (density coefficient).

- This information is fed into a computer, which translates the values into different shades of gray.

- These images are displayed on a television monitor and photographed as a series of two-dimensional images depicting a cross section of the part under examination.

Preparation

- You will be shown the CT machine and asked to express any concerns.

- If you experience claustrophobia in small, enclosed spaces, you may be given a mild sedative to quell your anxiety.

- If an intravenous contrast agent is to be used, you will be asked to abstain from ingesting food and water for at least four hours beforehand.

- Before entering the unit, you will be asked to remove any jewelry or other objects that may interfere with clear X-ray images.

- If CT scans of the abdomen and/or pelvis are being done, you may be asked to drink a flavored barium drink.

Test Procedure

- You will be asked to lie on a narrow examination table, which slides into the scanner.

- As you lie motionless as possible, the CT tube revolves slowly, taking multiple X-ray images, which are reconstructed into two-dimensional views of a cross section of the body.

- The table is then moved slightly to take another set of images through another plane of the body; typically, three to seven planes are imaged, but this varies according to the part of the body under examination.

- In some instances, the entire length of the body may be scanned; in others, only a relatively narrow section.

Variations

- CT scanning may be performed in conjunction with other imaging studies and diagnostic procedures, such as X-rays of the joint or spinal column (e.g., arthrography or myelography). This allows more detailed images of the entire joint structure than can be obtained from X-rays alone.

- A relatively new innovation is spiral CT imaging, which allows for continuous scanning as the gantry table slides through the unit. This technique cuts the amount of time needed for whole-body scanning.

After the Test

- You may be asked to wait while a radiologist quickly reviews the images to make sure that the part of the body under study has been adequately photographed.

- If necessary, you may be asked to return to the scanner for additional images. Otherwise, you will be able to resume normal activities.

- If an intravenous contrast medium was used, you will be instructed to drink extra fluids to speed its removal from the body.

- You should also watch for delayed allergic reactions, such as hives, a rash, itching, or perhaps a rapid heartbeat. Such symptoms usually appear within two to six hours; in severe cases, and antihistamine or steroid medication may be prescribed to ease discomfort.

Factors Affecting Results

- Obesity, movement during the examination, and the presence of metallic objects can interferer with obtaining clear images.

- In some cases, excessive gas or fecal material in the intestines can give misleading results in a abdominal CT scan.

Interpretation

The doctor studies the images and looks for abnormalities that may signal lung disease.

Advantages

- CT scanning provides a painless, noninvasive method of obtaining a detailed view of internal organs.

- In many instances, CT scanning eliminates the need for more invasive procedures, such as arteriography.

The Next Step

- A normal CT scan may require no further evaluation.

- An abnormal CT scan may require monitoring (observation), confirmation by another test such as an MRI or bronchoscopy, or a biopsy.

Chapter 48

Lung Scans

General Information

Where It's Done: Hospital or outpatient facility.

Who Does It: Doctor specializing in nuclear medicine and a nuclear medicine technologist.

How Long It Takes: 30-60 minutes.

Discomfort/Pain: Minor discomfort when radioactive material is injected intravenously.

Results Ready When: Within days.

Special Equipment: Radioactive material, oxygen mask, IV equipment, and gamma scintillation camera.

Risks/Complications: High blood pressure in the lungs may be temporarily worsened; a very small number of patients (less than 1%) may feel claustrophobic about camera.

Other Names: Perfusion lung scan, lung perfusion scintigraphy, radionuclide pulmonary scan, and ventilation-perfusion scan.

From *The Yale University School of Medicine: Patient's Guide to Medical Tests.* © 1997 by Yale University School of Medicine and G.S. Sharpe Communications, Inc. Reprinted by permission of Houghton Mifflin Company. All rights reserved.

Purpose

- To assess the ability of the lungs to ventilate (take in air) and the ability of the lungs' tiny arteries (arterioles) to receive blood.

- To detect a blood clot in an artery leading to the lung (pulmonary embolism).

- To assess the function of the lungs in anticipation of lung surgery.

How It Works

A gamma scintillation camera picks up radiation emitted by the radionuclide particles in your lung tissue or in the arterioles and produces an image showing which portions are receiving air and blood, which is displayed on the screen or printed out on film.

Preparation

- A regular chest X-ray is usually performed within 12 hours before this test or immediately afterward to identify any abnormalities that would alter the scan.

- Before the scan, you remove clothing and jewelry above the waist.

Test Procedure

For the ventilation part of the test, you are seated and a mask is placed over your nose and mouth. You follow specific instructions about inhaling and exhaling, and you breathe in a combination of air and radioactive gas.

A large scanning camera takes pictures of your chest. For the perfusion part of the test, radioactive material is injected intravenously through your hand or arm. You sit or lie down and breathe freely as the scanning camera takes pictures of your chest at various angles. Sometimes, SPECT (single photon emission computed tomography) technology may be used to produce a three-dimensional lung scan.

Patient Tip

A very small minority of patients feel claustrophobic when the camera is held close to their face. If this bothers you, ask if you can turn your head to the side.

After the Test

You dress and are free to leave.

Factors Affecting Results

- Traces of a radioactive substance remaining from a similar test recently performed.

- The presence of pneumonia, obstructive lung disease, or structural abnormalities in the chest.

- Movement during the test will distort the image.

Interpretation

If the blood flow through the lungs is normal, the radioactive material will be evenly distributed throughout the lungs. Areas where no radionuclide is seen may signal the presence of an abnormality, such as an obstruction to blood flow or a blood clot. If the airflow to the lungs is normal, radioactive gas will be evenly distributed throughout the lungs. Areas where no radionuclide is seen may signal a mechanical obstruction to airflow. Areas that retain radionuclide for a prolonged period usually indicate areas of trapped gas, such as occurs in obstructive lung disease. Results are expressed in terms of probability of a pulmonary embolism (blood clot), ranging from normal (less than 2% probability), to high (85% to 90%).

Calculation of the percent of blood flow to a given area of the lung may help your doctor predict lung function after lung surgery to remove a piece of lung or a whole lung.

Advantages

- Exposure to radiation from radionuclides is minimal.

- Adverse reactions to radionuclides are extremely rare.

- The test is helpful in the evaluation of pulmonary embolism. It is also helpful in preoperative evaluation of lung function.

Disadvantages

- It may detect an abnormality but fail to lead to a definitive diagnosis.

• It involves exposure, although minimal, to radiation.

The Next Step

If the patient's symptoms are suggestive of an embolism and the test shows a high probability, the scan is considered a reliable indicator that there is an embolism, and no further testing is needed. If the patient doesn't have definitive symptoms and the scan is normal, the test is a reliable indicator that there is no embolism. If the patient's symptoms and the test outcome are not consistent, pulmonary angiography or other diagnostic tests may be recommended to clarify the results.

Chapter 49

Mediastinoscopy

General Information

Where It's Done: Hospital.

Who Does It: Doctor (chest surgeon) and surgical team.

How Long It Takes: 1-2 hours.

Discomfort/Pain: Discomfort associated with general anesthesia and incision.

Results Ready When: 2 days.

Special Equipment: Mediastinoscope, general anesthetic, and biopsy instruments.

Risks/Complications: Risks associated with surgery and general anesthesia.

Other Names: Cervical or anterior mediastinoscopy.

Purpose

To examine the mediastinum (the space between the lungs) if imaging techniques suggest that it contains an abnormality but cannot determine its nature. To diagnose sarcoidosis, cancers, tuberculosis, and other infections. To determine to what extent the cancer has spread (staging of lung or other cancer).

How It Works

Fiber-optic technology allows direct viewing of the area between the lungs as well as removal of a biopsy sample.

Preparation

- Avoid eating or drinking for 12 hours before the test.
- You will receive general anesthesia. A soft breathing tube is usually inserted through your windpipe (called endotracheal intubation) to make sure you breathe properly during the procedure.

Test Procedure

- A small incision is made through your skin and tissues, usually between the area of the collarbones.
- A mediastinoscope, a long tube with a light source, is introduced into the area between the lungs.
- The doctor examines the mediastinum through the viewing instrument and removes tissue samples (biopsy) from any suspicious areas.

After the Test

After recovering from general anesthesia, a hospital stay of one to two days is typical. You should be able to return to regular activities within a few hours.

Factors Affecting Results

Accurate selection of the biopsy site.

Interpretation

The doctor observes the structures in the mediastinum. The biopsy Sample removed during the procedure is examined under a microscope and provides additional information. A diagnosis may be suggested by the appearance of the mediastinum.

Confirmation needs to be made pathologically. Biopsy material may also be sent for culture.

Advantages

- The test allows the doctor to make definitive diagnosis of several disorders of the lung and chest.

Disadvantages

- It's invasive.
- It requires hospitalization.

The Next Step

If a diagnosis is made by mediastinoscopy, decisions about treatment can be made. If a diagnosis is not made, further evaluation may be necessary, perhaps with other surgical biopsies.

Chapter 50

Mouth Pressure Test

General Information

Where It's Done: Doctor's office, commercial pulmonary function laboratory, or hospital.

Who Does It: Doctor, respiratory therapist, or pulmonary lab technician.

How Long It Takes: 5-10 minutes.

Discomfort/Pain: None.

Results Ready When: Immediately to 1-2 days.

Special Equipment: Electronic manometer equipped with a flexible hollow tube ending in a rubber mouthpiece, and a nose clip.

Risks/Complications: None.

Other Names: Maximum inspiratory pressure/maximum expiratory pressure or MIP/MEP.

Purpose

To assess the functioning and strength of respiratory muscles when they are suspected of causing symptoms arising from the respiratory system, or if pulmonary function tests show small lung volumes.

How It Works

Air pressure, determined by the force with which you inhale and exhale, is recorded by a device called a manometer and reflects the strength of your respiratory muscles.

Preparation

- You put on a nose clip to prevent air from escaping through your nostrils.

- Loose-fitting dentures may have to be removed.

Test Procedure

You insert the mouthpiece between your teeth, seal your lips tightly around it, take a deep breath, and then exhale, blowing the air out as forcefully as possible. The test also requires a forceful inhalation maneuver.

Chapter 51

Needle Biopsy of the Lung

General Information

Where It's Done: Hospital radiology department.

Who Does It: Radiologist and radiation technologist.

How Long It Takes: An hour or more, depending on the difficulty of reaching the right spot with the needle.

Discomfort/Pain: Stinging or burning associated with local anesthesia, discomfort from having to remain still, and a painful sensation when the pleura is penetrated by the needle.

Results Ready When: 2 days.

Special Equipment: A long needle and an imaging device, ultrasound equipment, a fluoroscope, or a CT scanner.

Risks/Complications: Collapsed lung (20% of cases) or coughing up blood.

Other Names: Fine-needle aspiration biopsy, transthoracic needle aspiration biopsy, transbronchial needle aspiration, and percutaneous needle aspiration. Purpose To obtain a tissue sample to diagnose or rule out causes of localized lung masses, such as lung cancer or infection.

How It Works: Samples of cells or fluid are obtained for microscopic examination.

Preparation

- You must avoid eating and drinking for six to 12 hours before the procedure.

- You remove all clothing above the waist and don a hospital gown.

- Local anesthesia is applied to your skin and tissue under the skin.

Test Procedure

- You lie on a scanning table on your stomach or back, depending on the location of the tissue to be biopsied.

- Local anesthesia is injected into the muscle of the chest wall.

- An imaging device such as a CT scanner or fluoroscope is used to guide appropriate placement of the needle.

- When the needle is about to penetrate the pleura, you are asked to hold your breath.

- Using a needle, the doctor aspirates (withdraws) a sample of tissue or fluid.

- The sample is sent to the laboratory for microscopic examination. A culture may be sent to detect infectious organisms.

After the Test

- A chest X-ray is taken to make sure you haven't developed pneumothorax (collapsed lung), which almost always goes away by itself but occasionally requires inserting a chest tube for drainage.

- You will remain in bed in the recovery area for up to three hours while your pulse, breathing, blood pressure, and temperature are monitored periodically.

- You are free to leave after the recovery period, but you should have someone drive you home. If there is a pneumothorax, observation in the hospital may be recommended.

- You may resume normal activities but should avoid heavy exertion for the first 24 hours.

- You may cough up small amounts of blood, but this should taper off and stop. If not, notify your doctor. Report to a hospital emergency department at once if you feel chest pain or have difficulty breathing.

Factors Affecting Results

- Accurate selection of the biopsy site.

- Ability to reach the abnormality with the needle.

Interpretation

Examination of tissue samples obtained with this biopsy may help to detect infection, to diagnose lung cancer and determine its type, and to diagnose inflammatory disease.

Advantages

- It's less invasive than surgical lung biopsy.

Disadvantages

- It yields minute amounts of tissue compared with surgical lung biopsy.

- The part of the abnormality that is likely to be most helpful for diagnosis is sometimes missed.

- There are potential complications.

The Next Step

- If a diagnosis is made by needle biopsy, decisions about treatment can be made.

- If a diagnosis is not made, further evaluation with bronchoscopy or open surgical biopsies may be necessary.

Chapter 52

Open Lung Biopsy

General Information

Where It's Done: Hospital.

Who Does It: Doctor (chest surgeon and surgical team).

How Long It Takes: 2-4 hours.

Discomfort/Pain: Discomfort associated with general anesthesia; chest discomfort afterward due to incision.

When Results Ready: 2 days.

Special Equipment: Surgical instruments; breathing and suction tubes; general anesthesia.

Risks/Complications: Risks of surgery and general anesthesia.

Other Names: Surgical lung biopsy.

Purpose

- To inspect abnormalities in the lung that require surgical biopsy.

- To obtain lung tissue for examination to confirm or rule out lung diseases, including cancer.

- To investigate causes of unexplained fluid in the pleural cavity.

How It Works

- A sample of lung tissue is obtained for analysis in the laboratory for the presence of abnormal cells, infection, or inflammation.

- Prior to the test, you will have a chest X-ray, electrocardiogram, and various blood tests.

- An arterial blood gas and a pulmonary function test may also be done.

Preparation

- Avoid eating and drinking for 12 hours before the procedure.

- General anesthesia is administered and preparations are made for chest.

- A soft breathing tube is inserted through your windpipe (a procedure known as endotracheal intubation) to make sure you breathe properly during the procedure.

Test Procedure

- An incision is made between two ribs near the breast bone.

- The abnormal area of the lung is identified.

- Small wedges of lung tissue are removed for microscopic and laboratory examination.

- A biopsy sample may be sent to the pathology lab for a frozen section. If the biopsy shows cancer, more extensive surgery may be performed to remove the tumor and all or part of the lung.

- A chest tube is placed in the pleural space to remove air and fluids, and will remain in place for several days. When drainage of air and fluids stops, the tube is removed.

Did You Know?

Improved imaging techniques and development of less invasive biopsy methods have greatly reduced the use of open lung biopsy.

After the Test

- You will be taken to a recovery room for observation and to recover from anesthesia.

- Depending on the underlying illness, you will return to your hospital room for 3 to 7 days (average) of recuperation.

Interpretation

The doctor may make the diagnosis by observing the structures in the chest. The biopsy sample will be studied microscopically; cultures may also be performed.

Advantages

- It provides definitive diagnosis of several disorders of the lung and chest.

Disadvantages

- It's invasive.

- It requires general anesthesia and several days of hospitalization.

The Next Step

- Treatment of underlying condition.

Chapter 53

Oxygen Saturation

General Information

Where It's Done: Doctor's office, commercial pulmonary function laboratory, hospital, or home.

Who Does It: Doctor, respiratory therapist, pulmonary lab technician, or patient.

How Long It Takes: About 1 minute.

Discomfort/Pain: None.

Results Ready When: Immediately.

Special Equipment: Pulse oximeter.

Risks/Complications: None.

Other Names: Pulse oximetry.

Purpose

To evaluate how well the lungs are providing oxygen to the blood during rest, exercise, or a medical procedure.

How It Works

Oxygen concentration determines the color of the blood, which in turn determines the refraction of light that passes through the skin. A device called an oximeter analyzes the refraction to determine the blood's oxygen saturation: Well-oxygenated blood is bright red, while blood carrying less oxygen is darker.

Preparation

None.

Test Procedure

- The probe is attached to your finger, earlobe, or toe.
- The probe emits a light signal, which passes through the finger, earlobe, or toe.
- Because some people have poor blood oxygenation only during activity, the test may be performed while you are exercising on a stationary bicycle or treadmill.

After the Test

The clip is removed, and you are free to return to previous activities. After exercise, cool down gradually by walking or pedaling slowly for a few minutes. Your pulse and blood pressure may be monitored during this time until they return to normal.

Patient Tip

Ask about the following in advance so you can be prepared:

- If exercise will be involved, wear comfortable walking or running shoes or sneakers, and loose-fitting shorts or exercise pants.
- If a finger probe will be done, do not wear nail polish.

Factors Affecting Results

- Poor circulation in the fingers, toes, or earlobe.
- Bright external light.
- Smoking can affect blood oxygenation.

Interpretation

It is considered abnormal if oxygen saturation declines by more than 5% during exercise or sleep. Normal resting oxygen saturation is usually greater than 90%.

Advantages

- It's noninvasive, quick, and simple.

Disadvantages

- It has limited diagnostic value because it evaluates only oxygen saturation.

The Next Step

Measurement of oxygen saturation will help your doctor evaluate the severity of your disease, and will determine if you need supplemental oxygen.

Chapter 54

Peak Flow Measurement

General Information

Where It's Done: At home, in a hospital, or virtually anywhere.

Who Does It: Patient.

How Long It Takes: Less than 1 minute.

Discomfort/Pain: None.

Results Ready When: Immediately.

Special Equipment: Peak flow meter.

Risks/Complications: May make you feel temporarily out of breath, but no real risk.

Other Names: Peak expiratory flow.

Purpose

To monitor the condition of the airways in order to monitor asthma, help predict an asthma attack, and determine when medication or emergency care is needed. Because it is self-test, it can be done at virtually any time.

From *The Yale University School of Medicine: Patient's Guide to Medical Tests.* © 1997 by Yale University School of Medicine and G.S. Sharpe Communications, Inc. Reprinted by permission of Houghton Mifflin Company. All rights reserved.

How It Works

The flow of air you are able to generate forcefully into a closed cylinder is an indication of whether or not your airways are constricted. Preparation Avoid eating a heavy meal for about three hours before taking the test.

Test Procedure

- Insert the mouthpiece of the peak flow meter between your teeth, and make sure your lips form a tight seal.

- Exhale strongly, with the greatest possible force.

- Repeat the maneuver at least twice, until results vary by no more than 10%.

- Record the maximum flow rate shown on the meter.

Did You Know?

Peak flow measurement is a simple test that asthmatics can do to monitor themselves, thus enabling them to take preventive medication and, perhaps avoid the need for emergency medical care. It is recommended for all asthmatics, and in particular for the following persons:

- People who experience severe asthma attacks with little warning.

- Those who require daily high-dose, or low-dose inhaled corticosteriods.

- Those with wide variations (20% or more) in the peak flow rate.

- Home peak flow meters are easy enough to use that they can be used for children with asthma. Many models are small, lightweight (less than 3 ounces) cylinders that can be carried in a purse or briefcase.

After the Test

If results are within 20% of your normal capacity, no special care is necessary.

Factors Affecting Results

- Insufficient effort on your part during the test.

- Lack of a tight seal over the mouthpiece.

- Improper handling of the peak flow meter (most devices must be held horizontally to achieve accurate measurements).

Interpretation

Compare the measurements with your usual results. If they drop 20% below your average, follow your doctor's orders for taking medication or getting medical help.

Advantages

- You and your physician may be able to use peak flows to help you monitor your asthma.

- It's quick, inexpensive, and noninvasive.

- It provides valuable information for asthmatics.

Disadvantages

- It's reliable only if performed properly.

The Next Step

You take your medication if it is indicated.

Chapter 55

Pulmonary Exercise Test

General Information

Where It's Done: Doctor's office, commercial pulmonary function laboratory, or hospital.

Who Does It: Respiratory therapist or pulmonary lab technician, under the supervision of a doctor.

How Long It Takes: 1-2 hours.

Discomfort/Pain: A high level of exertion; people may find the test intimidating.

Results Ready When: Several days.

Special Equipment: Bicycle ergometer or treadmill, oxygen and carbon dioxide analyzers, mouthpiece and nose clips, ECG equipment, pulse oximeter, sphygmomanometer, and a wave-form analyzer or computer to process signals from measuring devices.

Risks/Complications: May aggravate symptoms of the underlying lung or heart disease. Should not be done in people with unstable asthma, chest pain, high blood pressure, or heart failure that cannot be controlled with drugs, nor in people with high fever and several other lung or heart abnormalities.

Other Names: Incremental exercise testing or cardiopulmonary stress test.

Purpose

- To detect an abnormality causing unexplained shortness of breath or inability to exercise. In particular, to determine whether the shortness of breath and inability to exercise is due to a heart or lung problem.

- To identify the cause of shortness of breath not revealed by pulmonary function tests, electrocardiogram, or other procedures.

- To detect lung disease that is apparent only during exercise.

- In people seeking disability evaluation, to determine the level of physical exertion they are able to achieve.

How It Works

Your ability to exercise under controlled conditions is an indication of heart and lung fitness and capacity. It can be measured using equipment that records your heart rate, blood pressure, and respiration.

Preparation

- Wear loose-fitting, comfortable clothing and tennis or other comfort able shoes for pedaling on an exercise bike or walking on a treadmill.

- Avoid heavy meals for at least two hours before the test.

- Your medical history, height, and weight are recorded and used to calculate the workload you are expected to achieve during the test.

- ECG electrodes are attached to your chest (the area may be shaved if necessary), a blood pressure cuff is placed on your arm, and a pulse oximeter is placed on your finger, ear, or nose.

- A clip is placed on your nose to prevent air from leaking through the nostrils.

- You are given supporting headgear to keep the mouthpiece in place during the test.

Test Procedure

- You insert the mouthpiece between your teeth and make sure your lips form a tight seal (loose-fitting dentures may have to be removed).

- You start pedaling on a stationary bicycle at a given rate, or start walking on the treadmill.

- After two or three minutes, the workload is increased. The increases continue and are intended to bring you to the point of maximal exercise capacity within eight to 12 minutes.

- You stop exercising when you cannot reach maximal exercise capacity, cannot continue due to exhaustion, or because of medical reasons-for example, if the ECG shows an abnormality.

- The ECG recording is performed continuously during the test, and your blood pressure and the amount of oxygen in your blood are monitored.

- Measurements taken during the test include heart rate, breathing rate, oxygen uptake by the lungs, and the concentration of oxygen and carbon dioxide in the exhaled air. A sample of arterial blood may be drawn to determine the amounts of various gases it contains.

After the Test

- You slow down gradually to let your heart rate and breathing return to normal.

- All equipment that was attached to your body is removed, except the blood pressure cuff.

- Blood pressure is measured until it returns to normal.

Factors Affecting Results

- Failure to apply maximum effort during the test.
- Lack of a tight seal over the mouthpiece.

- Medications or the presence of disease.
- Ability to complete the test.

Interpretation

The doctor analyzes your oxygen consumption, carbon dioxide exhaled, and other measurements obtained during the test; correlates them with values expected for a person of your age, height, weight, and sex; and tries to establish the cause of any limitation in your ability to exercise. In disability evaluations, specific jobs are assigned levels of oxygen consumption that a worker must be able to achieve comfortably in order to be judged able to perform those jobs.

Advantages

- It's noninvasive.
- The risk of serious complications is extremely low (lower than in a cardiac stress test) because these patients normally do not have heart disease.

Disadvantages

- It cannot be performed in people who are unable to exercise.
- It detects the existence of a problem but not its cause.

The Next Step

An abnormal test result may help your doctor decide which system (lungs, heart, or other) should be further evaluated. A normal test indicates that your lungs are not the source of the shortness of breath or inability to exercise.

Chapter 56

Pulmonary Function Tests

General Information

Where It's Done: Doctor's office, commercial pulmonary function laboratory or hospital.

Who Does It: Doctor, respiratory therapist, or pulmonary lab technician.

How Long It Takes: 20-45 minutes.

Discomfort/Pain: Test can be tiring.

Results Ready When: Several hours to a few days.

Special Equipment: Pulmonary function analyzer (usually includes a spirometer).

Risks/Complications: May aggravate symptoms of lung disease. Should not be performed in people with unstable asthma or respiratory distress, recent heart attack or unstable heart disease, pneumothorax, coughing up large amounts of blood or active tuberculosis.

Other Names: Spirometry.

From *The Yale University School of Medicine: Patient's Guide to Medical Tests.* © 1997 by Yale University School of Medicine and G.S. Sharpe Communications, Inc. Reprinted by permission of Houghton Mifflin Company. All rights reserved.

Purpose

- To assess the ability of the lungs to receive, hold, and use air.
- To evaluate the severity of lung disease.
- To distinguish between restrictive and obstructive lung disease.
- To monitor the course of lung disease.
- To monitor the effectiveness of treatment.

How It Works

The volume of air you exhale through a tube can be measured with a device called a spirometer, and is an indication of how well your lungs are functioning.

Preparation

- You must refrain from smoking or heavy eating for four to eight hours before the test.
- If possible, avoid using bronchodilators or other drugs for 24 hours prior to the test or as specified by your doctor before this test.
- Wear loose, comfortable clothing that doesn't restrict breathing.
- Your age, sex, height, and weight are recorded in order to calculate expected test values.
- A clip is placed on your nose to prevent the air from escaping through the nostrils.
- Loose-fitting dentures may be removed.

Test Procedure

- You put a mouthpiece (made of cardboard or rubber, depending on the test) in your mouth and breathe normally while the technician makes sure the equipment is functioning properly (see Figure 56.1).
- You perform various breathing maneuvers: taking a deep breath, holding it briefly, and forcefully blowing the air out through the mouthpiece, which is attached to a flexible tube that leads to the spirometer.

- These tests are usually repeated at least three times to make sure similar values are obtained at each attempt. Values that vary widely may indicate a technical problem.

- Various measurements are taken of the volume of air that you are able to inhale and exhale. The ability of your lungs to deliver oxygen to blood may be measured by inhaling one breath of air with a high concentration of carbon monoxide.

After the Test

The nose clip is removed, and you are free to leave.

Factors Affecting Results

- Failure to follow instructions, such as not exhaling with maximum force. Anxiety or fatigue.

- Recent or current respiratory disease. Bronchodilators, sedatives, and other drugs that affect breathing or all body systems.

- Other procedures performed a few hours before the test, such as positive-pressure-breathing therapy.

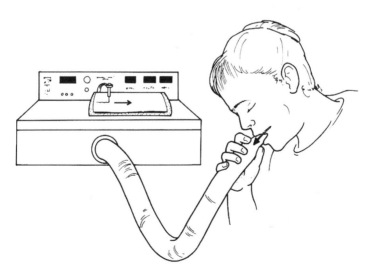

Figure 56.1. During pulmonary function tests (spirometry), the patient is asked to perform various breathing maneuvers by exhaling into a special mouthpiece attached to monitoring equipment.

Patient Tip

You may feel somewhat light-headed or dizzy after the test, if so, do not leave the test area alone until these symptoms disappear.

Time of Day

Pulmonary function tends to rise and then fall from morning to evening.

Portable spirometers used at bedside tend to be less reliable than stationary spirometry equipment.

Interpretation

Your test results, printed out as a table or a graph, are compared with average values for your age, sex, height, and weight.

Advantages

- It's noninvasive.
- It's reliable and reproducible.
- It produces few false-positive results.
- It provides information about pulmonary physiology.
- It provides a quantitative measure for the severity of lung disease.

Disadvantages

- Results may be affected by the patient's effort or understanding of instructions.

The Next Step

The pulmonary test will be interpreted by your physician. Decisions regarding further evaluation or treatment can then be made.

Chapter 57

Thoracentesis

General Information

Where It's Done: Hospital or doctor's office.

Who Does It: Doctor.

How Long It Takes: 15-60 minutes.

Discomfort/Pain: Discomfort associated with local anesthesia.

Results Ready When: 1-2 days.

Special Equipment: Needle, local anesthetics, and sometimes ultrasound or CT guidance equipment.

Risks/Complications: Collapsed lung, infection, or pain at the site of the test.

Other Names: Pleural fluid "tap."

Purpose

To determine the cause of abnormal accumulation of fluid in the pleural space. To drain large amounts of pleural fluid.

From *The Yale University School of Medicine: Patient's Guide to Medical Tests*. © 1997 by Yale University School of Medicine and G.S. Sharpe Communications, Inc. Reprinted by permission of Houghton Mifflin Company. All rights reserved.

How It Works

A sample of the pleural fluid is analyzed in the lab for the presence of certain cells, sugar content, protein content, and other substances.

Preparation

You remove all clothing from the waist up and don a hospital gown.

Test Procedure

- The doctor examines your chest to locate excess pleural fluid. Ultrasound or a CT scan may be used if localization is difficult or if the amount of fluid is small.

- Local anesthesia is administered at the site of the test.

- Fluid from the pleural space is withdrawn with a long, thin needle inserted between the ribs (see Figure 57.1).

- The sample is sent to a laboratory for analysis.

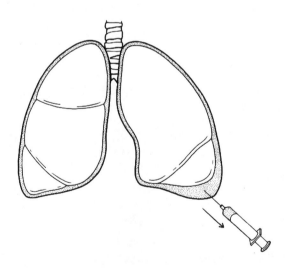

Figure 57.1. *To do thoracentesis—or a pleural fluid tap—a thin, hollow needle is inserted between two ribs and into the space between the pleura, the membranes surrounding the lungs. If there is fluid in this space, a sample can then be withdrawn for laboratory analysis.*

After the Test

- Pressure is applied to the puncture site to prevent bleeding.

- An X-ray is taken to be sure the lung has not been punctured or collapsed (a condition called pneumothorax).

Factors Affecting Results

- Bleeding from the puncture site may interfere with analysis of the sample.

Interpretation

The number and type of cells in the fluid, as well as the levels of glucose, acid, and various proteins, help establish whether the excess fluid is a result of infection, cancer, or other lung disease, or a complication of another disease such as congestive heart failure.

Advantages

- It's less invasive than open surgery.

- It's also easy to perform and minimally painful.

Disadvantage

- It doesn't always help diagnose disease inside the lung.

The Next Step

- If the pleural fluid analysis is diagnostic of the process causing it, treatment plans can be made.

- If the fluid is not diagnostic, further intervention—such as pleural biopsy, thoracoscopic evaluation, or lung biopsy—may be necessary.

Chapter 58

Thoracoscopy

General Information

Where It's Done: Hospital.

Who Does It: Doctor (chest surgeon or pulmonary specialist) and surgical team.

How Long It Takes: 2-4 hours.

Discomfort/Pain: Discomfort associated with general anesthesia; also chest discomfort after the procedure due to incision.

Results Ready When: 2 days.

Special Equipment: Thoracoscope and surgical instruments; general anesthesia.

Risks/Complications: Risks associated with general anesthesia and surgery.

Other Names: Pleuroscopy.

Purpose

- To inspect abnormalities in the lung that require a surgical biopsy.

- To obtain lung tissue for examination to confirm or rule out lung diseases, including lung cancer.

- To investigate causes of unexplained fluid in the pleural cavity.

How It Works

A flexible tube that resembles a miniature telescope, a tiny camera, and surgical instruments are inserted through three tiny incisions in the chest wall, allowing the surgeon to view and take samples from the lungs.

Preparation

- Prior to the test, you will have a chest X-ray, electrocardiogram (if you are over age 35), and various blood tests. An arterial blood gas and a pulmonary function test may also be done.

- You must fast for 12 hours before the procedure.

- General anesthesia is administered, and preparations for chest surgery are made.

Test Procedure

- The surgeon makes several incisions in your chest and inserts suction tubes that remove blood during the surgery.

- A bronchoscope is inserted into the airway to check for anatomical abnormalities.

- A Y-shaped endotracheal tube with two inner tubes connected to a ventilator (breathing machine) is passed down the throat, and one end is inserted into each bronchus.

- The lung to be examined is allowed to partially deflate (during the procedure you will breathe through the other lung). This creates a space between the lung and chest wall that provides the doctor with a good view of the lung and inner chest structures.

- The thoracoscope, a viewing tube that has a light source and may be flexible or rigid, is inserted into the space between the lung and the chest wall. The camera displays the image on TV screens.

- The doctor examines the surface of the lung, makes a cut through the pleura, and removes tissue samples of the pleura and the lung. Biopsies can also be taken of any accessible structures and tissues.

- If a cancerous tumor is suspected, a biopsy sample is sent to the pathology lab for a "frozen section," the results of which are 95% accurate. if it is positive for cancer, open chest surgery may be performed to remove the malignancy and part or all of the lung. (The final pathology report takes three to seven working days.)

Did You Know?

In the early 1990s, thoracoscopy began replacing surgical lung biopsy In many cases, except when the patient is too ill to function temporarily on only one lung. Like open surgical lung biopsy, it requires hospitalization and general anesthesia, but the recuperation time is usually measured in days rather than weeks.

After the Test

- The lung is reinflated, and two of the incisions are closed.

- A tube is placed in the third, which will remain in place for one to several days to remove air and fluids from the chest.

- When drainage of the fluid stops, the tube is removed.

- After one to two hours in the recovery room, you return to your hospital room for two to five days of recuperation.

- After discharge, refrain from lifting anything heavier than a phone book for two to three weeks.

Factors Affecting Results

- Accurate selection of the biopsy site.

Interpretation

The doctor may make the diagnosis by observing the structures in the chest. The biopsy sample removed during the procedure is examined under a microscope and provides additional information. Additionally, cultures may be performed.

Advantages

- It requires a smaller incision than open lung biopsy, and a shorter recuperation time.

- It may provide definitive diagnosis.

Disadvantages

- It's invasive.

- It requires hospitalization of several days.

- It's usually used only to evaluate lesions that are close to the surface of the lung.

- It yields a smaller tissue sample than open lung biopsy.

The Next Step

Treatment will be initiated if a disease is diagnosed.

Chapter 59

The Meaning of a Positive TB Test

The most commonly used skin test to check for tuberculosis is the PPD. If you have a positive PPD, it means you have been exposed to a person who has tuberculosis and you are now infected with the bacteria that causes the disease.

Do I have tuberculosis if I have a positive PPD test?

Not necessarily. A person can be infected with the bacteria that causes tuberculosis and not have tuberculosis disease. Many people are infected with the bacteria that causes tuberculosis, but only a few people (about 10 percent) go on to develop the disease. People who have the disease are said to have "active" tuberculosis.

Healthy people who get infected with the tuberculosis bacteria are able to fight off the infection and do not get tuberculosis disease. The bacteria is dormant (inactive) in their lungs. If the body is not able to fight off the infection and the bacteria continues to grow, active tuberculosis develops.

Would I know if I developed active tuberculosis?

You might not know that you have active tuberculosis. Tuberculosis bacteria can grow in your body without making you feel sick. Most people with active tuberculosis don't feel well. People with tuberculosis often feel tired and have a cough that won't go away. They may also lose weight, or have a fever, or break out in a sweat in bed (called "night sweats"). They may have trouble breathing.

If you have active tuberculosis, you will have to get regular checkups and chest x-rays for the rest of your life to make sure you stay free of disease, even after you have taken tuberculosis medicine.

Does a positive PPD test mean that I am contagious and can give tuberculosis to someone else?

Not necessarily. After you have a positive PPD skin test, you must have a chest x-ray and a physical exam to make sure that you don't have active disease and that you're not contagious. It usually takes only a few days to tell whether you're contagious. Most people with a positive skin test aren't contagious.

What will I have to do if my skin test is positive?

To be sure that you remain healthy, your doctor may recommend that you take medicine for six months to kill the tuberculosis infection. If you don't take the medicine, the bacteria will remain in your lungs, and you will always be in danger of getting active tuberculosis. The medicine used to treat tuberculosis infection is isoniazid, which is also called INH. You need to take one pill every day for six months.

People who take INH may have side effects, but not very often. Side effects include a skin rash, an upset stomach or liver disease. Ask your doctor about other side effects that might happen.

What if I forget to take my medicine?

It is very important that you take the medicine every day. Keep the medicine in a place where you will always see it. Take it at the same time every day.

Do I need to do anything else?

Every month you will need to visit your doctor to get another prescription of the medicine you are taking and to be sure you don't have any side effects or complications from the medicine. If you are feeling well, your doctor will give you a prescription for the next month. It is important that you stop drinking alcohol while taking isoniazid (INH). Alcohol increases the risk of liver damage if you drink while taking the medicine.

Could I still get active tuberculosis after I take the medicine for six months?

Even after you take the medicine every day for six months there is a small chance that you could develop active tuberculosis disease, because some organisms are resistant to the medicine. Staying healthy depends on having sensible living habits. You need adequate sleep and exercise and a nutritious diet to keep up your good health and resistance to the tuberculosis bacteria.

This information provides a general overview on tuberculosis and may not apply to everyone. Talk to your family doctor to find out if this information applies to you and to get more information on this subject.

Part Four

Treatment

Chapter 60

Guide to Choosing Medical Treatments

Medical treatments come in many shapes and sizes. There are "home remedies" shared among families and friends. There are prescription medicines, available only from a pharmacist, and only when ordered by a physician. There are over-the-counter drugs that you can buy—almost anywhere—without a doctor's order. Of growing interest and attention in recent years are so-called alternative treatments, not yet approved for sale because they are still undergoing scientific research to see if they really are safe and effective. And, of course, there are those "miracle" products sold through "back-of-the-magazine" ads and TV infomercials.

How can you tell which of these may really help treat your medical condition, and which will only make you worse off—financially, physically, or both?

Many advocates of unproven treatments and cures contend that people have the right to try whatever may offer them hope, even if others believe the remedy is worthless. This argument is especially compelling for people with life-threatening diseases with no known cure.

Clinical Trials

Before gaining Food and Drug Administration marketing approval, new drugs, biologics, and medical devices must be proven safe and effective by controlled clinical trials.

Excerpted from "An FDA Guide to Choosing Medical Treatments," *FDA Consumer*, Food and Drug Administration (FDA), June 1995; revised July 1996; current as of December 1999.

In a clinical trial, results observed in patients getting the treatment are compared with the results in similar patients receiving a different treatment or placebo (inactive) treatment. Preferably, neither patients nor researchers know who is receiving the therapy under study.

To the FDA, it doesn't matter whether the product or treatment is labeled alternative or falls under the auspices of mainstream American medical practice. (Mainstream American medicine essentially includes the practices and products the majority of medical doctors in this country follow and use.) It must meet the agency's safety and effectiveness criteria before being allowed on the market.

In addition, just because something is undergoing a clinical trial doesn't mean it works or FDA considers it to be a proven therapy, says Donald Pohl, of FDA's Office of AIDS and Special Health Issues. "You can't jump to that conclusion," he says. A trial can fail to prove that the product is effective, he explains. And that's not just true for alternative products. Even when the major drug companies sponsor clinical trials for mainstream products, only a small fraction are proven safe and effective.

Many people with serious illnesses are unable to find a cure, or even temporary relief, from the available mainstream treatments that have been rigorously studied and proven safe and effective. For many conditions, what's effective for one patient may not help another.

Real Alternatives

"It is best not to abandon conventional therapy when there is a known response [in the effectiveness of that therapy]," says Joseph Jacobs, M.D., former director of the National Institutes of Health's Office of Alternative Medicine, which was established in October 1992. As an example he cites childhood leukemia, which has an 80 percent cure rate with conventional therapy.

But what if conventional therapy holds little promise?

Many physicians believe it is not unreasonable for someone in the last stages of an incurable cancer to try something unproven. But, for example, if a woman with an early stage of breast cancer wanted to try shark cartilage (an unproven treatment that may inhibit the growth of cancer tumors, currently undergoing clinical trials), those same doctors would probably say, "Don't do it," because there are so many effective conventional treatments.

Jacobs warns that, "If an alternative practitioner does not want to work with a regular doctor, then he's suspect."

Alternative medicine is often described as any medical practice or intervention that:

- lacks sufficient documentation of its safety and effectiveness against specific diseases and conditions

- is not generally taught in U.S. medical schools

- is not generally reimbursable by health insurance providers.

According to a study in the January 28, 1993, *New England Journal of Medicine*, 1 in 3 patients used alternative therapy in 1990. More than 80 percent of those who use alternative therapies used conventional medicine at the same time, but did not tell their doctors about the alternative treatments. The study's authors concluded this lack of communication between doctors and patients "is not in the best interest of the patients, since the use of unconventional therapy, especially if it is totally unsupervised, may be harmful." The study concluded that medical doctors should ask their patients about any use of unconventional treatment as part of a medical history.

Many doctors are interested in learning more about alternative therapies, according to Brian Berman, M.D., a family practitioner with the University of Maryland School of Medicine in Baltimore. Berman says his own interest began when "I found that I wasn't getting all the results that I would have liked with conventional medicine, especially in patients with chronic diseases.

What I've found at the University of Maryland is a healthy skepticism among my colleagues, but a real willingness to collaborate. We have a lot of people from different departments who are saying, let's see how we can develop scientifically rigorous studies that are also sensitive to the particular therapies that we're working with."

Anyone who wants to be treated with an alternative therapy should try to do so through participation in a clinical trial. Clinical trials are regulated by FDA and provide safeguards to protect patients, such as monitoring of adverse reactions. In fact, FDA is interested in assisting investigators who want to study alternative therapies under carefully controlled clinical trials.

While many alternative therapies are the subject of scientifically valid research, it's important to remember that at this time their safety and effectiveness are still unproven.

347

Avoiding Fraud

FDA defines health fraud as the promotion, advertisement, distribution, or sale of articles, intended for human or animal use, that are represented as being effective to diagnose, prevent, cure, treat, or mitigate disease (or other conditions), or provide a beneficial effect on health, but which have not been scientifically proven safe and effective for such purposes. Such practices may be deliberately deceptive, or done without adequate knowledge or understanding of the article.

Health fraud costs Americans an estimated $30 billion a year. However, the costs are not just economic, according to John Renner, M.D., a Kansas City-based champion of quality health care for the elderly. "The hidden costs—death, disability—are unbelievable," he says.

To combat health fraud, FDA established its National Health Fraud Unit in 1988. The unit works with the National Association of Attorneys General and the Association of Food and Drug Officials to coordinate federal, state and local regulatory actions against specific health frauds.

Regulatory actions may be necessary in many cases because products that have not been shown to be safe and effective pose potential hazards for consumers both directly and indirectly. The agency's priorities for regulatory action depend on the situation; direct risks to health come first.

Unproven products cause direct health hazards when their use results in injuries or adverse reactions. For example, a medical device called the InnerQuest Brain Wave Synchronizer was promoted to alter brain waves and relieve stress. It consisted of an audio cassette and eyeglasses that emitted sounds and flashing lights. It caused epileptic seizures in some users. As a result of a court order requested by FDA, 78 cartons of the devices, valued at $200,000, were seized by U.S. marshals and destroyed in June 1993.

Indirectly harmful products are those that do not themselves cause injury, but may lead people to delay or reject proven remedies, possibly worsening their condition. For example, if cancer patients reject proven drug therapies in favor of unproven ones and the unproven ones turn out not to work, their disease may advance beyond the point where proven therapies can help.

How to Approach Alternative Therapies

The National Institutes of Health (NIH) Office of Alternative Medicine recommends the following before getting involved in any alternative therapy:

- Obtain objective information about the therapy. Besides talking with the person promoting the approach, speak with people who have gone through the treatment—preferably both those who were treated recently and those treated in the past. Ask about the advantages and disadvantages, risks, side effects, costs, results, and over what time span results can be expected.

- Inquire about the training and expertise of the person administering the treatment (for example, certification).

- Consider the costs. Alternative treatments may not be reimbursable by health insurance.

- Discuss all treatments with your primary care provider, who needs this information in order to have a complete picture of your treatment plan.

For everyone—consumers, physicians and other health-care providers, and government regulators—FDA has the same advice when it comes to weeding out the hopeless from the hopeful:

- Be open-minded, but don't fall into the abyss of accepting anything at all. For there are—as there have been for centuries—countless products that are nothing more than fraud.

Tip-Offs to Rip-Offs

New health frauds pop up all the time, but the promoters usually fall back on the same old clichés and tricks to gain your trust and get your money. According to FDA, some red flags to watch out for include:

- claims the product works by a secret formula. (Legitimate scientists share their knowledge so their peers can review their data.)

- publicity only in the back pages of magazines, over the phone, by direct mail, in newspaper ads in the format of news stories, or 30-minute commercials in talk show format. (Results of studies on bona fide treatments are generally reported first in medical journals.)

- claims the product is an amazing or miraculous breakthrough. (Real medical breakthroughs are few and far between, and when they happen, they're not touted as "amazing" or "miraculous" by any responsible scientist or journalist.)

349

- promises of easy weight loss. (For most people, the only way to lose weight is to eat less and exercise more.)

- promises of a quick, painless, guaranteed cure

- testimonials from satisfied customers. (These people may never have had the disease the product is supposed to cure, may be paid representatives, or may simply not exist. Often they're identified only by initials or first names.)

Chapter 61

Bronchodilators—Inhalation

In deciding to use a medicine, the risks of taking the medicine must be weighed against the good it will do. This is a decision you and your doctor will make. For inhalation adrenergic bronchodilators, the following should be considered:

- *Allergies* — Tell your doctor if you have ever had any unusual or allergic reaction to albuterol, bitolterol, epinephrine, fenoterol, isoetharine, isoproterenol, metaproterenol, pirbuterol, procaterol, salmeterol, terbutaline, or other inhalation medicines. Also tell your health care professional if you are allergic to sulfites, which may be used as a preservative in some of these medicines.

- *Pregnancy*—

    For albuterol, bitolterol, metaproterenol, and salmeterol: These medicines are used to treat asthma in pregnant women. Although there are no studies on birth defects in humans, problems have not been reported. Some studies in animals have shown that they cause birth defects when given in doses many times higher than the human dose.

    For epinephrine: Women given epinephrine subcutaneously (under the skin) during pregnancy have been studied. The

---

babies of these women had more birth defects than expected, although the severity of the mother's asthma may
have contributed to this result.

For fenoterol, isoproterenol, pirbuterol, procaterol, and
terbutaline: These medicines are used to treat asthma in
pregnant women. Although there are no studies on birth defects in humans, problems have not been reported. These
medicines have not been shown to cause birth defects in animal studies when given in doses many times higher than
the human dose.

For isoetharine: Studies on birth defects have not been done
in either humans or animals.

- *Breast Feeding*—It is not known whether these medicines pass
  into the breast milk. Although most medicines pass into breast
  milk in small amounts, many of them may be used safely while
  breast feeding. Mothers who are using these medicines and who
  wish to breast feed should discuss this with their doctor.

- *Children*—Appropriate studies performed to date have not demonstrated pediatrics-specific problems that would limit the usefulness of these medicines in children. However, isoetharine is
  not recommended for use in children.

- *Older Adults*—

  For albuterol, bitolterol, epinephrine, fenoterol, isoetharine,
  isoproterenol, metaproterenol, pirbuterol, procaterol, and
  terbutaline: These medicines have not been studied specifically in older people. Therefore, it may not be known
  whether they work exactly the same way they do in younger
  adults or if they cause different side effects or problems in
  older people. There is no specific information comparing use
  of inhalation adrenergic bronchodilators in the elderly with
  use in other age groups.

  For salmeterol: This medicine has been tested in a limited
  number of patients 65 years of age or older. It has not been
  shown to cause different side effects or problems in older
  people than it does in younger adults.

- *Other Medicines*—Although certain medicines should not be
  used together at all, in other cases two different medicines may

be used together even if an interaction might occur. In these cases, your doctor may want to change the dose, or other precautions may be necessary. When you are using inhalation adrenergic bronchodilators, it is especially important that your health care professional know if you are taking any of the following:

Beta-adrenergic blocking agents (acebutolol [e.g., Sectral], atenolol [e.g., Tenormin], betaxolol [e.g., Kerlone], carteolol [e.g., Cartrol], labetalol [e.g., Normodyne], metoprolol [e.g., Lopressor], nadolol [e.g., Corgard], oxprenolol [e.g., Trasicor], penbutolol [e.g., Levatol], pindolol [e.g., Visken], propranolol [e.g., Inderal], sotalol [e.g., Sotacor], timolol [e.g., Blocadren])—These medicines may make your condition worse and prevent the adrenergic bronchodilators from working properly

- *Other Medical Problems*—The presence of other medical problems may affect the use of inhalation adrenergic bronchodilators. Make sure you tell your doctor if you have any other medical problems, especially:

Heart or blood vessel disease—These medicines may make these conditions worse

High blood pressure, not well controlled—Epinephrine may make this condition worse

Overactive Thyroid—The chance of side effects may be increased

Proper Use of This Medicine

These medicines come with patient directions. Read them carefully before using the medicine. If you do not understand the directions or if you are not sure how to use the medicine, ask your health care professional to show you what to do. Also, ask your health care professional to check regularly how you use the medicine to make sure you are using it properly.

Use this medicine only as directed. Do not use more of it and do not use it more often than recommended on the label, unless otherwise directed by your doctor. Using the medicine more often may increase the chance of serious unwanted effects. Deaths have occurred when too much inhalation bronchodilator medicine was used.

Keep the spray away from your eyes because it may cause irritation.

Salmeterol is used to prevent asthma attacks. It is not used to relieve an attack that has already started. For relief of an asthma attack that has already started, you should use a medicine that starts working faster than salmeterol does. If you do not have another medicine to use for an attack or if you have any questions about this, check with your doctor. Because the effects of salmeterol usually last about 12 hours, doses should never be taken more than two times a day or less than 12 hours apart.

Some epinephrine preparations are available without a doctor's prescription. However, do not use this medicine unless you are seeing a doctor about asthma. Do not use this medicine if you have been hospitalized for asthma treatment or if you are taking a prescription medicine for asthma, unless you have been told to do so by a doctor.

When you use the inhaler for the first time, or if you have not used it in a while, the inhaler may not deliver the right amount of medicine with the first puff. Therefore, before using the inhaler, you may have to test or prime it.

To test or prime most inhalers

- Insert the medicine container (canister) firmly into the clean mouthpiece according to the manufacturer's directions. Check to make sure it is placed properly into the mouthpiece.

- Take the cap off the mouthpiece and shake the inhaler three or four times.

- Hold the inhaler well away from you at arm's length and press the top of the canister, spraying the medicine into the air two times. The inhaler will now be ready to provide the right amount of medicine when you use it.

To use most inhalers

- Using your thumb and one or two fingers, hold the inhaler upright, with the mouthpiece end down and pointing toward you.

- Take the cap off the mouthpiece. Check the mouthpiece to make sure it is clear. Then, gently shake the inhaler three or four times.

- Breathe out slowly to the end of a normal breath.

Use the inhalation method recommended by your doctor

- Open-mouth method—Place the mouthpiece about 1 to 2 inches (2 finger widths) in front of your widely opened mouth. Make sure the inhaler is aimed into your mouth so the spray does not hit the roof of your mouth or your tongue.

- Closed-mouth method—Place the mouthpiece in your mouth between your teeth and over your tongue with your lips closed tightly around it. Make sure your tongue or teeth are not blocking the opening.

- Start to breathe in slowly through your mouth. At the same time, press the top of the canister one time to get 1 puff of medicine. Continue to breathe in slowly for 3 to 5 seconds. Count the seconds while breathing in. It is important to press the canister and breathe in slowly at the same time so the medicine gets into your lungs. This step may be difficult at first. If you are using the closed-mouth method and you see a fine mist coming from your mouth or nose, the inhaler is not being used correctly.

- Hold your breath as long as you can up to 10 seconds. This gives the medicine time to settle into your airways and lungs.

- Take the mouthpiece away from your mouth and breathe out slowly.

- If your doctor has told you to inhale more than 1 puff of medicine at each dose, gently shake the inhaler again and take the next puff following exactly the same steps you used for the first puff. Press the canister one time for each puff of medicine.

- When you are done, wipe off the mouthpiece and replace the cap.

Your doctor, nurse, or pharmacist may want you to use a spacer or holding chamber with the inhaler. A spacer helps get the medicine into the lungs and reduces the amount of medicine that stays in your mouth and throat.

To use a spacer with the inhaler

- Attach the spacer to the inhaler according to the manufacturer's directions. There are different types of spacers available, but the method of breathing is the same with most spacers.

- Gently shake the inhaler and spacer three or four times.

- Hold the mouthpiece of the spacer away from your mouth and breathe out slowly to the end of a normal breath.

- Place the mouthpiece into your mouth between your teeth and over your tongue with your lips closed around it.

- Press down on the canister top one time to release 1 puff of medicine into the spacer. Within one or two seconds, begin to breathe in slowly through your mouth for three to five seconds. Do not breathe in through your nose. Count the seconds while inhaling.

- Hold your breath as long as you can up to ten seconds (count slowly to ten).

- Breathe out slowly. Do not remove the mouthpiece from your mouth. Breathe in and out slowly two or three times to make sure the spacer is emptied.

- If your doctor has told you to take more than 1 puff of medicine at each dose, gently shake the inhaler and spacer again, and take the next puff, following exactly the same steps you used for the first puff. Do not put more than 1 puff of medicine into the spacer at a time.

- If you rinse your mouth with water after you have finished, be sure to spit out the rinse water. Do not swallow it.

- When you are finished, remove the spacer from the inhaler. Wipe off the mouthpiece and replace the cap.

- Clean the inhaler and mouthpiece at least once a week.

To clean the inhaler

- Remove the canister from the inhaler and set the canister aside.

- Wash the mouthpiece and cap with warm, soapy water. Then, rinse well with warm, running water.

- Shake off the excess water and let the inhaler parts air dry completely before putting the inhaler back together.

- Save your inhaler. Refill units may be available.

For patients using the powder for inhalation dosage form

- These medicines are used with a special device. If you do not understand the directions that come with the inhaler or if you are not sure how to use the inhaler, ask your health care professional to show you how to use it. Also, ask your health care professional to check regularly how you use the inhaler to make sure you are using it properly.

For patients using the inhalation solution dosage form

- If you are using this medicine in a nebulizer, make sure you understand exactly how to use it. If you have any questions about this, check with your health care professional.

- Do not use if solution turns pinkish to brownish in color or if it becomes cloudy.

- Do not mix another inhalation medicine with an adrenergic bronchodilator medicine in the nebulizer unless told to do so by your health care professional.

Dosing

The dose of these medicines will be different for different patients. Follow your doctor's orders or the directions on the label. The following information includes only the average doses of these medicines. If your dose is different, do not change it unless your doctor tells you to do so.

The number of inhalations or the amount of medicine that you use depends on the strength of the medicine. Also, the number of doses you take each day, the time allowed between doses, and the length of time you take the medicine depend on the medical problem for which you are taking the adrenergic bronchodilator.

For Albuterol

For inhalation aerosol dosage form

- For preventing or treating bronchospasm:

  Adults and children 4 years of age and older—2 inhalations (puffs) every four to six hours.

  Children up to 4 years of age—Dose must be determined by your doctor.

- For preventing bronchospasm caused by exercise:

  Adults and children 4 years of age and older—2 inhalations (puffs) taken fifteen minutes before you start to exercise.

  Children up to 4 years of age—Dose must be determined by your doctor.

For inhalation solution dosage form

- For preventing or treating bronchospasm:

  Adults and children 12 years of age and older—This medicine is used in a nebulizer and is taken by inhalation over five to fifteen minutes. The usual dose is 2.5 milligrams (mg) of albuterol taken every four to six hours if needed.

  Children up to 12 years of age—This medicine is used in a nebulizer and is taken by inhalation over five to fifteen minutes. The usual dose is 1.25 to 2.5 milligrams (mg) of albuterol taken every four to six hours if needed.

For capsules (powder) for inhalation dosage form

- For preventing or treating bronchospasm:

  Adults and children 4 years of age and older—200 or 400 mcg taken by inhalation every four to six hours.

  Children up to 4 years of age—Dose must be determined by your doctor.

- For preventing bronchospasm caused by exercise:

  Adults and children 4 years of age and older—200 mcg taken by inhalation fifteen minutes before you start to exercise.

  Children up to 4 years of age-Dose must be determined by your doctor.

For Albuterol Sulfate

For inhalation aerosol dosage form

- For treating bronchospasm:

  Adults and children 12 years of age and older—2 inhalations (puffs) every four to six hours.

  Children up to 12 years of age—Dose must be determined by your doctor.

For Bitolterol

For inhalation aerosol dosage form

- For preventing or treating bronchospasm:

  Adults and children 12 years of age and older—2 inhalations (puffs) every eight hours or 2 inhalations (puffs) at first, allowing one to three minutes between each puff. This dose may be followed by another puff, if needed. However, the dose taken each day should not be more than 2 puffs every four hours or 3 puffs every six hours.

Children up to 12 years of age—Dose must be determined by your doctor.

- For preventing bronchospasm caused by exercise:

Adults and teenagers—2 inhalations (puffs) taken five minutes before you start to exercise.

Children—1 or 2 inhalations (puffs) taken five minutes before you start to exercise.

For inhalation solution dosage form

- For preventing or treating bronchospasm:

Adults and children 12 years of age and older—This medicine is used in a nebulizer and is taken by inhalation over ten to fifteen minutes. The usual dose is 1 to 2.5 milligrams (mg) of bitolterol taken three or four times a day. Doses should be taken at least four hours apart.

Children up to 12 years of age—Dose must be determined by your doctor.

For Epinephrine

For treating bronchospasm

- For inhalation aerosol dosage form:

Adults and children 4 years of age and older—1 inhalation (puff). The dose may be repeated after at least one minute, if needed. Doses should be taken at least three hours apart.

Children up to 4 years of age—Dose must be determined by your doctor.

- For inhalation solution dosage form:

Adults and children 4 years of age and older—This medicine should be used in a hand-bulb nebulizer. The usual dose is 1 to 3 inhalations (puffs) of a 1% solution. Doses should be taken at least three hours apart.

Children up to 4 years of age—Dose must be determined by your doctor.

For Fenoterol

For inhalation aerosol dosage form

- For preventing or treating bronchospasm:

  Adults and children 12 years of age and older—100 or 200 micrograms (mcg), repeated three or four times a day if needed. This medicine should not be taken more often than every four hours. The total dose should not be more than 8 puffs a day of the 100 mcg per spray product or 6 puffs of the 200 mcg per spray product.

  Children up to 12 years of age—Dose must be determined by your doctor.

For inhalation solution dosage form

- For preventing or treating bronchospasm:

  Adults and children 12 years of age and older—This medicine is used in a nebulizer and is taken by inhalation over ten to fifteen minutes. The usual dose is 0.5 to 1 milligram (mg) of fenoterol taken every six hours if needed.

  Children up to 12 years of age—Dose must be determined by your doctor.

For Isoetharine

For inhalation solution dosage form

- For treating bronchospasm:

  Adults—This medicine is used in a nebulizer and is taken by inhalation over fifteen to twenty minutes. The amount of medicine you use and whether it requires dilution depends on the product ordered by your doctor. The usual dose is 2.5 to 10 milligrams (mg). This medicine usually should not be used more often than every four hours.

  Children—Use is not recommended.

For inhalation aerosol dosage form

- For treating bronchospasm:

  Adults and teenagers—1 or 2 inhalations (puffs). This dose may be repeated every four hours as necessary.

  Children—Use is not recommended.

For Isoproterenol

For inhalation solution dosage form

- For treating bronchospasm:

    Adults and teenagers—This medicine is used in a nebulizer and is taken by inhalation over ten to twenty minutes. The usual dose is 2.5 milligrams (mg). This medicine usually should not be used more often than every four hours.

    Children—This medicine is used in a nebulizer and is taken by inhalation over ten to twenty minutes. The usual dose is 0.05 to 0.1 milligram (mg) per kilogram (kg) of body weight, up to 1.25 mg, diluted. The dose may be repeated every four hours, if needed.

For Isoproterenol Hydrochloride

For inhalation aerosol dosage form:

- For treating bronchospasm:

    Adults and children 12 years of age and older—1 inhalation (puff), repeated after two to five minutes if needed. This dose is taken every three to four hours.

    Children up to 12 years of age—Use is not recommended.

For Isoproterenol Sulfate

For inhalation aerosol dosage form

- For treating bronchospasm:

    Adults and children 12 years of age and older—1 inhalation (puff), repeated after two to five minutes if needed. This dose is taken every four to six hours.

    Children up to 12 years of age—Dose must be determined by your doctor.

For Metaproterenol

For inhalation aerosol dosage form

- For preventing and treating bronchospasm:

    Adults and children 12 years of age and older—2 or 3 inhalations (puffs) every three to four hours. The total dose should not be more than 12 puffs a day.

Children up to 12 years of age—1 to 3 inhalations (puffs) every three to four hours. The total dose should not be more than 12 puffs a day.

For inhalation solution dosage form

- For preventing or treating bronchospasm:

  Adults and children 6 years of age and older—This medicine is used in a nebulizer and is taken by inhalation. The amount of medicine you use and whether it requires dilution depends on the product ordered by your doctor. The usual dose is 10 to 15 milligrams (mg) taken three or four times a day. Doses should be taken at least four hours apart.

  Children up to 6 years of age—This medicine is used in a nebulizer and is taken by inhalation. The amount of medicine you use and whether it requires dilution depends on the product ordered by your doctor. The usual dose is 5 to 15 milligrams (mg) taken three or four times a day, at least four hours apart.

For Pirbuterol

For inhalation aerosol dosage form

- For preventing and treating bronchospasm:

  Adults and children—1 or 2 inhalations (puffs) every four to six hours. The total dose should not be more than 12 puffs a day.

- For preventing bronchospasm caused by exercise:

  Adults and children—2 inhalations (puffs) taken five minutes before you start to exercise.

For Procaterol

For inhalation aerosol dosage form

- For preventing and treating bronchospasm:

  Adults and children 12 years of age and older—1 or 2 inhalations (puffs) three times a day.

  Children up to 12 years of age—Dose must be determined by your doctor.

- For preventing bronchospasm caused by exercise:

  Adults and children 12 years of age and older—1 or 2 inhalations (puffs) taken at least fifteen minutes before you start to exercise.

For Salmeterol

For the inhalation aerosol dosage form

- For preventing bronchospasm:

  Adults and children 12 years of age and older—2 inhalations (puffs) two times a day, in the morning and evening. Doses should be taken about twelve hours apart.

  Children up to 12 years of age—Dose must be determined by your doctor.

- For preventing bronchospasm caused by exercise:

  Adults and children 12 years of age and older—2 inhalations (puffs) taken at least thirty to sixty minutes before you start to exercise. If you are already using salmeterol two times a day to treat your asthma, you do not need to use additional salmeterol before you exercise.

  Children up to 12 years of age—Dose must be determined by your doctor.

For the powder for inhalation dosage form

- For preventing bronchospasm:

  Adults and children 12 years of age and older—1 inhalation (the contents of one blister) two times a day, in the morning and evening. Doses should be taken about twelve hours apart.

  Children up to 12 years of age—Dose must be determined by your doctor.

For Terbutaline

For inhalation aerosol dosage form

- For preventing or treating bronchospasm:
  Adults and children—
  - For the 200 microgram (mcg) per metered spray product: 2 inhalations (puffs) every four to six hours.
  - For the 500 mcg per metered spray product: 1 inhalation (puff), repeated after five minutes if needed. The total dose should not be more than 6 puffs a day.

- For preventing bronchospasm caused by exercise:

363

Adults and children—

- For the 200 microgram (mcg) per metered spray product: 2 inhalations (puffs) taken five to fifteen minutes before you start to exercise.

Missed Dose

For salmeterol: If you use salmeterol inhalation regularly and you miss a dose of this medicine, use it as soon as possible. Then go back to your regular schedule. Do not double doses. If you have wheezing or breathlessness before the next dose is due, you should use another inhaled bronchodilator that starts to work faster than salmeterol does to relieve the attack.

For all other adrenergic bronchodilators: If you are using one of these medicines regularly and you miss a dose, use it as soon as possible. Then use any remaining doses for that day at regularly spaced intervals. Do not double doses.

To Store This Medicine

- Keep out of the reach of children.

- Store away from heat.

- Store the solution form of this medicine away from direct light. Store the inhalation aerosol form of this medicine away from direct sunlight.

- Keep the medicine from freezing.

- Store canister with the nozzle end down.

- Do not store the powder for inhalation forms of these medicines in the bathroom, near the kitchen sink, or in other damp places. Moisture may cause the medicine to break down.

- Do not puncture, break, or burn the inhalation aerosol container, even if it is empty.

- Do not keep outdated medicine or medicine no longer needed. Be sure that any discarded medicine is out of the reach of children.

Precautions While Using This Medicine

It is important that your doctor check your progress at regular intervals to make sure that your medicine is working properly.

If you still have trouble breathing after using one of these medicines, or if your condition becomes worse, check with your doctor at once.

You may also be taking an anti-inflammatory medicine for asthma along with this medicine. Do not stop taking the anti-inflammatory medicine even if your asthma seems better, unless you are told to do so by your doctor.

For patients using salmeterol, check with your doctor

- If you need to use 4 or more inhalations (puffs) a day of a fast-acting inhaled bronchodilator for 2 or more days in a row to relieve asthma attacks.

- If you need to use more than 1 canister (a total of 200 inhalations per canister) of a fast-acting inhaled bronchodilator in a 2-month period to relieve asthma attacks.

For patients using any of these medicines except salmeterol, check with your doctor:

- If you need more inhalations (puffs) than usual of a fast-acting beta-adrenergic bronchodilator to relieve an acute attack

- If not using an anti-inflammatory medicine and using a fast-acting beta-adrenergic bronchodilator to relieve symptoms more than two times per week

- If you are using an anti-inflammatory medicine and you also are using more than 1 canister per month of a fast-acting beta-adrenergic bronchodilator to relieve symptoms

Side Effects of This Medicine

Along with its needed effects, a medicine may cause some unwanted effects. Although not all of these side effects may occur, if they do occur they may need medical attention.

Check with your doctor immediately if any of the following side effects occur:

- **Rare:** Dizziness, severe; feeling of choking, irritation, or swelling in throat; flushing or redness of skin; hives; increased shortness of breath; skin rash; swelling of face, lips, or eyelids; tightness in chest or wheezing, troubled breathing

Other side effects may occur that usually do not need medical attention. These side effects may go away during treatment as your body adjusts to the medicine. However, check with your doctor if any of the following side effects continue or are bothersome:

- **More common:** Fast heartbeat; headache; nervousness; trembling

- **Less common:** Coughing or other bronchial irritation; dizziness or lightheadedness; dryness or irritation of mouth or throat

- **Rare:** Chest discomfort or pain; drowsiness or weakness; irregular heartbeat; muscle cramps or twitching; nausea and/or vomiting; restlessness; trouble in sleeping

Not all of the side effects listed above have been reported for each of these medicines, but they have been reported for at least one of them. All of the adrenergic bronchodilators are similar, so any of the above side effects may occur with any of these medicines.

While you are using an adrenergic bronchodilator, you may notice an unusual or unpleasant taste. This may be expected and will go away when you stop using the medicine.

Isoproterenol may cause the saliva to turn pinkish to red. This is to be expected while you are taking this medicine.

Other side effects not listed above may also occur in some patients. If you notice any other effects, check with your doctor.

Commonly Used Brand Names

In the U.S.

- Adrenalin Chloride
- Airet
- Alupent
- Arm-a-Med Isoetharine
- Arm-a-Med Metaproterenol
- Asthmahaler Mist
- AsthmaNefrin
- Beta-2
- Brethaire
- Bronkaid Mist
- Bronkaid Suspension Mist
- Bronkometer
- Bronkosol
- Dey-Lute Isoetharine
- Dey-Lute Metaproterenol
- Isuprel
- Isuprel Mistometer
- Maxair
- Maxair Autohaler
- Medihaler-Iso
- microNefrin
- Nephron
- Primatene Mist
- Proventil
- Proventil HFA
- S-2
- Serevent
- Tornalate
- Vaponefrin
- Ventolin
- Ventolin Nebules
- Ventolin Rotacaps

In Canada

- Alupent
- Apo-Salvent
- Berotec
- Bricanyl
  Turbuhaler
- Bronkaid
  Mistometer

- Gen-Salbutamol
  Sterinebs P.F.
- Isuprel
- Isuprel
  Mistometer
- Maxair
- Novo-Salmol
- Pro-Air

- Serevent
- Vaponefrin
- Ventodisk
- Ventolin
- Ventolin Nebules
  P.F.
- Ventolin
  Rotacaps

Other commonly used names are:

- Adrenaline
- Orciprenaline
- Salbutamol

Description

Adrenergic bronchodilators are medicines that are breathed in through the mouth to open up the bronchial tubes (air passages) of the lungs. Some of these medicines are used to treat the symptoms of asthma, chronic bronchitis, emphysema, and other lung diseases, while others are used to prevent the symptoms.

Salmeterol is a long-acting bronchodilator that is used with anti-inflammatory medication to prevent asthma attacks. Salmeterol is different from the other adrenergic bronchodilators because it does not act quickly enough to relieve an asthma attack that has already started.

Some of these medicines are also breathed in through the mouth to prevent bronchospasm (wheezing or difficulty in breathing) caused by exercise. Also, epinephrine may be used in the treatment of croup.

All of these medicines, except some epinephrine preparations, are available only with your doctor's prescription. Although some of the epinephrine preparations are available without a prescription, your doctor may have special instructions on the proper dose of epinephrine for your medical condition.

These medicines are available in the following dosage forms:

Inhalation

- Albuterol
  Inhalation aerosol (U.S. and Canada)
  Inhalation solution (U.S. and Canada)
  Powder for inhalation (U.S. and Canada)

- Bitolterol
    Inhalation aerosol (U.S.)
    Inhalation solution (U.S.)

- Epinephrine
    Inhalation aerosol (U.S. and Canada)
    Inhalation solution (U.S. and Canada)

- Fenoterol
    Inhalation aerosol (Canada)
    Inhalation solution (Canada)

- Isoetharine
    Inhalation aerosol (U.S.)
    Inhalation solution (U.S.)

- Isoproterenol
    Inhalation aerosol (U.S. and Canada)
    Inhalation solution (U.S. and Canada)

- Metaproterenol
    Inhalation aerosol (U.S. and Canada)
    Inhalation solution (U.S. and Canada)

- Pirbuterol
    Inhalation aerosol (U.S. and Canada)

- Procaterol
    Inhalation aerosol (Canada)

- Salmeterol
    Inhalation aerosol (U.S. and Canada)
    Powder for inhalation (Canada)

- Terbutaline
    Inhalation aerosol (U.S. and Canada)

Chapter 62

Bronchodilators— Oral/Injection

In deciding to use a medicine, the risks of taking the medicine must be weighed against the good it will do. This is a decision you and your doctor will make. For adrenergic bronchodilators taken by mouth or given by injection, the following should be considered:

- *Allergies:* Tell your doctor if you have ever had any unusual or allergic reaction to albuterol, ephedrine, epinephrine, isoproterenol, metaproterenol, or terbutaline. Also, tell your doctor if you are allergic to any other substances, such as foods, preservatives, or dyes.

- *Pregnancy:* Some of these medicines can increase blood sugar, blood pressure, and heart rate in the mother, and may increase the heart rate and decrease blood sugar in the infant. Before taking any of these medicines, make sure your doctor knows if you are pregnant or may become pregnant.

  Some of these medicines also relax the muscles of the uterus and may delay labor.

  For albuterol: Albuterol has not been studied in pregnant women. Studies in animals have shown that albuterol causes birth defects when given in doses many times the usual human dose.

Reprinted from *Advice for the Patient: Drug Information in Lay Language, Volume II*; © 2000 Micromedex Thomson Healthcare. Reprinted with permission.

For ephedrine: Ephedrine has not been studied in pregnant women or in animals.

For epinephrine: Epinephrine has been shown to cause birth defects in humans. However, this medicine may be needed during allergic reactions that threaten the mother's life.

For isoproterenol: Studies on birth defects with isoproterenol have not been done in humans. However, there is some evidence that it causes birth defects in animals.

For metaproterenol: Metaproterenol has not been studied in pregnant women. However, studies in animals have shown that metaproterenol causes birth defects and death of the animal fetus when given in doses many times the usual human dose.

For terbutaline: Terbutaline has not been shown to cause birth defects in humans using recommended doses or in animal studies when given in doses many times the usual human dose.

- *Breast feeding:* For albuterol, isoproterenol, and metaproterenol: It is not known whether albuterol, isoproterenol, or metaproterenol passes into breast milk. Although most medicines pass into breast milk in small amounts, many of them may be used safely while breast feeding. Mothers who are taking this medicine and who wish to breast feed should discuss this with their doctor.

  For ephedrine: Ephedrine passes into breast milk and may cause unwanted side effects in babies of mothers using ephedrine.

  For epinephrine: Epinephrine passes into breast milk and may cause unwanted side effects in babies of mothers using epinephrine.

  For terbutaline: Terbutaline passes into breast milk but has not been shown to cause harmful effects in the infant. Mothers who are taking this medicine and who wish to breast-feed should discuss this with their doctor.

- *Children:* There is no specific information comparing use of isoproterenol, metaproterenol, or terbutaline in children with use in other age groups.

  Excitement and nervousness may be more common in children 2 to 6 years of age who take albuterol than in adults and older children.

  Infants and children may be especially sensitive to the effects of epinephrine.

- *Older adults:* Older adults may be more sensitive to the side effects of these medicines, such as trembling, high blood pressure, or fast or irregular heartbeats.

- *Other medicines:* Although certain medicines should not be used together at all, in other cases two different medicines may be used together even if an interaction might occur. In these cases, your doctor may want to change the dose, or other precautions may be necessary. When you are taking adrenergic bronchodilators, it is especially important that your health care professional know if you are taking any of the following:

- *For all adrenergic bronchodilators:* Amphetamines or Appetite suppressants (diet pills) or Medicine for colds, sinus problems, or hay fever or other allergies (including nose drops or sprays) or Other medicines for asthma or other breathing problems— The chance for side effects may be increased

  Beta-adrenergic blocking agents taken orally or by injection (acebutolol [e.g., Sectral], atenolol [e.g., Tenormin], betaxolol [e.g., Kerlone], bisoprolol [e.g., Zebeta], carteolol [e.g., Cartrol], labetalol [e.g., Normodyne], metoprolol [e.g., Lopressor, Toprol XL], nadolol [e.g., Corgard], oxprenolol [e.g., Trasicor], penbutolol [e.g., Levatol], pindolol [e.g., Visken], propranolol [e.g., Inderal], sotalol [e.g., Sotacor], timolol [e.g., Blocadren])— These medicines may prevent the adrenergic bronchodilators from working properly.

  Beta-adrenergic blocking agents used in the eye (betaxolol [e.g., Betoptic], levobunolol [e.g., Betagan], metipranolol [e.g., OptiPranolol], timolol [e.g., Timoptic]—Enough of these medicines may be absorbed from the eye into the blood stream to prevent the adrenergic bronchodilators from working properly.

  Cocaine—Unwanted effects of both medicines on the heart may be increased.

  Digitalis medicines (e.g., Lanoxin) or Quinidine (e.g., Quinaglute Dura-Tabs, Quinidex)—The risk of heart rhythm problems may be increased.

  Monoamine oxidase (MAO) inhibitors (furazolidone [e.g., Furoxone], isocarboxazid [e.g., Marplan], phenelzine [e.g., Nardil], procarbazine [e.g., Matulane], selegiline [e.g., Eldepryl], tranylcypromine [e.g., Parnate])—Taking adrenergic bronchodilators while you are taking or within 2 weeks of taking monoamine oxidase (MAO) inhibitors may dramatically increase the effects of MAO inhibitors.

Thyroid hormones—The effect of this medicine may be increased.

Tricyclic antidepressants (amitriptyline [e.g., Elavil], amoxapine [e.g., Asendin], clomipramine [e.g., Anafranil], desipramine [e.g., Norpramin], doxepin [e.g., Sinequan], imipramine [e.g., Tofranil], nortriptyline [e.g., Aventyl, Pamelor], protriptyline [e.g., Vivactil], trimipramine [e.g., Surmontil])— The effects of these medicines on the heart and blood vessels may be increased.

Other medical problems—The presence of other medical problems may affect the use of these medicines. Make sure you tell your doctor if you have any other medical problems, especially:

- Convulsions (seizures)—These medicines may make this condition worse.

- Diabetes mellitus (sugar diabetes)—These medicines may increase blood sugar, which could change the amount of insulin or other diabetes medicine you need.

- Enlarged prostate—Ephedrine may make the condition worse.

- Gastrointestinal narrowing—Use of the extended-release dosage form of albuterol may result in a blockage in the intestines.

- Glaucoma—Ephedrine or epinephrine may make the condition worse.

- High blood pressure or Overactive thyroid—Use of ephedrine or epinephrine may cause severe high blood pressure and other side effects may also be increased.

- Parkinson's disease—Epinephrine may make stiffness and trembling worse.

- Psychiatric problems—Epinephrine may make problems worse.

- Reduced blood flow to the brain—Epinephrine further decreases blood flow, which could make the problem worse.

- Reduced blood flow to the heart or Heart rhythm problems—These medicines may make these conditions worse.

Proper Use of This Medicine

Use this medicine only as directed. Do not use more of it and do not use it more often than your doctor ordered, do not use more than recommended on the label unless otherwise directed by your doctor. To do so may increase the chance of side effects.

If you are using this medicine for asthma, you should use another medicine that works faster than this one for an asthma attack that has already started. If you do not have another medicine to use for an attack or if you have any questions about this, check with your doctor.

For patients taking albuterol extended-release tablets:

- Swallow the tablet whole.
- Do not crush, break, or chew before swallowing.

For patients using epinephrine injection:

- This medicine is for injection only. If you will be giving yourself the injections, make sure you understand exactly how to give them. If you have any questions about this, check with your health care professional.
- When injected into the muscle (intramuscular) this medicine should be injected into the thigh. It should not be injected into the buttocks.
- Do not use the epinephrine solution or suspension if it turns pinkish to brownish in color or if the solution becomes cloudy.
- Keep this medicine ready for use at all times. Also, keep the telephone numbers for your doctor and the nearest hospital emergency room readily available.
- Check the expiration date on the injection regularly. Replace the medicine before that date.

For patients using epinephrine injection for an allergic reaction emergency:

- If a severe allergic reaction occurs, use the epinephrine injection immediately.
- After using the epinephrine injection, notify your doctor immediately or go to the nearest hospital emergency room. Be sure to tell your doctor that you have used the epinephrine injection.

- If you have been stung by an insect, remove the insect's stinger with your fingernails, if possible. Be careful not to squeeze, pinch, or push it deeper into the skin. Ice packs or sodium bicarbonate (baking soda) soaks, if available, may then be applied to the area stung.

If you are using the epinephrine auto-injector (automatic injection device):

- The epinephrine auto-injector comes with patient directions. Read them carefully before you actually need to use this medicine. Then, when an emergency arises, you will know how to inject the epinephrine.

- It is important that you do not remove the safety cap on the auto-injector until you are ready to use it. This prevents accidental activation of the device during storage and handling.

To use the epinephrine auto-injector:

- Remove the gray safety cap.
- Place the black tip on the thigh, at a right angle (90-degree angle) to the leg.
- Press hard into the thigh until the auto-injector functions. Hold in place for several seconds. Then remove the auto-injector and discard.
- Massage the injection area for 10 seconds.

Dosing

The dose of these medicines will be different for different patients. Follow your doctor's orders or the directions on the label. The following information includes only the average doses of these medicines. If your dose is different, do not change it unless your doctor tells you to do so.

The number of capsules or tablets or teaspoonfuls of solution or syrup that you take, or the amount of injection that you use, depends on the strength of the medicine. Also, the number of doses you take each day, the time allowed between doses, and the length of time you take the medicine depend on the medical problem for which you are taking it.

For Albuterol

For symptoms of asthma, chronic bronchitis, emphysema, or other lung disease:

- For oral dosage form (solution):

  Adults and children 12 years of age and older—2 to 4 milligrams (mg) (1 to 2 teaspoonfuls) three or four times a day.

  Children 6 to 12 years of age—2 mg (1 teaspoonful) three or four times a day.

  Children 2 to 6 years of age—Dose is based on body weight and must be determined by your doctor. The usual dose is 0.1 mg per kg (0.045 mg per pound) of body weight up to a maximum dose of 2 mg (1 teaspoonful) three or four times a day.

  Children up to 2 years of age—Use and dose must be determined by your doctor.

- For oral dosage form (syrup):

  Adults and children 14 years of age and older—2 to 4 mg (1 to 2 teaspoonfuls) three or four times a day. Then your doctor may increase your dose, if needed.

  Children 6 to 14 years of age—At first, 2 mg (1 teaspoonful) of albuterol three or four times a day. Then your doctor may increase your dose, if needed.

  Children 2 to 6 years of age—Dose is based on body weight and must be determined by your doctor. The usual dose is 0.1 mg per kg (0.045 mg per pound) of body weight up to a maximum dose of 2 mg (1 teaspoonful) three or four times a day.

  Children up to 2 years of age—Use and dose must be determined by your doctor.

- For oral dosage form (tablets):

  Adults and children 12 years of age and older—At first, 2 to 4 mg three or four times a day. Then your doctor may increase your dose, if needed.

  Children 6 to 12 years of age—2 mg three or four times a day.

  Children up to 6 years of age—Use and dose must be determined by your doctor.

- For oral dosage form (extended-release tablets):

  Adults and children 12 years of age and older—4 to 8 mg every twelve hours.

Children 6 to 12 years of age—4 mg every twelve hours.

Children up to 6 years of age—Use and dose must be determined by your doctor.

- For injection dosage form: Dose is usually based on body weight and must be determined by your doctor. Depending on your condition, this medicine is injected into either a muscle or vein or injected slowly into a vein over a period of time.

For Epinephrine

For injection dosage form:

- For allergic reactions:

  Adults—At first, 300 to 500 micrograms (mcg) (0.3 to 0.5 mg) injected into a muscle or under the skin. Then the dose may be repeated, if needed, every ten to twenty minutes for up to three doses. In some cases, it may be necessary for 100 to 250 mcg to be injected slowly into a vein by your doctor instead of injecting the dose into a muscle or under the skin.

  Children—Dose is based on body weight and must be determined by your doctor. The usual dose is 10 mcg per kg (4.5 mcg per pound) of body weight, up to 300 mcg (0.3 mg) a dose, injected into a muscle or under the skin. The dose may be repeated, if needed, every fifteen minutes for up to three doses.

- For symptoms of bronchial asthma, chronic bronchitis or other lung disease:

  Adults—Dose is based on body weight and must be determined by your doctor. The usual dose is 10 mcg per kg (4.5 mcg per pound) of body weight, up to 300 to 500 mcg (0.3 to 0.5 mg) a dose, injected under the skin. The dose may be repeated, if needed, every twenty minutes for up to three doses.

  Children—Dose is based on body weight and must be determined by your doctor. The usual dose is 10 mcg per kg (4.5 mcg per pound) of body weight, up to 300 mcg (0.3 mg) a dose, injected under the skin. The dose may be repeated, if needed, every fifteen minutes for three or four doses or every four hours.

For Isoproterenol

For injection dosage form:

- For symptoms of asthma, chronic bronchitis, emphysema, or other lung disease: Isoproterenol is given by intravenous injection in a doctor's office or hospital.

For Metaproterenol

For oral dosage forms (syrup or tablets):

- For symptoms of asthma, chronic bronchitis, emphysema, or other lung disease:

  Adults and children 9 years of age and older or weighing 27 kilograms (kg) (59 pounds) or more—20 milligrams (mg) three or four times a day.

  Children 6 to 9 years of age or weighing up to 27 kg (59 pounds)—10 mg three or four times a day.

  Children up to 6 years of age—Dose must be determined by your doctor.

For Terbutaline

For symptoms of asthma, chronic bronchitis, emphysema, or other lung disease:

- For oral dosage form (tablets):

  Adults and adolescents 15 years of age and older—5 milligrams (mg) three times a day. The medicine may be taken about every six hours while you are awake, until three doses have been taken.

  Children 12 to 15 years of age—2.5 mg three times a day, taken about every six hours.

  Children 6 to 11 years of age—Dose is based on body weight and must be determined by your doctor.

  Children up to 6 years of age—Use and dose must be determined by your doctor.

- For injection dosage form:

  Adults and children 12 years of age or older—250 micrograms (mcg) injected under the skin. The dose may be repeated after fifteen to thirty minutes, if needed. However, not more than 500 mcg should be taken within a four-hour period.

Children 6 to 12 years of age—Dose is based on body weight and must be determined by your doctor. The usual dose is 5 to 10 mcg per kg (2.3 to 4.5 mcg per pound) of body weight injected under the skin. The dose may be repeated after fifteen to twenty minutes for up to a total of three doses.

Children up to 6 years of age—Use and dose must be determined by your doctor.

Missed Dose

If you are using this medicine regularly and you miss a dose, use it as soon as possible. Then use any remaining doses for that day at regularly spaced intervals. Do not double doses.

To Store This Medicine

- Keep out of the reach of children.
- Store away from heat and direct light.
- Do not store the capsule or tablet form of this medicine in the bathroom, near the kitchen sink, or in other damp places. Heat or moisture may cause the medicine to break down.
- Keep the injection or syrup form of this medicine from freezing.
- Do not keep outdated medicine or medicine no longer needed. Be sure that any discarded medicine is out of the reach of children.

Precautions While Using This Medicine

It is important that your doctor check your progress at regular visits to make sure that this medicine is working properly and to check for unwanted effects.

Do not take other medicines unless they have been discussed with your doctor. This especially includes over-the-counter (nonprescription) medicines for appetite control, asthma, colds, cough, hay fever, or sinus problems, since they could increase the unwanted effects of this medicine.

For patients with diabetes

- This medicine may cause your blood sugar levels to rise, which could change the amount of insulin or diabetes medicine that you need to take.

For patients taking this medicine for asthma

- If you still have trouble breathing or if your condition becomes worse (for example, if you have to use an inhaler more frequently to relieve asthma attacks), check with your doctor right away.

For patients who are using epinephrine injection

- Because epinephrine reduces blood flow to the area where it is injected, it is possible that it could cause damage to the tissues if it is injected in one spot too often. Check with your doctor right away if you notice severe pain at the place of injection.

For patients who are using the epinephrine auto-injector

- Do not inject this medicine into your hands or feet. There is already less blood flow to the hands and feet, and epinephrine could make that worse and cause damage to these tissues. If you accidentally inject epinephrine into your hands or feet, check with your doctor or go to the hospital emergency room right away.

Side Effects of This Medicine

Along with its needed effects, a medicine may cause some unwanted effects. Although not all of these side effects may occur, if they do occur they may need medical attention.

Check with your doctor immediately if any of the following side effects occur:

- **Rare:** Possible signs of an allergic reaction; hoarseness; large hive-like swellings on eyelids, face, genitals, hands or feet, lips, throat, tongue; sudden trouble in swallowing or breathing; tightness in throat

  Possible signs of a severe reaction that has occurred in children taking albuterol by mouth; Bleeding or crusting sores on lips; chest pain; chills; fever; general feeling of illness; muscle cramps or pain; nausea; painful eyes; painful sores, ulcers, or white spots in mouth or on lips; red or irritated eyes; skin rash or sores, hives, and/or itching; sore throat; vomiting

Check with your doctor as soon as possible if any of the following side effects occur:

- **More common:** Fast heartbeat; irregular heartbeat

- **Rare:** Chest pain; convulsions (seizures); fainting (with isoproterenol); hives; increase in blood pressure (more common with ephedrine or epinephrine); mental problems; muscle cramps or pain; nausea or vomiting; trouble in urinating; unusual tiredness or weakness

Other side effects may occur that usually do not need medical attention. These side effects may go away during treatment as your body adjusts to the medicine. However, check with your doctor if any of the following side effects continue or are bothersome:

- **More common:** Anxiety (with epinephrine); headache; nervousness; tremor

- **Less common:** Dizziness; feeling of constant movement of self or surroundings; sweating; trouble in sleeping

Although not all of the side effects listed above have been reported for each of these medicines, they have been reported for at least one of them. All of these medicines are similar, so many of the above side effects may occur with any of the medicines.

Other side effects not listed above may also occur in some patients. If you notice any other effects, check with your doctor.

Additional Information

Once a medicine has been approved for marketing for a certain use, experience may show that it is also useful for other medical problems. Although these uses are not included in product labeling, some of the adrenergic bronchodilators are used in certain patients with the following medical conditions:

- Premature labor (terbutaline)

- Bleeding of gums and teeth during dental procedures (epinephrine)

- Priapism (prolonged abnormal erection of penis) (epinephrine)

Other than the above information, there is no additional information relating to proper use, precautions, or side effects for these uses.

Some Commonly Used Brand Names

In the U.S.

- Adrenalin
- Alupent
- Ana-Guard
- Brethine
- Bricanyl

- EpiPen Auto-Injector
- EpiPen Jr. Auto-Injector
- Isuprel

- Proventil
- Proventil Repetabs
- Ventolin
- Volmax

In Canada

- Adrenalin
- Alupent
- Bricanyl

- EpiPen Auto-Injector
- EpiPen Jr. Auto-Injector

- Isuprel
- Ventolin

Other commonly used names are:

- Adrenaline
- Salbutamol
- Orciprenaline

Description

Adrenergic bronchodilators are medicines that stimulate the nerves in many parts of the body, causing different effects.

Because these medicines open up the bronchial tubes (air passages) of the lungs, they are used to treat the symptoms of asthma, bronchitis, emphysema, and other lung diseases. They relieve cough, wheezing, shortness of breath, and troubled breathing by increasing the flow of air through the bronchial tubes.

Epinephrine injection (including the auto-injector but not the sterile suspension) is used in the emergency treatment of allergic reactions to insect stings, medicines, foods, or other substances. It relieves skin rash, hives, and itching; wheezing; and swelling of the lips, eyelids, tongue, and inside of the nose.

These medicines may be also used for other conditions as determined by your doctor.

Ephedrine capsules are available without a prescription. However, check with your doctor before taking ephedrine.

All of the other adrenergic bronchodilators are available only with your doctor's prescription.

These medicines are available in the following dosage forms:

Oral

- Albuterol
  Oral solution (Canada)
  Syrup (U.S.)
  Tablets (U.S.)
  Extended-release tablets (U.S.)

- Ephedrine
  Capsules (U.S.)

- Metaproterenol
  Syrup (U.S. and Canada)
  Tablets (U.S. and Canada)

- Terbutaline
  Tablets (U.S. and Canada)

Parenteral

- Albuterol
  Injection (Canada)

- Ephedrine
  Injection (U.S. and Canada)

- Epinephrine
  Injection (U.S. and Canada)

- Isoproterenol
  Injection (U.S. and Canada)

- Terbutaline
  Injection (U.S.)

Chapter 63

Antihistamines and Decongestants

If you are taking this medicine without a prescription, carefully read and follow any precautions on the label. For antihistamine and decongestant combinations, the following should be considered:

- *Allergies:* Tell your doctor if you have ever had any unusual or allergic reaction to antihistamines or to amphetamine, dextro-amphetamine (e.g., Dexedrine), ephedrine (e.g., Ephed II), epinephrine (e.g., Adrenalin), isoproterenol (e.g., Isuprel), metaproterenol (e.g., Alupent), methamphetamine (e.g., Desoxyn), norepinephrine (e.g., Levophed), phenylephrine (e.g., Neo-Synephrine), pseudoephedrine (e.g., Sudafed), PPA (e.g., Dexatrim), or terbutaline (e.g., Brethine).

- *Diet:* It is very important that you do not take terfenadine-containing medicines (e.g., Seldane-D) with grapefruit juice. Studies have shown that taking terfenadine and grapefruit juice may cause heart rhythm problems.

- *Pregnancy:* The occasional use of antihistamine and decongestant combinations is not likely to cause problems in the fetus or in the newborn baby. However, when these medicines are used at higher doses and/or for a long time, the chance that problems might occur may increase. For the individual ingredients of these combinations, the following apply:

Reprinted from *Advice for the Patient: Drug Information in Lay Language, Volume II*; © 2000 Micromedex Thomson Healthcare. Reprinted with permission.

Alcohol: Some of these combination medicines contain alcohol. Too much use of alcohol during pregnancy may cause birth defects.

Antihistamines: Antihistamines have not been shown to cause problems in humans.

Phenylephrine: Studies on birth defects have not been done in either humans or animals with phenylephrine.

Phenylpropanolamine: Studies on birth defects have not been done in either humans or animals with phenylpropanolamine. However, it seems that women who take phenylpropanolamine in the weeks following delivery are more likely to suffer mental or mood changes.

Promethazine: Phenothiazines, such as promethazine (contained in some of these combination medicines [e.g., Phenergan-D]), have been shown to cause jaundice and muscle tremors in a few newborn infants whose mothers received phenothiazines during pregnancy. Also, the newborn baby may have blood clotting problems if promethazine is taken by the mother within 2 weeks before delivery.

Pseudoephedrine: Studies on birth defects with pseudoephedrine have not been done in humans. In animal studies pseudoephedrine did not cause birth defects but did cause a decrease in average weight, length, and rate of bone formation in the animal fetus when administered in high doses.

- *Breast-feeding:* Small amounts of antihistamines and decongestants pass into the breast milk. Use is not recommended since the chances are greater for this medicine to cause side effects, such as unusual excitement or irritability, in the nursing baby. Also, since antihistamines tend to decrease the secretions of the body, it is possible that the flow of breast milk may be reduced in some patients. It is not known yet whether loratadine or terfenadine causes these same side effects.

- *Children:* Very young children are usually more sensitive to the effects of this medicine. Increases in blood pressure, nightmares or unusual excitement, nervousness, restlessness, or irritability may be more likely to occur in children. Also, mental changes may be more likely to occur in young children taking combination medicines that contain phenylpropanolamine. Before giving any of these combination medicines to a child, check the package label very carefully. Some of these medicines are too strong for use in children. If you are not certain whether a specific product can be given to a child, or if you have any questions about the amount to give, check with your health care professional.

- *Older adults:* Confusion, difficult and painful urination, dizziness, drowsiness, dryness of mouth, or convulsions (seizures) may be more likely to occur in the elderly, who are usually more sensitive to the effects of this medicine. Also, nightmares or unusual excitement, nervousness, restlessness, or irritability may be more likely to occur in elderly patients.

- *Other medicines:* Although certain medicines should not be used together at all, in other cases different medicines may be used together even if an interaction might occur. In these cases, your doctor may want to change the dose, or other precautions may be necessary. When you are taking antihistamines it is especially important that your health care professional know if you are taking any of the following:

  Anticholinergics (medicine for abdominal or stomach spasms or cramps)—Side effects, such as dryness of mouth, of antihistamines or anticholinergics may be more likely to occur.

  Azithromycin (e.g., Zithromax) or Clarithromycin (e.g., Biaxin) or Erythromycin (e.g., E-Mycin) or Itraconazole (e.g., Sporanox) or Ketoconazole (e.g., Nizoral)—Use of these medicines with the terfenadine-containing combination may cause heart problems, such as an irregular heartbeat; these medicines should not be used together

  Central nervous system (CNS) depressants—Effects, such as drowsiness, of CNS depressants or antihistamines may be worsened.

  Cisapride (e.g., Propulsid) or HIV protease inhibitors (indinavir [e.g., Crixivan], nelfinavir [e.g., Viracept], ritonavir [e.g., Norvir], saquinavir [e.g., Invirase]) or Mibefradil (e.g., Posicor) or Serotonin reuptake inhibitors (fluvoxamine [e.g., Luvox], nefazodone [e.g., Serzone], sertraline [e.g., Zoloft]) or Sparfloxacin (e.g., Zagam) or Zileuton (e.g., Zyflo)—Use of these medicines with terfenadine may cause heart problems; these medicines should not be used with terfenadine.

  Maprotiline (e.g., Ludiomil) or Tricyclic antidepressants (amitriptyline [e.g., Elavil], amoxapine [e.g., Asendin], clomipramine [e.g., Anafranil], desipramine [e.g., Pertofrane], doxepin [e.g.,

Sinequan], imipramine [e.g., Tofranil], nortriptyline [e.g., Aventyl], protriptyline [e.g., Vivactil], trimipramine [e.g., Surmontil])—Effects, such as drowsiness, of CNS depressants or antihistamines may be worsened; also, taking these medicines together may cause some of their side effects, such as dryness of mouth, to become more severe.

Monoamine oxidase (MAO) inhibitors (furazolidone [e.g., Furoxone], isocarboxazid [e.g., Marplan], phenelzine [e.g., Nardil], procarbazine [e.g., Matulane], selegiline [e.g., Eldepryl], tranylcypromine [e.g., Parnate])—If you are now taking, or have taken within the past 2 weeks, any of the MAO inhibitors, the side effects of the antihistamines may become more severe; these medicines should not be used together.

Rauwolfia alkaloids (alseroxylon [e.g., Rauwiloid], deserpidine [e.g., Harmonyl], rauwolfia serpentina [e.g., Raudixin], reserpine [e.g., Serpasil])—These medicines may increase or decrease the effect of the decongestant.

Also, if you are taking one of the combinations containing phenylpropanolamine or pseudoephedrine and are also taking:

- Amantadine (e.g., Symmetrel) or Amphetamines or Appetite suppressants (diet pills), except fenfluramine (e.g., Pondimin) or Caffeine (e.g., NoDoz) or Chlophedianol (e.g., Ulone) or Medicine for asthma or other breathing problems or Medicine for colds, sinus problems, or hay fever or other allergies (including nose drops or sprays) or Methylphenidate (e.g., Ritalin) or Nabilone (e.g., Cesamet) or Pemoline (e.g., Cylert)—Using any of these medicines together with an antihistamine and decongestant combination may cause excessive stimulant side effects, such as difficulty in sleeping, heart rate problems, nervousness, and irritability.

- Beta-adrenergic blocking agents (acebutolol [e.g., Sectral], atenolol [e.g., Tenormin], betaxolol [e.g., Kerlone], bisoprolol [e.g., Zebeta], carteolol [e.g., Cartrol], labetalol [e.g., Normodyne], metoprolol [e.g., Lopressor], nadolol [e.g., Corgard], oxprenolol [e.g., Trasicor], penbutolol [e.g., Levatol], pindolol [e.g., Visken], propranolol [e.g., Inderal], sotalol [e.g., Sotacor], timolol [e.g., Blocadren])—Using any of these medicines together with an antihistamine and decongestant combination may cause high blood pressure and heart problems (e.g., unusually slow heartbeat).

- Other medical problems—The presence of other medical problems may affect the use of antihistamine and decongestant combinations. Make sure you tell your doctor if you have any other medical problems, especially:

Diabetes mellitus (sugar diabetes)—The decongestant in this medicine may put diabetic patients at a greater risk of having heart or blood vessel disease.

Enlarged prostate or Urinary tract blockage or difficult urination—Some of the effects of antihistamines may make urinary problems worse.

Glaucoma—A slight increase in inner eye pressure may occur.

Heart or blood vessel disease or High blood pressure—The decongestant in this medicine may cause the blood pressure to increase and may also speed up the heart rate.

Kidney disease—Higher blood levels of loratadine may result, which may increase the chance of side effects. The dosage of loratadine-containing combination may need to be reduced.

Liver disease—Higher blood levels of terfenadine may result, which may increase the chance of heart problems (for terfenadine-containing combination only; higher blood levels of loratadine may result, which may increase the chance of side effects).

Overactive thyroid—If the overactive thyroid has caused a fast heart rate, the decongestant in this medicine may cause the heart rate to speed up further.

Proper Use of This Medicine

Take this medicine only as directed. Do not take more of it and do not take it more often than recommended on the label, unless otherwise directed by your doctor. To do so may increase the chance of side effects.

If this medicine irritates your stomach, you may take it with food or a glass of water or milk, to lessen the irritation.

For patients taking the extended-release capsule or tablet form of this medicine:

- Swallow it whole.

- Do not crush, break, or chew before swallowing.

- If the capsule is too large to swallow, you may mix the contents of the capsule with applesauce, jelly, honey, or syrup and swallow without chewing.

Dosing

There is a large variety of antihistamine and decongestant combination products on the market. Some products are for use in adults only, while others may be used in children. If you have any questions about this, check with your health care professional.

The dose of antihistamines and decongestants will be different for different products. The number of capsules or tablets or teaspoonfuls of liquid or granules that you take depends on the strengths of the medicines. Also, the number of doses you take each day and the time between doses depend on whether you are taking a short-acting or long-acting form of antihistamine and decongestant. Follow your doctor's orders if this medicine was prescribed. Or, follow the directions on the box if you are buying this medicine without a prescription.

Missed Dose

If you are taking this medicine regularly and you miss a dose, take it as soon as possible. However, if it is almost time for your next dose, skip the missed dose and go back to your regular dosing schedule. Do not double doses.

To Store This Medicine

- Keep out of the reach of children.
- Store away from heat and direct light.
- Do not store in the bathroom, near the kitchen sink, or in other damp places. Heat or moisture may cause the medicine to break down.
- Keep the liquid form of this medicine from freezing.
- Do not keep outdated medicine or medicine no longer needed. Be sure that any discarded medicine is out of the reach of children.

Precautions While Using This Medicine

Before you have any skin tests for allergies, tell the doctor in charge that you are taking this medicine. The results of the test may be affected by the antihistamine in this medicine.

When taking antihistamines (contained in this combination medicine) on a regular basis, make sure your doctor knows if you are taking large amounts of aspirin at the same time (as for arthritis or rheumatism). Effects of too much aspirin, such as ringing in the ears, may be covered up by the antihistamine.

Terfenadine-containing combination should not be taken with clarithromycin (e.g., Biaxin), erythromycin (e.g., E-Mycin), itraconazole (e.g., Sporanox), ketoconazole (e.g., Nizoral), or mibefradil (e.g., Posicor). Using these medicines together may increase the risk of serious side effects affecting the heart.

The antihistamine in this medicine will add to the effects of alcohol and other CNS depressants (medicines that slow down the nervous system, possibly causing drowsiness). Some examples of CNS depressants are other antihistamines or medicine for hay fever, other allergies, or colds; sedatives, tranquilizers, or sleeping medicine; prescription pain medicine or narcotics; barbiturates; medicine for seizures; muscle relaxants; or anesthetics, including some dental anesthetics. Check with your doctor before taking any of the above while you are taking this medicine.

The antihistamine in this medicine may cause some people to become drowsy, dizzy, or less alert than they are normally. Some antihistamines are more likely to cause drowsiness than others (loratadine and terfenadine, for example, rarely produce this effect). Make sure you know how you react before you drive, use machines, or do anything else that could be dangerous if you are dizzy or are not alert.

The decongestant in this medicine may add to the central nervous system (CNS) stimulant and other effects of phenylpropanolamine (PPA)-containing diet aids. Do not use medicines for diet or appetite control while taking this medicine unless you have checked with your doctor.

The decongestant in this medicine may cause some people to be nervous or restless or to have trouble in sleeping. If you have trouble in sleeping, take the last dose of this medicine for each day a few hours before bedtime. If you have any questions about this, check with your doctor.

Antihistamines may cause dryness of the mouth, nose, and throat. Some antihistamines are more likely to cause dryness of the mouth than others (loratadine and terfenadine, for example, rarely produce this effect). For temporary relief, use sugarless candy or gum, melt bits of ice in your mouth, or use a saliva substitute. However, if your mouth continues to feel dry for more than 2 weeks, check with your dentist. Continuing dryness of the mouth may increase the chance of dental disease, including tooth decay, gum disease, and fungus infections.

For patients using promethazine-containing medicine

- This medicine controls nausea and vomiting. For this reason, it may cover up the signs of overdose caused by other medicines or the symptoms of intestinal blockage. This will make it difficult for your doctor to diagnose these conditions. Make sure your doctor knows that you are taking this medicine if you have other symptoms such as stomach or lower abdominal pain, cramping, or soreness. Also, if you think you may have taken an overdose of any medicine, tell your doctor that you are taking this medicine.

Side Effects of This Medicine

Along with its needed effects, a medicine may cause some unwanted effects. Although serious side effects occur rarely when this medicine is taken as recommended, they may be more likely to occur if:

- too much medicine is taken
- it is taken in large doses
- it is taken for a long period of time

Get emergency help immediately if any of the following symptoms of overdose occur

- Clumsiness or unsteadiness; convulsions (seizures); drowsiness (severe); dryness of mouth, nose, or throat (severe); flushing or redness of face; hallucinations (seeing, hearing, or feeling things that are not there); headache (continuing); shortness of breath or troubled breathing; slow, fast, or irregular heartbeat; trouble in sleeping

For promethazine only

- Muscle spasms (especially of neck and back); restlessness; shuffling walk; tic-like (jerky) movements of head and face; trembling and shaking of hands.

Also, check with your doctor as soon as possible if any of the following side effects occur:

- **Rare:** Mood or mental changes; sore throat and fever; tightness in chest; unusual bleeding or bruising; unusual tiredness or weakness.

Other side effects may occur that usually do not need medical attention. These side effects may go away during treatment as your body adjusts to the medicine. However, check with your health care professional if any of the following side effects continue or are bothersome:

- **More common** (rare with loratadine or terfenadine-containing combination): Drowsiness; thickening of the bronchial secretions

- **Less common** (more common with high doses): Blurred vision; confusion; difficult or painful urination; dizziness; dryness of mouth, nose, or throat; headache; loss of appetite; nightmares; pounding heartbeat; ringing or buzzing in ears; skin rash; stomach upset or pain (more common with pyrilamine and tripelennamine); unusual excitement, nervousness, restlessness, or irritability.

Other side effects not listed may also occur in some patients. If you notice any other effects, check with your doctor.

Some Commonly Used Brand Names

In the U.S

- Actagen
- Actifed
- Actifed Allergy Nighttime Caplets
- Alcomed
- Allent
- Allercon
- Allerest Maximum Strength
- Allerfrim
- Allerphed
- Amilon
- Anamine
- Anamine T.D.
- Andec
- Andec-TR
- Aprodrine
- A.R.M. Maximum Strength Caplets
- Atrofed
- Atrohist Pediatric
- Atrohist Pediatric Suspension Dye Free
- Banophen
- Benadryl Allergy Decongestant Liquid Medication
- Biohist-LA
- Brexin L.A.
- Brofed Liquid
- Bromadrine PD
- Bromadrine TR
- Bromaline
- Bromanate
- Bromatapp
- Bromfed
- Bromfed-PD
- Bromfenex
- Bromfenex PD
- Bromophen T.D.
- Brompheril
- Carbiset
- Carbiset-TR
- Carbodec
- Carbodec TR
- Cardec
- Cardec-S
- Cenafed Plus

- Chemdec
- C-Hist-SR
- Chlorafed
- Chlorafed H.S. Timecelles
- Chlorafed Timecelles
- Chlordrine S.R.
- Chlorfed
- Chlorfed II
- Chlorphedrine SR
- Chlor-Rest
- Chlortox
- Chlor-Trimeton 4 Hour Relief
- Chlor-Trimeton 12 Hour Relief
- Chlor-Trimeton Allergy-D 12 Hour
- Claritin-D 12 Hour
- Claritin-D 24 Hour
- Codimal-L.A.
- Codimal-L.A. Half
- Cold and Allergy
- Cold-Gest Cold
- Colfed-A
- Comhist
- Comhist LA
- Contac 12-Hour
- Contac Maximum Strength 12-Hour Caplets
- Cophene No. 2
- Co-Pyronil 2
- CP Oral
- Dallergy Jr
- Deconamine
- Deconamine SR
- Decongestabs
- Deconomed SR
- Delhistine D
- Demazin
- Demazin Repetabs
- Dexaphen SA
- Dexophed
- Dimaphen
- Dimaphen S.A.
- Dimetane Decongestant
- Dimetane Decongestant Caplets
- Dimetapp
- Dimetapp Cold and Allergy
- Dimetapp Cold & Allergy Quick Dissolve
- Dimetapp Extentabs
- Dimetapp 4-Hour
- Disobrom
- Disophrol Chronotabs
- Dorcol Children's Cold Formula
- Drixomed
- Drixoral Cold and Allergy
- Drize
- Duralex
- Dura-Tap PD
- Dura-Vent/A
- Ed A-Hist
- Endafed
- E.N.T.
- Fedahist
- Fedahist Gyrocaps
- Fedahist Timecaps
- Genac
- Genamin
- Genatap
- Gencold
- Hayfebrol
- Histalet
- Histalet Forte
- Histatab Plus
- Histatan
- Hista-Vadrin
- Histor-D
- Iofed
- Iofed PD
- Iohist-D
- Klerist-D
- Kronofed-A Jr. Kronocaps
- Kronofed-A Kronocaps
- Linhist-L.A.
- Liqui-Histine-D
- Liqui-Minic Infant Drops
- Lodrane LD
- Lodrane Liquid
- Med-Hist
- Metahistine D
- M-Hist
- Mooredec
- Myphetapp
- Nalda-Relief Pediatric Drops
- Naldecon
- Naldecon Pediatric Drops
- Naldecon Pediatric Syrup
- Naldelate
- Naldelate Pediatric Drops

- Naldelate Pediatric Syrup
- Nalex-A
- Nalfed
- Nalfed-PD
- Nalgest
- Nalgest Pediatric
- Nalphen
- Nalphen Pediatric
- ND Clear T.D.
- Nolamine
- Novafed A
- Novahistine
- Ornade Spansules
- PediaCare Cold-Allergy
- PediaCare Cold Formula
- Phenergan VC
- Pherazine VC
- Poly D
- Poly-D
- Poly Hist Forte
- Poly-Histine-D
- Poly-Histine-D Ped
- Promethazine VC
- Prometh VC Plain
- Prop-a-Hist
- Pseudo-Chlor
- Pseudo-gest Plus
- Q-Hist LA
- Resaid S.R.
- Rescon
- Rescon-ED
- Rescon JR
- Respahist

- Rhinatate
- Rhinolar-EX
- Rhinosyn
- Rhinosyn-PD
- Ricobid
- Ricobid Pediatric
- Rinade B.I.D.
- Rolatuss Plain
- Rondamine
- Rondec
- Rondec Chewable
- Rondec Drops
- Rondec-TR
- R-Tannamine
- R-Tannamine Pediatric
- R-Tannate
- R-Tannate Pediatric
- Ru-Tuss
- Ryna
- Rynatan
- Rynatan Pediatric
- Rynatan-S Pediatric
- Seldane-D
- Semprex-D
- Shellcap
- Shellcap PD
- Silafed
- Silaminic
- Sinucon
- Sinucon Pediatric Drops
- Sudafed Plus
- Tamine S.R.
- Tanafed
- Tanoral
- Tavist-D

- Teldrin 12 Hour Allergy Relief
- Temazin Cold
- Touro A&H
- Triaminic
- Triaminic-12
- Triaminic Allergy
- Triaminic Chewables
- Triaminic Cold
- Triaminic Oral Infant Drops
- Triaminic TR
- Trihist-D
- Trinalin Repetabs
- Tri-Nefrin Extra Strength
- Triofed
- Triotann
- Triotann Pediatric
- Triotann-S Pediatric
- Tri-Phen-Chlor
- Tri-Phen-Chlor Pediatric
- Tri-Phen-Chlor T.R.
- Tri-Phen-Mine Pediatric Drops
- Tri-Phen-Mine Pediatric Syrup
- Tri-Phen-Mine S.R. 14
- Triphenyl
- Triposed
- Tritan
- Tri-Tannate
- Tri-Tannate Pediatric

- ULTRAbrom
- ULTRAbrom PD
- Uni-Decon
- Uni-Multihist D
- Vanex Forte Caplets

- Vicks Children's DayQuil Allergy Relief
- Vicks DayQuil 4 Hour Allergy Relief

- Vicks DayQuil 12 Hour Allergy Relief
- West-Decon

In Canada

- Actifed
- Chlor-Tripolon Decongestant
- Chlor-Tripolon N.D.
- Claritin Extra
- Coricidin D Long Acting
- Corsym
- Dimetapp

- Dimetapp Chewables
- Dimetapp Clear
- Dimetapp Extentabs
- Dimetapp Liqui-Fills
- Dimetapp Oral Infant Drops
- Drixoral
- Drixoral Night

- Drixtab
- Neo Citran A
- Novahistex
- Ornade
- Ornade-A.F.
- Ornade Spansules
- Triaminic
- Trinalin Repetabs
- Vasofrinic

Note: Seldane-D (terfenadine and pseudoephedrine) was withdrawn from the U.S. market by the Food and Drug Administration in February 1998.

Description

Antihistamine and decongestant combinations are used to treat the nasal congestion (stuffy nose), sneezing, and runny nose caused by colds and hay fever.

Antihistamines work by preventing the effects of a substance called histamine, which is produced by the body. Histamine can cause itching, sneezing, runny nose, and watery eyes. Antihistamines contained in these combinations are:

- acrivastine, azatadine, brompheniramine, carbinoxamine, chlorpheniramine, clemastine, dexbrompheniramine, diphenhydramine, loratadine, pheniramine, phenyltoloxamine, promethazine, pyrilamine, terfenadine, and triprolidine.

The decongestants, such as phenylephrine, phenylpropanolamine (also known as PPA), and pseudoephedrine, produce a narrowing of blood vessels. This leads to clearing of nasal congestion, but it may also cause an increase in blood pressure in patients who have high blood pressure.

Some of these combinations are available only with your doctor's prescription. Others are available without a prescription; however, your doctor may have special instructions on the proper dose of the medicine for your medical condition. They are available in the following dosage forms:

Oral

- Acrivastine and Pseudoephedrine
      Capsules (U.S.)

- Azatadine and Pseudoephedrine
      Extended-release tablets (U.S. and Canada)

- Brompheniramine and Phenylephrine
      Elixir (U.S.)
      Tablets (U.S.)

- Brompheniramine, Phenylephrine, and Phenylpropanolamine
      Elixir (U.S. and Canada)
      Oral solution (Canada)
      Tablets (Canada)
      Extended-release tablets (U.S. and Canada)

- Brompheniramine and Phenylpropanolamine
      Capsules (Canada)
      Elixir (U.S.)
      Oral solution (U.S. and Canada)
      Tablets (U.S.)
      Chewable tablets (U.S. and Canada)
      Extended-release tablets (U.S.)

- Brompheniramine and Pseudoephedrine
      Extended-release capsules (U.S.)
      Oral solution (U.S.)
      Syrup (U.S.)
      Tablets (U.S.)
      Chewable tablets (U.S.)

- Carbinoxamine and Pseudoephedrine
    Oral solution (U.S.)
    Syrup (U.S.)
    Tablets (U.S.)
    Extended-release tablets (U.S.)

- Chlorpheniramine, Phenindamine, and Phenylpropanolamine
    Extended-release tablets (U.S.)

- Chlorpheniramine and Phenylephrine
    Elixir (U.S.)
    Oral solution (U.S.)
    Oral suspension (U.S.)
    Syrup (U.S.)
    Tablets (U.S.)
    Extended-release tablets (U.S.)

- Chlorpheniramine, Phenylephrine, and Phenylpropanolamine
    Tablets (U.S.)

- Chlorpheniramine and Phenylpropanolamine
    Extended-release capsules (U.S. and Canada)
    Oral solution (U.S. and Canada)
    Extended-release oral suspension (Canada)
    Syrup (U.S. and Canada)
    Tablets (U.S.)
    Extended-release tablets (U.S. and Canada)

- Chlorpheniramine, Phenyltoloxamine, and Phenylephrine
    Extended-release capsules (U.S.)
    Tablets (U.S.)
    Extended-release tablets (U.S.)

- Chlorpheniramine, Phenyltoloxamine, Phenylephrine, and Phenylpropanolamine
    Oral solution (U.S.)
    Syrup (U.S.)
    Extended-release tablets (U.S.)

- Chlorpheniramine and Pseudoephedrine
    Capsules (U.S.)
    Extended-release capsules (U.S. and Canada)

Oral solution (U.S. and Canada)
Oral suspension (U.S.)
Syrup (U.S.)
Tablets (U.S.)
Chewable tablets (U.S.)
Extended-release tablets (U.S.)

- Chlorpheniramine, Pyrilamine, and Phenylephrine
  Oral suspension (U.S.)
  Tablets (U.S.)

- Chlorpheniramine, Pyrilamine, Phenylephrine, and Phenylpro-
  panolamine
  Tablets (U.S.)
  Extended-release tablets (U.S.)

- Clemastine and Phenylpropanolamine
  Extended-release tablets (U.S. and Canada)

- Dexbrompheniramine and Pseudoephedrine
  Tablets (U.S. and Canada)
  Extended-release tablets (U.S. and Canada)

- Diphenhydramine and Pseudoephedrine
  Capsules (U.S.)
  Oral solution (U.S.)
  Tablets (U.S. and Canada)

  Loratadine and Pseudoephedrine
  Extended-release tablets (U.S. and Canada)

- Pheniramine and Phenylephrine
  for Oral solution (Canada)

- Pheniramine, Phenyltoloxamine, Pyrilamine, and Phenylpro-
  panolamine
  Extended-release capsules (U.S.)
  Elixir (U.S.)

- Pheniramine, Pyrilamine, and Phenylpropanolamine
  Oral solution (U.S.)
  Extended-release tablets (U.S. and Canada)

- Promethazine and Phenylephrine
    Syrup (U.S.)

- Terfenadine and Pseudoephedrine
    Withdrawn from the U.S. market by the Food and Drug Administration in February 1998

- Triprolidine and Pseudoephedrine
    Syrup (U.S. and Canada)
    Tablets (U.S. and Canada)

Chapter 64

Managing Your Medication Supply

Managing your medications is a very important task. When you take medications prescribed, your disease can be controlled. Your health care provider will give you specific information about your medications. Learning about your medications and following the guidelines listed below will help you more effectively manage your disease.

Understanding Your Medications

1. Learn about the medications you are taking. Know the brand name and generic name of your medications. Learn the medication's action, dose, when to take it and what side effects to watch for. In addition, ask about any potential drug or food interactions.

2. Talk with your health care provider about the use of generic (non-brand name) substitutions. Some generic medications are not recommended.

3. If your prescription does not look right, ask your health care provider.

4. Keep your medications in the original bottle. The original bottle has the correct label and instructions. But for the times you cannot, ask your pharmacist for an extra labeled container.

School health policies require that all medications have an original pharmacy label.

5. Do not substitute over-the-counter (OTC) medications for the medications your health care provider has prescribed. These medications can be dangerous. For example OTC bronchodilators (i.e., Primatine Mist, Bronkaid) may contain epinephrine and/or theophylline which can interact with the medications your health care provider has prescribed.

6. Most people with respiratory or allergic diseases can use over-the-counter decongestants and anti-histamines safely. It is important to talk with your health care provider, he or she can make specific recommendations about these types of medications.

7. When your medications change, be sure to keep your old medications separate.

8. If you have difficulty swallowing medications, ask about different ways to take your medications.

Remembering to Take Your Medications

1. Develop a daily routine for taking your medications. Pick something you do everyday (i.e., waking, brushing your teeth, eating meals, bedtime) and plan your medication schedule around that activity.

2. Use a medication checklist or worksheet to record when you take medications. Place the checklist someplace visible to use as a reminder. Children may enjoy using stars or stickers.

3. Pill boxes can help you remember to take your medications. By packing a day or a week's worth of medication you will know exactly if you took your medication or not. However, once the medication leaves the original bottle, it loses its identification and instruction label. You may want to have someone double check your pill box to make sure it is packed correctly.

Refilling Your Prescriptions

1. When you first receive your medication, make sure the number of refills on the label matches the number on the original prescription. Ask the pharmacist at the time if you notice a

problem. Plan to get a new prescription when you are on your last refill—or sooner.

2. Contact your pharmacy well in advance of the time you need your medication. The pharmacist may need time to telephone the physician, check the medication supply, order the medication, then package and label the medication.

3. Most prescriptions, including refills, are only good for 12 months. At that time, a new prescription is necessary and any unused refills cannot be filled.

4. Date the canister of your metered dose inhaler (MDI) so you know how long the medication lasts. Plan ahead to get the quantities you need.

Checking for Expiration Dates

1. Note the expiration date on all medication packages.

2. Make sure you check expiration dates on the medications you may have stored in different locations (i.e., work desk, school, purse, backpack, kitchen cabinet).

3. Do not use any medications after they expire.

Storing Your Medications

1. Temperature changes and humidity can cause medication to become ineffective or dangerous.

2. Humidity can cause a tablet to become moist and powdery. Do not store medications in places with high humidity, like gym lockers, bathrooms and above the stove.

3. Do not store medications in the glove compartment of your car. The temperature can range from -20 degrees F to 120 degrees F. When too cold to too hot, your MDI will not deliver a good spray and may burst. Check your MDI label for the recommended temperature range.

Traveling with Medications

1. When you travel, make sure you have more than adequate supply of medications.

2. Put your medications in your carry-on luggage.

3. Be cautious about using foreign purchased medications.

Chapter 65

Immunotherapy (Allergy Shots)

Immunotherapy (commonly called allergy shots) is a form of treatment to reduce your allergic reaction to allergens. Allergens are substances to which you are allergic. Research has shown that allergy shots can reduce symptoms of allergic rhinitis (hay fever) and allergic asthma. Remember, not all asthma is due to allergies. Allergy shots can be effective against grass, weed and tree pollens, house dust mites, cat and dog dander and insect stings. Allergy shots are less effective against molds and are not a useful method for the treatment of food allergy.

Immunotherapy consists of a series of injections (shots) with a solution containing the allergens that cause your symptoms. Treatment usually begins with a weak solution given once or twice a week. The strength of the solution is gradually increased with each dose. Once the strongest dosage is reached, the injections are usually given once a month to control your symptoms. At this point, you have decreased your sensitivity to the allergens and have reached your maintenance level. Allergy shots should always be given at your health care provider's office.

When Is Immunotherapy Recommended?

If you are considering allergy shots, talk to your health care provider about a referral to board certified allergist. A board certified allergist will follow a number of steps to evaluate if allergy shots are appropriate for you.

First, the allergist will ask you questions about your environment and symptoms to determine if skin testing is necessary. Typically, prick skin testing is conducted to identify the specific allergens that are causing your symptoms. Skin testing should only be administered under the supervision of a board certified allergist.

Once an allergy has been identified, the next step is to decrease or eliminate exposure to the allergen. This is called environmental control. Evidence shows that allergy and asthma symptoms may improve over time, if the recommended environmental control changes are made. For example, removing furry or feathered pets or following control measures for house dust mites and cockroaches may decrease symptoms. Preventing your contact with grasses, weeds and tree pollen may be more difficult but possible by keeping outside doors and windows closed and using air conditioning.

Next, your health care provider may recommend antihistamines and nasal medications as remedies. In general, allergy shots are recommended only for persons with a history of severe or prolonged allergic rhinitis and for persons with allergic asthma when the allergen cannot be avoided. Allergy shots should be prescribed only by a board certified allergist.

How Long Are Allergy Shots Given?

Six months to a year of immunotherapy may be required before you experience any improvement in symptoms. If your symptoms do not improve after this time, your allergist should review your overall treatment program. If the treatment is effective, the shots usually continue three to five years, until the individual is symptom-free or until symptoms can be controlled with mild medications for one year. In general, allergy shots should be stopped if they are not effective within two to three years.

Rush Immunotherapy

Rush immunotherapy is a variation of allergy shots which "rushes" the initial phase of the treatment. Steadily increasing doses of allergen extract are given every few hours instead of every few days or weeks. There is an increased risk of a reaction with this procedure. Therefore, rush immunotherapy should only be done in a hospital under very close supervision.

Other Therapies

There are a number of alternative treatments which claim to "cure" allergies. These methods are not supported by scientific studies and are not approved by the American Academy of Allergy and Immunology. Unapproved alternative treatments include:

- Desensitization to foods, chemicals and environmental allergens with sublingual (under the tongue) drops.

- High-dose vitamin and mineral therapy.

- Urine injections.

- Bacterial vaccines.

- Exotic diets.

It is easy to feel overwhelmed or confused by the many different methods of allergy testing and treatment. We encourage you to work with a board certified allergist to evaluate and determine what is appropriate for you.

Chapter 66

Use and Care of Home Humidifiers

Humidifiers are commonly used in homes to relieve the physical discomforts of dry nose, throat, lips, and skin. The moisture they add to dry air also helps alleviate common nuisances brought on by winter heating, such as static electricity, peeling wallpaper, and cracks in paint and furniture. However, excess moisture can encourage the growth of biological organisms in the home. These organisms include dust mites, which are microscopic animals that produce materials causing allergic reactions to household dust, and molds.

Recent studies by the Environmental Protection Agency (EPA) and the Consumer Product Safety Commission (CPSC) have shown that ultrasonic and impeller (or "cool mist") humidifiers can disperse materials, such as microorganisms and minerals, from their water tanks into indoor air. At present, only limited information is available on the growth of microorganisms and the dispersal of microorganisms and minerals by home humidifiers.

Proper care and cleaning of ultrasonic and impeller humidifiers are important for reducing potential exposures to microorganisms, such as bacteria and molds. Microorganisms often grow in humidifiers which are equipped with tanks containing standing water. Breathing mist containing these pollutants has been implicated as causing a certain type of inflammation of the lungs.

The Federal government has not concluded that the dispersal of minerals by home humidifiers poses a serious health risk. Nevertheless,

"Indoor Air Facts No. 8: Use and Care of Home Humidifiers," U.S. Environmental Protection Agency (EPA), modified April 7, 1998.

using water with lower mineral content will reduce exposures to these materials.

The young, the elderly, and those people with lung diseases or respiratory allergies may be particularly susceptible to certain types of airborne pollutants. However, if you follow the recommendations for the use and care of home humidifiers provided in this fact sheet, the potential for dispersal of microorganisms and minerals from your humidifier should be reduced.

Can I Use Tap Water in My Ultrasonic or Impeller Humidifier?

The Federal government has not concluded that using tap water in ultrasonic or impeller humidifiers poses a serious health risk. However, researchers have documented that these humidifiers are very efficient at dispersing minerals in tap water into the air. In addition, some consumers are bothered by a "white dust" that may appear on surfaces during use of these devices. Most importantly, minerals in tap water may increase the development of crusty deposits, or scale, in humidifiers. Scale can be a breeding ground for microorganisms.

Retarding the growth of scale is the most compelling reason to find alternatives to tap water. For this reason, or if white dust is a problem or you wish to minimize your exposure to minerals in the tap water as a matter of prudence, you should either:

1. Use bottled water labeled "distilled." While distilled water still contains some mineral content, it will likely contain lower mineral content than most tap water. Distillation is the most effective method for removing minerals from water.

    Two additional demineralization processes, deionization and reverse osmosis, remove most of the minerals from water, but are generally less effective than distillation. Water demineralized by these two processes would, on the average, be expected to contain a higher mineral content than distilled waters. "Purified" water may be produced by any of these three or other similar processes.

    Be aware, however, that not all bottled water is produced using demineralization processes. Bottled waters labelled "spring", "artesian" or "mineral" have not been treated to remove mineral content.

2. Consider using demineralization cartridges, cassettes, or filters if supplied or recommended for use with your humidifier.

Be aware, however, that the ability of these devices to remove minerals may vary widely. Further research is needed to determine how well, and how long, these devices work. Watch for the appearance of "white dust," which would indicate that minerals are not being removed.

Also, in areas of the country where the mineral content in the tap water is high, using distilled water may be less expensive than cartridges, cassettes, or filters.

Types of Humidifiers and Associated Pollutants

Console humidifiers are encased in cabinets which are designed for floor use. Portable humidifiers are smaller and more readily moved. Central humidifiers are built into heating and air conditioning systems, and humidify the whole house.

The two types of humidifiers which generally appear to produce the greatest dispersions of both microorganisms and minerals are:

- Ultrasonic, which create a cool mist by means of ultrasonic sound vibrations.

- Impeller, or "cool mist," which produce a cool mist by means of a high speed rotating disk.

Two additional types of humidifiers can allow for growth of microorganisms if they are equipped with a tank that holds standing water, but generally disperse less, if any, of these pollutants into the air. These are:

- Evaporative, which transmit moisture into the air invisibly by using a fan to blow air through a moistened absorbent material, such as a belt, wick, or filter.

- Steam vaporizer, which create steam by heating water with an electrical heating element or electrodes. "Warm mist" humidifiers are a type of steam vaporizer humidifier in which the steam is cooled before exiting the machine.

Note: Steam vaporizer and evaporative humidifiers are not expected to disperse substantial amounts of minerals. A steam vaporizer tested by EPA did not disperse measurable amounts of minerals;

409

evaporative humidifiers have not been tested by EPA for mineral dispersal.

Recommendations for Use and Care

It is important to use a humidifier only when conditions require it, to use the correct moisture setting for existing conditions, and to clean it thoroughly.

The possible health effects resulting from the dispersal of microorganisms and minerals by home humidifiers are not fully understood. Meanwhile, it may be prudent to reduce the potential for personal exposures to these materials by taking the following precautions, particularly when using ultrasonic and impeller humidifiers.

- Empty the tank, wipe all surfaces dry, and refill the water in portable humidifiers daily to reduce any growth of microorganisms; follow the manufacturer's instructions for changing water in console humidifiers. Be sure you unplug the unit from the electrical socket first.

- Use water with low mineral content to prevent the build-up of scale and the dispersal of minerals into the air. See the box on the left for information on using water with low mineral content.

- Clean portable humidifiers every third day. Empty the tank and use a brush or other scrubber to clean it. Remove any scale, deposits, or film that has formed on the sides of the tank or on interior surfaces, and wipe all surfaces dry. Again, be sure you unplug the unit.

- Follow the manufacturer's suggestions on the use of cleaning products or disinfectants. In the absence of specific recommendations, clean all surfaces coming in contact with water with a 3% solution of hydrogen peroxide. If you use any cleaning or disinfecting agent, rinse the tank thoroughly with several changes of tap water to prevent dispersal of chemicals into the air during use.

- Follow the manufacturer's directions on cleaning and maintaining console and central (furnace mounted) humidifiers. In particular, if the humidifier contains a tank, do not allow water to stand in the tank for extended periods of time, and keep the water clean.

- Keep steam vaporizer humidifiers out of the reach of children. Steam and boiling water may cause burns.

- Do not humidify to indoor relative humidity levels exceeding 50 percent. Higher humidity levels may encourage the growth of biological organisms in the home. Hygrometers, available at local hardware stores, may be used to measure humidity levels. Some humidifiers contain a built-in humidistat which may be adjusted to the proper moisture level. If water condenses on windows, walls, or pictures, either relocate the humidifier, lower its humidistat setting, or reduce its use.

- Do not permit the area around the humidifier to become damp or wet. If dampness occurs, turn the output volume of the humidifier down. If the humidifier output volume cannot be turned down, use the, humidifier intermittently. Do not allow absorbent materials, such as carpeting, drapes, or tablecloths, to become damp.

- Follow the manufacturer's instructions regarding the use, maintenance, and replacement of any materials supplied with the humidifier. Use appropriate materials as recommended by the product manufacturer.

- Clean the humidifier, as directed, at the end of the humidifying season or when the product will not be in frequent use. Before storage, make sure all the parts are dry. Dispose of all used demineralization cartridges, cassettes, or filters. Store the unit in a dry location. After storage, clean the unit again and remove any dust on the outside.

- Stop using your humidifier and contact your physician if you have respiratory symptoms which you believe are associated with periods of use of your home humidifier, even if you are following maintenance directions.

Chapter 67

Noninvasive Ventilation

Noninvasive ventilation may improve the breathing of some patients with chronic obstructive pulmonary disease (COPD). A trial of noninvasive ventilation is worth considering in COPD patients with high PaCO2 who are doing poorly, have disrupted sleep, and require frequent doctor or hospital visits for shortness of breath despite otherwise optimal medical care.

Noninvasive ventilation helps to rest a patient's chest muscles, thereby helping a patient to breathe better.

Ventilation Is Not Oxygen Therapy

Noninvasive ventilation and oxygen therapy have certain features in common, most notably the ability to improve a patient's blood gasses. However, the two therapies differ significantly in their physiological action. An understanding of what noninvasive ventilation tries to accomplish is critical to understanding which patients should receive this therapy and what benefits they may gain from it.

Oxygen therapy and ventilation correspond to two distinct functions of the lungs: transfer of oxygen to blood and removal of carbon dioxide from blood

Although patients with COPD may have deficits in both function, they don't always fail in tandem. A patient with lung parenchymal damage secondary to severe pneumonia, for example, may have problems achieving adequate oxygenation, but usually has a normal ability to "blow off" carbon dioxide. Such a patient only requires oxygen therapy. On the other hand, some patients cannot breath sufficiently, which leads to an increased blood level of carbon dioxide. Noninvasive ventilation can help these patients get rid of excess carbon dioxide.

Benefits from Ventilation

Although the basis of the benefits that ventilatory support provides to patients is somewhat uncertain, noninvasive ventilation appears to allow patients to rest their breathing muscles.

Ventilation may reset the carbon dioxide "thermostat" of a patient's brainstem, the central nervous system structure that controls breathing.

COPD patients have an abnormally increased breathing workload because of their underlying lung disease. Patients with COPD face the risk of overtaxing their breathing muscles by the increased work of breathing. In addition COPD causes abnormal changes in the shape and configuration of breathing muscles that make them less functional. Finally, many COPD patients have breathing muscles that are reduced in size because of malfunction and metabolic problems. The sum of these effects is that the strength and endurance of the breathing muscles are clearly reduced in COPD patients, and these patients face an increased risk of developing muscle fatigue.

Some patients cannot breathe sufficiently, which leads to an increased blood level of carbon dioxide. Noninvasive ventilation can help these patients get rid of carbon dioxide.

Although the risk of muscle fatigue in COPD patients is great, few patients with elevated carbon dioxide levels have overt respiratory muscle fatigue. We hypothesize that in many patients the development of breathing muscle fatigue is avoided by a messenger-like-factor that originates in the over-worked breathing muscles. This factor signals the brainstem to reduce the patient's breathing and tolerate a higher blood CO_2 level, thereby avoiding overt fatigue and failure of the breathing muscles.

Noninvasive ventilation helps rest a patient's breathing muscles, thereby helping a patient to breath better. The blood CO_2 level drops, and the brainstem's sensitivity to CO_2 is reset back toward normal. As a result, most patients feel better, have less dyspnea, and appear to have fewer problems sleeping.

Who Benefits from Ventilation

Despite the theoretical benefits that ventilation can achieve in COPD patients, in practice the therapy has had mixed results. Some research efforts are aimed at determining why some COPD patients respond to ventilation and others don't. Most of the medical literature that documents success using ventilation consists of anecdotal reports of series of perhaps 5-20 patients who underwent negative-pressure therapy.

Noninvasive ventilation provides clinical benefit to only a small percentage of COPD patients. About three quarters of the COPD population won't benefit from ventilation because they do not have the appropriate indications, and should not even be started on therapy. A trial of ventilation should be limited to the COPD patients who have a elevated blood CO_2 level, and severe dyspnea or a general failure to thrive.

At National Jewish, we usually identify candidates for ventilatory support in our pulmonary rehabilitation clinic. We flag patients who have not responded to their rehabilitation program, medications, and oxygen therapy. Any patient with a PCO_2 of more than 45mmHg is a potential candidate for ventilation therapy; the normal value for PCO_2 is less than 40mmHg. In general, the higher a patient's PCO_2 the better are the chances that the patient will respond to ventilation.

However, even patients who meet the elevated CO_2 criteria may not always respond, and no well-established criteria currently exist for distinguishing likely responders from those who will fail. It appears that the best responders are patients whose bodies do not like living with an elevated PCO_2. This manifests as dyspnea, disrupted sleep, and the need for frequent hospital or physician visits.

Patients who tend to fail are those whose bodies seem to have adjusted to a high PCO_2 by breathing slower. These patients feel fine the way they are, derive little benefit from ventilation therapy, and are unlikely to comply with such therapy if it prescribed. In contrast, symptomatic patients are more likely to respond, and tend to be more compliant.

Types of Noninvasive Ventilation

Noninvasive ventilation is a family of methods that, as the name suggest, helps patients draw air into their lungs without introducing any tubing or other device into the patient's body.

Noninvasive ventilators fall into two broad categories: those that rely on negative pressure and positive-pressure device. Negative pressure units act externally on the chest and abdomen, cyclically expanding the chest wall so that the pressure inside the chest becomes less than the ambient atmospheric pressure, thereby helping to inflate the patient's lungs. Expiration is a passive event that results from the elastic recoil of the lungs and chest wall. The best-known negative pressure machine

415

is the iron lung, which was widely used several decades ago to treat polio patients. Polio patients were, in fact, the first population to undergo treatment with noninvasive ventilation.

About three quarters of the COPD population won't benefit from ventilation because they do not have the appropriate indications, and should not even be started on therapy.

The most common negative-pressure apparatus used today is the pneumowrap. It consists of an open mesh cage that surrounds the patient's chest, and which in turn is covered by a large shirt that fits over the cage and chest. A small vacuum device that is attached to the shirt periodically exerts negative pressure on the exterior of the chest cavity, thereby causing inspiration for into the lungs.

Until the late 1980's, negative-pressure devices offered the only form of noninvasive ventilation available. More recently, doctors have also had the option of using positive-pressure ventilators, which rely on a compressor to push air into a patient's lungs. These units are small, easy to use, and may be used with a nasal mask rather than the endotracheal or tracheotomy tubes of invasive ventilators.

Selecting the Ventilation Device

Although the concept has only gained acceptance in the last five years, the noninvasive use of positive-pressure ventilators has now superseded negative-pressure treatment for COPD Positive-pressure units are simpler to operate. After learning how to use the machinery, patients can manage their therapy themselves with only maintenance visit from a technician every couple of months. The nasal masked used with positive-pressure devices is easy for patients to put on and take off, and it provides superior ventilation compared to negative-pressure units. Negative-pressure ventilation may be useful inpatients who cannot tolerate a nasal mask, such as patients who are claustrophobic.

Patients may derive significant clinical benefit from ventilation support even if their PCO2 does not return to normal.

Two types of positive-pressure machines are available: a volume-cycled ventilator, and the newer, pressure-support, or BiPap ventilator. A volume-cycled unit is adjusted to deliver a specific volume of air, such as500ml, to the patient during each breath. Another setting for this machine specifies the breathing rate, such as 20 times a minute. The pressure-support devise is set to deliver a specific air pressure, such as 10 cm of water, at a certain rate. The patient determines the volume of each breath by deciding when to stop inspiration.

The decision for which type of positive-pressure device to initially prescribe for a patient is arbitrary. Some patients will feel more comfortable with one device or the other, but it is difficult to predict.

We tend to start patients with the pressure support unit, because it is somewhat simpler and easier to maintain. All a patient has to do is strap on the nasal mask and flip a switch. If patients don't feel comfortable on pressure support, we try a volume-cycled unit.

The medical literature indicates that negative-pressure devices, such as the pneumowrap, are generally less effective for resting breathing muscle compared to positive-pressure units. If a patient fails treatment with both pressure-support and volume-cycled units, a trial of negative pressure may be called for, but the chances that it will succeed are low.

Using Ventilation Therapy

Patients may derive significant clinical benefit from ventilation support even if their PCO2 does not return to normal, especially if they have severe hypercapnia when starting treatment. For example, a patient who starts with aPCO2 of 60 mmHg will notice significant improvements in function and dyspnea when, after several weeks of positive pressure ventilation, the PCO2 is lowered to only 47 mmHg. In fact, it is better for the severely hypercapnic patient not to return to normal too quickly.

Ventilation support is most often used only at night, while the patient is asleep. In fact, an issue that is now under study is whether most patients need treatment every night, or whether they can derive almost as much benefit from using their device only once or twice a week. Until this question is answered, nightly treatment remains the standard of care. However, it is usually acceptable for patients to stop using their ventilator when they go on a brief trip, so that they do not need to carry the machinery with them.

Patients who need ventilatory support should understand that they may have to continue to use a machine for the rest of their lives. So far there is little data available on patient outcome if ventilation is withdrawn.

The noninvasive use of positive pressure ventilators has now superseded negative pressure treatment for COPD.

Because a ventilator is only used at night, its use may cause less psychologic trauma than oxygen therapy, which patients also need to use during the day. Indeed, patients often have an improved mental state after starting ventilation because of the benefits of reducing their

PCO2. The cost of ventilation support is generally covered by insurers, including Medicare and Medicaid. A typical rental fee is $1,000-1,500 per month, which means that an insured patient's out-of-pocket expense may be $200-$300monthly.

The introduction of pressure-support devices has made these traditional rental fees controversial, because new pressure-support unit only costs about $6,000.Patients may therefore want to consider buying their device. This route will, of course, preclude the availability of technical support and upgrade to newer models, but pressure-support units are very simple to use and require little maintenance.

It is important to reemphasize that ventilator therapy is not a first-line therapy, and should only be considered for COPD patients who continue to have dyspnea and do poorly despite pulmonary rehabilitation, medication, and oxygen therapy. Another point to remember is that only a fraction of COPD patients can be expected to improve with ventilation. About a quarter of patients with severe COPD have the elevated PCO2 that makes them candidates for ventilation. Among this 23% of patients, perhaps half would tolerate, and clinically improve with, ventilation. And for these responders, about half will do best with a pressure-support device; the other half will prefer a volume-cycled unit.

References

1. Fernandez, E.Tanchoco-Tan, M., Make, B. Methods to improve respiratory muscle function. *Sem Resp Med* in press, 1993.

2. Elliott, M.W., Simonds, A.K., Carroll, M.P., Wedzicha, J.A., Branthwaite, M.A. Domiciliary nocturnal nasal intermittent positive pressure ventilation in hypercapnic respiratory failure due to chronic obstructive lung disease: effects on sleep and quality of life. *Thorax* 47:342-48, 1992.

3. Marin, J.C., Levy, R.D.Respiratory muscle rest. Prob Resp Care 3:534-41, 1990.

4. Belman, M.J., Hoo, G.W.S., Kuei, J.H., Shadmehr, R, Efficacy of positive vs. negative pressure ventilation in unloading the respiratory muscles. *Chest* 98:850-56, 1990.

5. Carrey, Z., Gottfried, S.B., Levy, R.D.Ventilatory muscle support in respiratory failure with nasal positive pressure ventilation. *Chest* 97:150-58,1990.

6. Braun, N.M.T. Intermittent mechanical ventilation. *Clin Med* 9:153-161, 1988.

Chapter 68

Use and Care of a Nebulizer

A nebulizer is a device driven by a compressed air machine. It allows you to take asthma medicine in the form of a mist (wet aerosol). It consists of a cup, a mouthpiece attached to a T-shaped part or a mask, and thin, plastic tubing to connect to the compressed air machine. It is used mostly by three types of patients:

- Young children under age 5
- Patients who have problems using metered dose inhalers
- Patients with severe asthma

A nebulizer helps make sure they get the right amount of medicine.

A routine for cleaning the nebulizer is important because an unclean nebulizer may cause an infection. A good cleaning routine keeps the nebulizer from clogging up and helps it last longer. Directions for using the compressed air machine may vary (check the machine's directions), but generally the tubing has to be put into the outlet of the machine before it is turned on.

How to Use a Nebulizer

1. Measure the correct amount of normal saline solution using a clean dropper and put it into the cup. If your medicine is premixed, go to step 3.

"Worksheet No. 14: Use and Care of a Nebulizer," © 2000 Loyola University Health System; reprinted with permission.

2. Draw up the correct amount of medicine using a clean eyedropper or syringe and put it into the cup with the saline solution. Once you know your number of drops, you can count them as a check on yourself.

3. Fasten the mouthpiece to the T-shaped part and then fasten this unit to the cup OR fasten the mask to the cup. For a child over the age of 2, use a mouthpiece unit because it will deliver more medicine than a mask.

4. Put the mouthpiece in your mouth. Seal your lips tightly around it OR place the mask on your face.

5. Turn on the air compressor machine.

6. Take slow, deep breaths in through the mouth.

7. Hold each breathe 1 to 2 seconds before breathing out.

8. Continue until the medicine is gone from the cup (approximately 10 minutes).

9. Store the medicine as directed after each use.

Cleaning the Nebulizer

Don't forget: Cleaning and getting rid of germs prevents infection. Cleaning keeps the nebulizer from clogging up and helps it last longer.

After Each Use

1. Remove the mask or the mouthpiece and T-shaped part from the cup. Remove the tubing and set it aside. The tubing should not be washed or rinsed. Rinse the mask or mouthpiece and T-shaped part—as well as the eyedropper or syringe—in warm running water for 30 seconds. Use distilled or sterile water for rinsing, if possible.

2. Shake off excess water. Air dry on a clean cloth or paper towel.

3. Put the mask or the mouthpiece and T-shaped part, cup, and tubing back together and connect the device to the compressed air machine. Run the machine for 10 to 20 seconds to dry the inside of the nebulizer.

4. Disconnect the tubing from the compressed air machine. Store the nebulizer in a zip lock plastic bag.

5. Place a cover over the compressed air machine.

Once Every Day

1. Remove the mask or the mouthpiece and T-shaped part from the cup. Remove the tubing and set it aside. The tubing should not be washed or rinsed.

2. Wash the mask or the mouthpiece and T-shaped part as well as the eyedropper or syringe with a mild dish washing soap and warm water.

3. Rinse under a strong stream of water for 30 seconds. Use distilled (or sterile) water if possible.

4. Shake off excess water. Air dry on a clean cloth or paper towel.

5. Put the mask or the mouthpiece and T shaped part, cup, and tubing back together and connect the device to the compressed air machine. Run the machine for 10 to 20 seconds to dry the inside of the nebulizer.

6. Disconnect the tubing from the compressed air machine. Store the nebulizer in a zip lock plastic bag.

7. Place a cover over the compressed air machine.

Once or Twice a Week

1. Remove the mask or the mouthpiece and T-shaped part from the cup. Remove the tubing and set it aside. The tubing should not be washed or rinsed. Wash the mask or the mouthpiece and T-shaped part as well as the eyedropper or syringe with a mild dish washing soap and warm water.

2. Rinse under a strong stream of water for 30 seconds.

3. Soak for 30 minutes in a solution that is one part distilled white vinegar and two parts distilled water. Throw out the vinegar water solution after use; do not reuse it.

4. Rinse the nebulizer parts and the eyedropper or syringe under warm running water for 1 minute. Use distilled or sterile water, if possible.

5. Shake off excess water. Air dry on a clean cloth or paper towel.

6. Put the mask or the mouthpiece and T-shaped part, cup, and tubing back together and connect the device to the compressed air machine. Run the machine for 10 to 20 seconds to dry the inside of the nebulizer thoroughly.

7. Disconnect the tubing from the compressed air machine. Store the nebulizer in a zip lock plastic bag.

8. Clean the surface of the compressed air machine with a well-wrung, soapy cloth or sponge. You could also use an alcohol or disinfectant wipe. NEVER PUT THE COMPRESSED AIR MACHINE IN WATER.

9. Place a cover over the compressed air machine.

Chapter 69

Frequently Asked Questions about Inhalers

What Kinds of Inhalers Are There?

Aerosol Inhalers

- *MDI:* metered-dose inhaler, consisting of an aerosol unit and plastic mouthpiece. This is currently the most common type of inhaler, and is widely available.

- *Autohaler:* MDI made by 3M, which is activated by one's breath, and doesn't need the breath-hand coordination that a regular MDI does. Available in U.S., UK, and NZ.

- *Integra:* MDI with compact spacer device. Available in UK.

- *Respihaler:* aerosol inhaler for Decadron. Unknown how this differs from the usual MDI. Available in the U.S.

- *Syncroner:* MDI with elongated mouthpiece, used as training device to see if medication is being inhaled properly. Available in Canada for Intal.

Dry Powder Inhalers

- *Accuhaler:* dry powder inhaler for use with Serevent. It contains a foil strip with 60 blisters, each containing one dose of the drug. Pressing the lever punctures the blister, allowing the drug to be inhaled through the mouthpiece. Available in the UK.

- *Diskhaler:* dry powder inhaler. The drug is kept in a series of little pouches on a disk; the diskhaler punctures the pouch and drug is inhaled through the mouthpiece. Currently available in Canada, South Africa, and UK, not in U.S.

- *Insufflator:* dry powder nasal inhaler used with Rynacrom cartridges. Each cartridge contains one dose; the inhaler opens the cartridge, allowing the powder to be blown into the nose by squeezing the bulb. Available in Canada.

- *Rotahaler:* dry powder inhaler used with Rotacaps capsules. Each capsule contains one dose; the inhaler opens the capsule such that the powder may be inhaled through the mouthpiece. Available in the U.S., Canada, and UK for Ventolin. In Canada, Beclovent Rotacaps are also available, as are Becotide Rotacaps in the UK.

- *Spinhaler:* dry powder inhaler used with Intal capsules for spinhaler. Each capsule contains one dose; the inhaler opens the capsule such that the powder may be inhaled through the mouthpiece. Available in Canada, UK, and the Netherlands. No longer manufactured in the U.S.

- *Turbuhaler:* dry powder inhaler. The drug is in form of a pellet; when body of inhaler is rotated, prescribed amount of drug is ground off this pellet. The powder is then inhaled through a fluted aperture on top. Available in Australia, Canada, Denmark, Switzerland, and the UK (spelled 'turbohaler' in the UK).

Do Inhaler Propellants Bother Some Asthmatics?

Some asthmatics find the dry powder inhalers more effective than their MDI (aerosol) counterparts. It is suspected that the aerosol or propellant in the MDI may act as an irritant to some asthmatics, as in the following article:

J.R.W. Wilkinson et al., "Paradoxical bronchoconstriction in asthmatic patients after salmeterol by metered dose inhaler", *British Medical Journal* 305 (1992) 931.

The first sentence in the conclusion is: "Bronchoconstriction after both salmeterol and placebo by metered dose inhaler but not after salmeterol by diskhaler suggests that the irritant is not the salmeterol itself." . . . "The similarity in characteristics of bronchoconstriction after beclomethasone by metered dose inhalers implicates one or both chlorofluorocarbons . . . as the irritant. That salbutamol caused no bronchoconstriction was attributed to its faster onset of action opposing any bronchoconstrictor effects of the propellants."

However, according to the 1994 *Physicians' Desk Reference*, Intal Spinhaler capsules are "contraindicated in those patients who have shown hypersensitivity to . . . lactose." So asthmatics who are lactose-intolerant may not have this form of cromolyn sodium as an option.

What Is a Spacer? What Is a Holding Chamber?

Metered dose inhalers (MDIs) for asthma medications typically consist of a metal aerosol canister (containing the medication and a propellant) in a plastic sleeve with a mouthpiece. The patient inhales one or more metered doses of a medication through the mouthpiece. Most people find it difficult (at least initially) to time the spraying of an MDI and the inhalation of the medicine: the patient must exhale fully and inhale and release the metered dose just at the beginning of the inhalation so as to draw the medication as fully and deeply into the lungs as possible.

All too often the puffs are mistimed and only make it part of the way into the airways, and some of the medication is invariably deposited into the mouth and on the back of the throat instead of into their lungs. In addition to being less effective, this can lead to other side effects (e.g., for inhaled steroids, an increased potential for thrush, an oral fungal).

Several devices have become available that address these difficulties to varying degrees. The devices are generally referred to as "spacers" since they place additional space between the patient and the MDI. The medication is sprayed into the spacer instead of the mouth. As the patient inhales, the column of medication passes through the mouth and throat relatively quickly, leaving little opportunity for the medication to be deposited in the mouth or throat. This is a more efficient means of delivering the medication to the airways where it's most needed.

The simplest kind of spacer is basically a tube. The patient sprays the medication in one end of the tube and inhales it out the other end. Azmacort has a simple spacer attached to it. A cardboard tube from the core of a roll of bathroom tissue can be used as a spacer (as long as it's clean, lint-free and germ-free). While a simple spacer reduces the amount of medication that gets deposited in the mouth and throat, it still requires you to carefully time your inhalation with the discharge of the medication to minimize the amount of the medication that escapes from the spacer.

A "holding chamber" is a more sophisticated device. It is a sealed chamber (once the inhaler is inserted) that traps and holds the medication, allowing the patient to spray the medication into the chamber and take a few seconds to inhale the medication. Since the medication is temporarily suspended in the holding chamber, the timing of the inhalation is not nearly as critical as with simple spacers or no spacer. AeroChamber is a brand of holding chamber. It's a plastic tube with a mouthpiece on one end and a place to insert the MDI on the other. The mouthpiece has a one-way valve built in that temporarily contains the sprayed medication, and also allows the patient to exhale without displacing the medication in the chamber (as without a spacer, the patient should exhale as completely as possible before taking in any medication, so that the medication can be inhaled as deeply as possible).

In addition to improving the timing of the inhalation, a holding chamber makes it possible to take in the medication more slowly than is possible without a spacer or with a simple spacer. This is important for the symptomatic patient, since rapid inhalation of the medication is more likely to trigger coughing and cause the patient to lose the medication before it has had a chance to be absorbed.

Some spacers are clear so that you can see the puff of medicine, and so that you can see when the medication is building up on the inside, indicating that the spacer needs cleaning. Spacers and holding chambers need periodic cleaning; clean carefully, following the manufacturer's instructions so as not to damage any delicate internal parts or allow molds or other contaminants to be introduced.

There are special holding chambers for younger children. There's a pediatric AeroChamber that has a mask built in; the child breathes normally for a few seconds with the mask held over his/her mouth and nose. This is typically used when a nebulizer is not available or not required, and for medications that are not available in a nebulized form, such as Beclovent or Vanceril.

There is also a device for children (and for people that have trouble holding their breath) called an InspirEase. It's kind of like a plastic bellows or balloon with a plastic mouthpiece. The patient inflates it, the medicine is sprayed into it, and the patient inhales, holds his/her breath for the count of 5 (or whatever the doctor recommends), exhales into the device, and then repeats. Some patients are instructed to breath slowly in and out several times instead of holding their breath. The InspirEase really helpful for younger children who yet aware of the difference between breathing in and breathing out or don't yet know how to hold their breath or breathe evenly and slowly. It gives them immediate physical feedback, and it also has a whistle built in to tell them when they're breathing too fast (although they seem to like making it whistle, so it's positive reinforcement for something that they shouldn't be doing). As the child grows, the Inspirease becomes less effective, since it has a limited capacity, although I've been told that it is available in different capacities.

Knowing the difference between a simple spacer and a holding chamber can help you use each in its proper way. If you use both a holding chamber and a simple spacer (e.g., a holding chamber for your Ventolin and the simple spacer attached to your Azmacort), you need to remember which you're using and adjust your style accordingly.

Spacers and holding chambers are sometimes provided by some HMOs and covered by some insurers.

What Is "Thrush Mouth" and How Can I Avoid It?

Thrush, or thrush mouth, is the popular term for a yeast infection (*candida albicans*) in the back of throat. The major symptom of thrush is a white film located at the back of the throat and tonsil area. It is usually cured by the use of an antifungal mouthwash.

Thrush is a very common side effect of taking inhaled corticosteroids, since steroids alter the local bacteria and fungal population of the mouth, enhancing fungal growth. The way to avoid this complication is to ensure that the back of the throat doesn't remain coated with corticosteroid after use of the inhaler, either by using a spacer or by rinsing the mouth very thoroughly afterwards. Unfortunately, some people still get it even when they are very thorough about rinsing.

Is Fisons Still Making the Intal Spinhaler?

In the US, Fisons is no longer manufacturing either the Intal Spinhaler (a dry powder inhaler for cromolyn sodium) or the capsules for it. However, the Spinhaler and capsules are still available in Canada and the United Kingdom. For further information, Fisons Corporation's number in the US for Rx Customer Service is 800-334-6433.

What's the Difference between Spinhalers and Rotahalers?

The Rotahaler and the Spinhaler are very different animals. The Rotahaler is a pussycat, the Spinhaler a ferocious lion.

The Rotahaler is a two-part mouthpiece that you snap apart, put a capsule in, twist, and inhale. When you twist the device, the capsule breaks open. When you inhale, the medicine lands in your lungs.

The Spinhaler is a three-piece device: a mouthpiece, a tiny fan, and a cap to cover the fan. You open it, put the capsule in a space on the fan, close it, push down then up on the cap (this breaks the capsule) and then tilt your head back, put the mouthpiece in your mouth, and inhale. The fan throws the medicine into the back of your throat. Then you gag.

Another difference: The Spinhaler comes in a little container like a medicine bottle, but the lid doesn't stay on very well in a purse. The Rotahaler comes in a little plastic case sort of like a compact and stays shut (i.e. clean) in a purse, backpack, or jeans pocket.

Why Are So Many Asthma Drugs Taken Via Inhaler?

Medications taken orally almost always have a much higher systemic concentration (concentration in your entire body) than inhaled medications. So if the side effects are due to systemic concentrations, then an inhaled drug is less likely to have these side effects, or may have them much less severely.

The idea behind an inhaler is that the full dose is delivered to the lungs, where it is immediately absorbed by the lung tissue, and starts to take effect locally. Excess drug may be absorbed by the bloodstream and delivered to the rest of your body, but this amount tends to be minimal. So your lungs receive an immediate, high concentration of the drug, and the rest of your body receives very little.

If you take the drug orally in tablet or capsule form, then you need a much higher dose. The reason is that for the same amount of drug to reach the lungs through the bloodstream, you need the same concentration of drug in the rest of your body. For example, most people take one or two puffs of albuterol (Ventolin or Proventil) every four to six hours, and each puff is 90 micrograms of albuterol. The usual dosage of Ventolin in tablets is 2-4 milligrams three or four times a day, which is something like 200 times the amount inhaled.

However, one advantage that tablets have is that the medication may be available in a time-release format. So for a short-acting medication like albuterol, the inhaled version might need to be taken every four to six hours, while a extended-release tablet such as Volmax would need to be taken only every twelve hours.

How Can I Tell When My MDI Is Empty?

The float test (in which you take the MDI canister out of the mouthpiece and place it in a container of water to see if it sinks) is no longer the recommended way to determine whether your MDI (metered dose inhaler) is empty. Glaxo, the manufacturer of Ventolin and Beclovent, claims that the float test is inaccurate, and recommends that doses be counted instead. Other manufacturers agree: the triamcinolone acetonide (Azmacort) package insert recommends dose counting also and the cromolyn sodium (Intal) inhaler package insert states that the metal cylinder should never be immersed in water. The number of doses per canister should be clearly written on the canister label.

One variation of dose counting, for medications that are taken regularly, is to calculate the date on which the medication will be used up, and discard the old canister for a new one on that date.

Are My Aerosol Inhalers Going to Disappear?

As you may know, CFC (chlorofluorocarbon) chemicals, which are used as propellants in aerosol products including asthma inhalers (MDIs), damage the ozone layer. As a result, there has been a worldwide ban on the production of these chemicals for all but essential uses.

Products which relied on CFCs, such as air conditioning units, refrigerators, and most aerosol products, have been modified to use alternative chemicals which do not damage the ozone layer.

Due to their nature, however, metered dose inhalers have been granted an "essential use" exemption to the worldwide ban, which grants the manufacturers an extra few years to develop alternatives.

Since the inactive ingredients (i.e., everything but the drug itself) must be changed, it's not as simple as using a different chemical for the propellant—the new device must go through much the same approval process as the original inhaler did, to ensure that the same dosage is delivered to the patient, that there are no side effects, that patients tolerate the new formulation well, etc.

The FDA has already approved one new non-CFC inhaler, Proventil HFA (albuterol), which uses hydrofluoralkane instead of CFC propellants. Other non-CFC devices are currently in the works. It is expected that future non-CFC inhalers may be reviewed and approved more quickly than the earlier ones.

CFC-based MDIs will continue to be available for some time. Proposed guidelines for final phaseout include that there be at least 3 multi-use (see below) non-CFC devices available in a drug class (i.e., bronchodilators, corticosteroids), providing at least 2 different drugs, before all CFC inhalers in that class are banned. As an example, CFC-based bronchodilators would be permitted as long as Proventil HFA is the only alternative; if Ventolin (also albuterol) and Alupent (metaproterenol) had non-CFC versions, then all CFC formulations might be banned.

The term "multi-use" refers both to aerosol inhalers and multi-use dry-powder inhalers such as the diskhaler. It does not include single-use dry-powder inhalers such as the rotahaler, which requires insertion of a new capsule of medication with each use.

Chapter 70

Metered-Dose Inhalers

How Can I Keep Track of How Much Medicine I've Used?

It's important to keep track of how much medicine you've used so you can plan ahead and replace your inhaler before you run out of medicine. One way to do this is to write a refill date on the canister itself. To figure out when you'll need to get a refill, start with a brand new inhaler.

Divide the number of puffs in the canister—the canister will usually have this number printed on it—by the number of puffs you take each day. The number you get will be the number of days the canister should last. (For example, if you take 4 puffs each day from a 200-puff canister, you will need to have a new canister every 50 days.) Using a calendar, count forward that many days to see when your medicine will run out. So you won't run out of the medicine that you use every day, choose a day 1 or 2 days before this date to have your prescription refilled. Using a permanent marker, write the refill date on the canister. If you use your inhaler for rescue medicine, you probably won't be using it regularly enough for this method to work. In that case, ask your doctor if he or she will write a prescription for two

---

Text in this chapter is from "How to Use Your Metered-Dose Inhaler" Reprinted with permission from http://www.familydoctor.org/handouts/040.html. American Academy of Family Physicians © 2001. All rights reserved. Text is also included from an undated fact sheet produced by the National Heart, Lung, and Blood Institute (NHLBI), available online at http://www.nhlbi.nih.gov, cited October 2001.

inhalers at a time. Then get your prescription filled when the first inhaler is empty. This way, you'll always have enough rescue medicine on hand when you need it most.

How Do I Use the Inhaler?

- Open mouth. Hold inhaler 1 to 2 inches away.

- Use spacer attached to inhaler.

- Hold inhaler in your mouth.

- Remove the cap and hold the inhaler upright.

- Shake the inhaler.

- Tilt your head back slightly and breathe out.

- Press down on the inhaler to release the medicine as you start to breathe in slowly.

- Breathe in slowly for 3 to 5 seconds.

- Hold your breath for 10 seconds to allow medicine to go deeply into your lungs.

- Repeat puffs as directed. Wait 1 minute between puffs to allow the second puff to get into the lungs better.

NOTE: Inhaled dry powder capsules are used differently. To use a dry powder inhaler, close your mouth tightly around the mouthpiece of the inhaler and breathe in quickly.

Answers to Questions about CFCs and Inhalers

Metered-dose inhalers (MDIs) are devices that people with asthma and chronic obstructive pulmonary disease (chronic bronchitis and emphysema) use to deliver medicine to their lungs. The medication is delivered by a propellant in the MDI whenever it is used. For most MDIs, the propellant is one or more gases called chlorofluorocarbons (CFCs).

Over the next few years, MDIs that contain CFCs are expected to be replaced by new inhaler devices that do not contain CFCs (non-CFC inhalers). This change has just begun and will continue for several years as more non-CFC options become available.

Patients and health care providers need to learn about the change to non-CFC inhalers. This fact sheet will help answer many of the questions that you may have about the change.

Why Will CFC MDIs Be Changing?

Although CFCs in medicines are safe for patients to inhale, CFCs are harmful to the environment. Scientists have found that when CFCs get into the upper regions of the earth's atmosphere (stratosphere), they reduce the amount of ozone in the ozone layer that surrounds the earth. The ozone layer acts as a shield to protect the earth against the sun's harmful rays. With less ozone in the ozone layer, too many of these harmful rays reach the earth and can increase the risk of potentially serious health problems, such as skin cancer and cataracts, as well as other health and environmental problems. To lower the risk of health and environmental problems caused by ozone depletion and to help restore the ozone layer, most countries have agreed to stop using CFCs. The agreement was made in 1987 and is known as the Montreal Protocol.

CFCs are used in many types of products (such as air conditioners, refrigerators, etc.), not just MDIs. However, in response to the Montreal Protocol, the manufacture of CFCs for these purposes has already been stopped. Nonetheless, CFC MDIs have been given a special exemption because they are so important for treating asthma and chronic obstructive pulmonary disease. The manufacture of CFCs for use in MDIs will not be stopped until safe and effective replacements are available. But the goal is to one day replace CFC MDIs with alternatives that do not contain CFCs.

What Are the Benefits of Changing to Non-CFC Inhalers?

The change to non-CFC inhalers is one of many steps being taken worldwide to restore the ozone layer. A clear benefit of these efforts will be to help reduce the health and environmental risks caused by the sun's harmful rays.

The change is stimulating the development of many new types of non-CFC inhalers. Some of these will be new MDIs that have non-CFC propellants. Other inhalers are being developed that do not use propellants, such as dry powder inhalers and mini-nebulizers. This means that physicians may have several options to prescribe and patients may have additional choices in how their medicine is delivered. The safety and effectiveness of every new non-CFC inhaler will be reviewed by the U.S. Food and Drug Administration (FDA) before it is approved.

What Steps Have Been Taken to Change from CFC to Non-CFC Inhalers?

Many professional, public, and private groups are working to ensure that medicines are available to properly care for patients during the change from CFC to non-CFC inhalers. Although the conversion has been challenging, there has been a worldwide drive to develop non-CFC inhalers.

- The pharmaceutical industry has been working very hard to develop non-CFC MDIs. Companies around the world are testing inhalers containing new propellants instead of CFCs. These new propellants have been shown to be just as safe for patients as CFCs.

- Other non-CFC options not requiring propellants are being developed, including dry powder inhalers, mini-nebulizers, and other devices.

- The FDA and the U.S. Environmental Protection Agency (EPA) are working together to ensure that CFC MDIs remain available until safe and effective replacements are available.

- The National Asthma Education and Prevention Program (NAEPP), in collaboration with the International Pharmaceutical Aerosol Consortium, is developing educational materials regarding the change to non-CFC inhalers. Several NAEPP member organizations are also involved in patient education efforts, including the Allergy and Asthma Network/Mothers of Asthmatics, Inc.; the American Academy of Allergy, Asthma, and Immunology; the American Lung Association; the Asthma and Allergy Foundation of America; and representatives from the FDA and the EPA.

Which MDIs Will Be Available to Patients During the Change to Non-CFC Inhalers?

Concerns about patient health are important in the change from CFC to non-CFC inhalers. In order for patients and health care providers to have time to prepare for these changes, CFC MDIs will remain available until an adequate number of safe and effective non-CFC inhalers are available. However, we do not know how long this will take. All patients should have adequate choices of medicines during the change.

How Will the New Inhalers Differ from CFC MDIs?

There may be some differences in how CFC and non-CFC MDIs work, look, taste, or feel. Many new products will be produced and approved over time. It will be important for patients to talk with their doctor, nurse, pharmacist, respiratory therapist, or other health care provider when they get a new inhaler to make sure they know the correct way to use it. One non-CFC MDI for the medicine albuterol is available. Although patients may notice some minor differences in the feel or taste of the new product, the FDA has found it comparable in safety and effectiveness to the albuterol CFC MDIs. As with any change in therapy, patients should talk to their health care provider about non-CFC medication and other alternatives when they become available.

Will All Patients Have to Use Non-CFC Inhalers?

Yes. The goal is to phase out and ultimately eliminate the use of CFCs in MDIs. Although it will likely take a few years for this to happen, the process has already begun. It is important for patients and their health care providers to start making plans for the change now.

Where Can I Get More Information?

For information about asthma, other respiratory diseases, the Montreal Protocol, and the change to non-CFC inhalers, contact:

Allergy and Asthma Network/Mothers of Asthmatics, Inc.
814 W. Diamond Ave., Suite 150
Gaithersburg, MD 20878
Phone: 301-590-2770
Fax: 301-590-2776
Internet address: http://www.podi.com

American Academy of Allergy, Asthma, and Immunology
611 East Wells Department
Milwaukee, WI 53202
Phone: 800-822-ASMA
Internet address: http://www.aaaai.org

American Association for Respiratory Care
11030 Ables Lane
Dallas, TX 75229
Phone: 972-243-2272
Fax: 972-484-2720
Internet address: http://www.aarc.org
E-Mail: info@aarc.org

American College of Allergy, Asthma, and Immunology
85 West Algonquin Road
Suite 550
Arlington Heights, IL 60005
Phone: 800-842-7777
Internet address: http://allergy.mcg.edu
E-Mail: mail@acaai.org

American College of Chest Physicians
3300 Dundee Rd.
Northbrook, IL 60062-2348
Phone: 847-498-1400
Fax: 847-498-5460
Internet address: http://www.chestnet.org
E-Mail: accp@chestnet.org

American Lung Association
1740 Broadway
New York, NY 10019
Toll Free: 800-LUNG USA
Phone: 212-315-8700
Internet address: http://www.lungusa.org
E-Mail: info@lungusa.org

American Pharmaceutical Association
2215 Constitution Avenue, N.W.
Washington, DC 20037-2985
Phone: 202-628-4410
Fax: 202-783-2351
Internet address: http://www.aphanet.org
E-Mail: membership@mail.aphanet.org

American Society of Health-System Pharmacists
7272 Wisconsin Avenue
Bethesda, MD 20814
Phone: 301-657-3000
Internet address: http://www.ashp.org

American Thoracic Society
1740 Broadway
New York, NY 10019
Phone: 212-315-8700
Fax: 212-315-6498
Internet address: http://www.thoracic.org

Asthma and Allergy Foundation of America
1233 20th Street, NW, Suite 402
Washington, D.C., 20036
Toll Free: 800-7-ASTHMA
Phone: 202-466-7643
Fax: 202-466-8940
Internet address: http://www.aafa.org

European Federation of Asthma and Allergy Associations
Internet address: http://www.efanet.org

International Pharmaceutical Aerosol Consortium
1301 K. Street, N.W.
Suite 900, East Tower
Washington, D.C. 20005-3317
Phone: 202-289-1504
Internet address: http://www.ipacmdi.com
E-Mail: comments@ipacmdi.com

National Association of School Nurses
P.O. Box 1300
Scarborough, ME 04070-1300
Toll Free: 877-627-6476
Phone: 207-883-2117
Fax: 207-883-2683
Internet address: http://www.nasn.org
E-Mail: nasn@nasn.org

National Asthma Education and Prevention Program
P.O. Box 30105
Bethesda, Maryland 20824-0105
Phone: 301-592-8573
Fax: 301-8563
Internet address: http://www.nhlbi.nih.gov/about/naepp

U.S. Environmental Protection Agency
1200 Pennsylvania Avenue, N.W.
Washington, D.C. 20460-0001
Toll Free: 800-296-1996
Fax: 202-565-2155
Internet address: http://www.epa.gov/ozone

U.S. Food and Drug Administration
5600 Fishers Lane
Rockville, MD 20857-0001
Toll Free: 888-463-6332
Phone: 301-827-4420
Internet address: http://www.fda.gov

Chapter 71

Heart-Lung Transplant

In the three decades since the performance of the first human heart transplant in December 1967, the procedure has changed from an experimental operation to an established treatment for advanced heart disease. Approximately 2,300 heart transplants are performed each year in the United States.

In 1981, combined heart and lung transplants began to be used to treat patients with conditions that severely damage both these organs. As of 1995, about 500 people in the United States and 2,000 worldwide have received heart-lung transplants.

There have been two main barriers to increasing the number of successful operations. In 1983, the first barrier to successful transplantations—rejection of the donor organ by the patient—was overcome. The drug cyclosporine was introduced to suppress rejection of a donor heart or heart-lung by the patient's body. Cyclosporine and other medications to control rejection have significantly improved the survival of transplant patients. About 80 percent of heart transplant patients survive 1 year or more. About 60 percent of heart-lung transplants live at least 1 year after surgery. Research is under way to develop even better ways to control transplant rejection and improve survival.

Organ availability is the second barrier to increasing the number of successful transplantations. Hospitals and organizations nationwide are trying to increase public awareness of this problem and improve organ distribution.

Excerpted from "The Lungs in Health and Disease," National Heart, Lung, and Blood Institute (NHLBI), NIH Publication Number 97-2990, 1997.

What happens during a heart or heart-lung transplant?

A transplant is the replacement of a patient's diseased heart or heart and lungs with a normal organ(s) from someone—called a donor—who has died. The donor's organ(s) is completely removed and quickly transported to the patient, who may be located across the country. Organs are cooled and kept in a special solution while being taken to the patient.

During the operation, the patient is placed on a heart-lung machine. This machine allows surgeons to bypass the blood flow to the heart and lungs. The machine pumps the blood throughout the rest of the body, removing carbon dioxide (a waste product) and replacing it with oxygen needed by body tissues. Doctors remove the patient's heart except for the back walls of the atria, the heart's upper chambers. The backs of the atria on the new heart are opened and the heart is sewn into place. A similar process is followed in heart-lung transplants, except doctors remove the heart and lungs as a unit from the donor; the new lungs are attached first, followed by the heart.

Surgeons then connect the blood vessels and allow blood to flow through the heart and lungs. As the heart warms up, it begins beating. Sometimes, surgeons must start the heart with an electrical shock. Surgeons check all the connected blood vessels and heart chambers for leaks before removing the patient from the heart-lung machine.

Patients are usually up and around a few days after surgery, and if there are no signs of the body immediately rejecting the organ(s), patients are allowed to go home within 2 weeks.

Why are transplants done?

A transplant is considered when the heart is failing and does not respond to all other therapies, but health is otherwise good. The leading reasons why people receive heart transplants are:

- Cardiomyopathy—a weakening of the heart muscle.
- Severe coronary artery disease—in which the heart's blood vessels become blocked and the heart muscle is damaged.
- Birth defects of the heart.

Heart-lung transplants are performed on patients who will die from end-stage lung disease that also involves the heart. Alternative therapies for these patients have been tried or considered.

Leading reasons people receive heart-lung transplants are:

- Severe pulmonary hypertension—a large increase in blood pressure in the vessels of the lungs that limits blood flow and delivery of oxygen to the rest of the body.

- A birth defect of the heart that results in Eisenmenger's complex—another name for acquired pulmonary hypertension.

Who can have a transplant?

Patients under age 60 are the most likely heart transplant candidates. Patients under age 45 are generally accepted for heart-lung transplants. In both cases, patients must be suffering from end-stage disease and be in good health otherwise. The doctor, patient, and family must address the following four basic questions to determine whether a transplant should be considered:

- Have all other therapies been tried or excluded?

- Is the patient likely to die without the transplant?

- Is the person in generally good health other than the heart or heart and lung disease?

- Can the patient adhere to the lifestyle changes—including complex drug treatments and frequent examinations—required after a transplant?

Patients who do not meet the above considerations or who have additional problems—other severe diseases, active infections, or severe obesity—are not good candidates for a transplant.

How are donors found?

Donors are individuals who are brain dead, meaning that the brain shows no signs of life while the person's body is being kept alive by a machine. Donors have often died as a result of an automobile accident, a stroke, a gunshot wound, suicide, or a severe head injury. Most hearts come from those who die before age 45. Donor organs are located through the United Network for Organ Sharing (UNOS).

Not enough organs are available for transplant. At any given time, almost 3,500 to 4,000 patients are waiting for a heart or heart-lung transplant. A patient may wait months for a transplant. More than 25 percent do not live long enough. Yet, only a fraction of those who could donate organs actually do.

441

Does a person lead a normal life after a transplant?

After a heart or heart-lung transplant, patients must take several medications. The most important are those to keep the body from rejecting the transplant. These medications, which must be taken for life, can cause significant side effects, including hypertension, fluid retention, tremors, excessive hair growth, and possible kidney damage. To combat these problems, additional drugs are often prescribed.

A transplanted heart functions differently from the old one. Because the nerves leading to the heart are cut during the operation, the transplanted heart beats faster (about 100 to 110 beats per minute) than the normal heart (70 beats per minute). The new heart also responds more slowly to exercise and doesn't increase its rate as quickly as before.

A patient's prognosis depends on many factors, including age, general health, and response to the transplant. Recent figures show that 73 percent of heart transplant patients live at least 3 years after surgery. Nearly 85 percent of patients return to work or other activities they like. Many patients enjoy swimming, cycling, running, or other sports.

As noted, 60 percent of patients who receive combined heart-lung transplants survive at least 1 year. Fifty percent live at least 3 years.

What are the risks from transplants?

The most common causes of death following a transplant are infection or rejection of the heart. Patients on drugs to prevent transplant rejection are at risk for developing kidney damage, high blood pressure, osteoporosis (a severe thinning of the bones, which can cause fractures), and lymphoma (a type of cancer that affects cells of the immune system).

Coronary artery disease (atherosclerosis) is a problem that develops in almost half the patients who receive transplants. Normally, patients with this disease experience chest pain and/or other symptoms when their hearts are under stress. This is called angina and is an early warning sign of a blocked heart artery. However, transplant patients may have no early pain symptoms of a blockage building up because they have no sensations in their new hearts.

Thirty to fifty percent of patients who receive a heart-lung transplant develop bronchiolitis obliterans, in which there are obstructive changes in the airways of the lungs.

What does rejection mean?

The body's immune system protects the body from infection. Cells of the immune system move throughout the body, checking for anything that looks foreign or different from the body's own cells. Immune cells recognize the transplanted organ(s) as different from the rest of the body and attempt to destroy it—this is called rejection. If left alone, the immune system would damage the cells of a new heart and eventually destroy it. In a heart-lung transplant, immune cells may also destroy healthy lung tissue.

To prevent rejection, patients receive immunosuppressants, drugs that suppress the immune system so that the new organ(s) is not damaged. Because rejection can occur anytime after a transplant, immunosuppressive drugs are given to patients the day before their transplant and thereafter for the rest of their lives. To avoid complications, patients must strictly adhere to their drug regimen. The three main drugs now being used are cyclosporine, azathioprine, and prednisone. Researchers are working on safer, more effective immunosuppressants for future testing. Some of the more promising drugs are FK-506 and mycophenolate mofetil.

Doctors must balance the dose of immunosuppressive drugs so that a patient's transplanted organ(s) is protected, but his or her immune system is not completely shut down. Without an active enough immune system, a patient can easily develop severe infections. For this reason, medications are also prescribed to fight any infections.

To carefully monitor transplant patients for signs of heart rejection, small pieces of the transplanted organ are removed for inspection under a microscope. Called a biopsy, this procedure involves advancing a thin tube called a catheter through a vein to the heart. At the end of the catheter is a bioptome, a tiny instrument used to snip off a piece of tissue. If the biopsy shows damaged cells, the dose and kind of immunosuppressive drug may be changed. Biopsies of the heart muscle are usually performed weekly for the first 3 to 6 weeks after surgery, then every 3 months for the first year, and then yearly thereafter.

How much do transplants cost?

According to the UNOS, the estimated first year charges for a heart transplant is $209,100, and annual followup charges are $15,000. In most cases these costs are paid by private insurance companies. More than 80 percent of commercial insurers and 97 percent of Blue Cross/Blue Shield plans offer coverage for heart transplants. Medicaid programs in 33 states and the District of Columbia also reimburse for transplants. Heart transplants are covered by Medicare for Medicare-eligible patients if the operation is performed at an approved center.

Approximately 70 percent of commercial insurance companies and 92 percent of Blue Cross/Blue Shield plans cover heart-lung transplants. Medicaid coverage for heart-lung transplants is available in 20 states. According to the UNOS, estimated first year charges for a heart-lung transplant is $246,000, and annual followup charges are $18,400.

What will transplants be like in 5 to 10 years?

Hospitals nationwide are trying to set up a better system for distributing organs to patients in need. Researchers are looking for easier methods to monitor rejection to replace the regular biopsies that are needed now. Work is progressing to make immunosuppressive drugs with fewer long-term side effects so that coronary artery disease development and lung destruction may by prevented.

Chapter 72

Oxygen Therapy

Long-term oxygen therapy is now widely accepted as the standard treatment for chronic hypoxia caused by chronic obstructive pulmonary disease or other disorders such as interstitial lung disease. Oxygen therapy has also become much more versatile in recent years, as several different types of oxygen delivery devices have become available. The diversity of these devices makes it easier for physicians to select a mode of oxygen therapy that suits the patient's lifestyle.

Many patients require long-term oxygen therapy. The American Lung Association estimates that more than 800,000 Americans are maintained on long-term, chronic oxygen therapy. Oxygen therapy is a significant national health care expenditure; it is the most expensive non-surgical treatment reimbursed by Medicare. The typical monthly cost of oxygen therapy is $300. Patients with private insurance or Medicare coverage usually pay 20% of the cost, or about $60 a month.

Because most patients on supplemental oxygen must receive it continuously, and in most cases for the rest of their lives, they may erroneously view oxygen therapy as a treatment of last resort. In reality, it is an important adjunct to other modes of treatment for chronic hypoxia.

Liquid oxygen systems provide the greatest degree of portability and versatility, but they are the most costly option, and are not available to all patients.

The American Lung Association estimates that more than 800,000 Americans are maintained on long-term, chronic oxygen therapy.

Oxygen therapy reduces pulmonary artery pressure and pulmonary vascular resistance, increases exercise capacity, improves oxygenation during sleep, improves neuropsychological performance, and prolongs patient survival.

Many primary care physicians are capable of identifying which patients need oxygen therapy, determining a patient's appropriate oxygen prescription, and establishing an oxygen therapy program. However, there are advantages to having these steps performed by oxygen therapy specialists.

An adequate oxygen supply maintains an oxygen saturation of 90%.

Who Needs Oxygen?

Physicians should assess the need for oxygen therapy patients with chronic lung disease, especially those who complain of dyspnea and are not completely responsive to medical management. A general rule is that an analysis of resting blood gases is mandatory for patients with a forced expiratory volume (FEV1) of one liter or less despite receiving optimal medical treatment. At high altitudes, such as in the Rocky Mountain region, the minimum FEV1 that should trigger a blood gas analysis is 1.2 to 1.25 liters.

Chronic hypoxia can be documented in patients who are already receiving optimal medical therapy by drawing an arterial blood specimen for analysis of arterial blood gases. The blood should be drawn from patients at rest, in the seated position. The patient is considered hypoxic and in need of supplemental oxygen if the arterial oxygen pressure (PaO2) at rest is at or below 59 mmHg or less if the patient also has a hematocrit of 55% or more, "p" pulmonale on an ECG, or peripheral edema that indicates right-sided heart failure. A normal PaO2 at rest does not rule out abnormally low oxygenation during exercise or sleep; oxygen saturation can be measured during these times using an oximeter.

Selecting the System

The companies that supply oxygen therapy may provide a patient with the least expensive system unless otherwise directed by the physician's prescription. It is therefore critical that a doctor be as specific as possible in defining the parameters of oxygen therapy. Of particular importance is specification of a supply system that provides the patient with the maximum degree of mobility that is consistent with the patient's lifestyle.

A complete oxygen prescription must also specify the oxygen flow at rest, during activity, and during sleep. The appropriate oxygen dose during activity is determined by having the patient engage in these activities while measuring the patient's blood oxygen level with a fingertip oximeter. An adequate oxygen supply maintains an oxygen saturation of 90%.

Other prescription parameters include the frequency of oxygen use each day, the duration of use, and the way by which the oxygen therapy company should monitor whether the patient is correctly using the therapy equipment.

The least expensive and least portable device for oxygen therapy is an oxygen concentrator, which concentrates atmospheric oxygen and provides this as supplemental oxygen to the patient.

These devices are usually powered electrically, and are outfitted with an oxygen tube that is, at most, 50 feet long. This design makes the concentrator suitable only for patients who are confined to home. In addition to their low cost, concentrators have the advantage of requiring the lowest number of maintenance visits. A monthly visit to check the operation of the concentrator is typical.

Portable systems, which dispense oxygen from cylinders, are of two basic types based on whether the oxygen is stored as a liquid or gas. Gas cylinders are readily available and of moderate cost. Although more portable than a concentrator, the patient's mobility is still somewhat restricted by the bulkiness of these cylinders. These systems are feasible for patients who require a low oxygen flow.

Because they rely on smaller cylinders that are readily refilled at home from a reservoir, liquid oxygen systems provide the greatest degree of portability and versatility. Liquid oxygen systems are the most costly option, and are not available to all patients, particularly those who live in rural areas. Liquid oxygen is usually available in most large towns, and within a 50-60 mile radius of most cities. Liquid oxygen cylinders are easier to fill from stationary reservoirs than tanks that hold gas oxygen.

Oxygen Conservers

Oxygen delivery systems may be augmented with an oxygen conservation device, which allows a reduction in the oxygen flow rate while maintaining adequate oxygenation. Three types of oxygen conservation devices are available: reservoir devices, demand delivery devices, and transtracheal oxygen catheters.

Reservoir devices store oxygen during the expiratory phase of ventilation, and deliver the stored oxygen during inspiration. These devices can achieve a 50-60% oxygen savings in patients with chronic obstructive pulmonary disease, and they are effective whether the patient is at rest or exercising. Although reservoir conservers are inexpensive and easy to use, patients often dislike them because they are more unsightly than standard nasal prongs. This may interfere with optimal patient compliance.

Demand oxygen conservers provide oxygen only during inspiration, and save oxygen by shutting off flow during expiration. These units work by detecting negative pressure at the nose, at which time they trigger oxygen flow into the nasal cannula. Although several demand conservers are available, only four have been proven effective in rigorous studies. These are the Oxymatic, Companion Oxygen Saver, Pulsair, and Companion 550.

The transtracheal catheter delivers oxygen directly to the lungs. This diagram shows where it is placed and how it works. The simple procedure to place the catheter is done on an outpatient basis (no hospital stay) and causes very little discomfort.

Transtracheal oxygen (TTO2) delivery involves percutaneously inserting a thin catheter directly into the trachea in the anterior neck. The most widely used catheter for this purpose is the SCOOP system, which is available in two types of designs.

The SCOOP-1 catheter contains only an end port, and is suitable for low flow rates. The SCOOP-2 catheter has side ports in addition to the end port, and is suited to higher flow rates. The SCOOP-2 catheter requires daily removal and cleaning by the patient. The SCOOP-1 catheter can be cleaned in place, although it can also be removed for cleaning.

Studies have documented that transtracheal catheters conserve oxygen and improve compliance with the oxygen prescription. In addition, transtracheal oxygen can provide important physiologic benefits by decreasing the patient-generated inspired volume and dead space. This effect results in reduced work of breathing for the patient. In addition, transtracheal oxygen may improve the patient's exercise capacity.

The disadvantages of transtracheal delivery are the need for daily catheter cleaning, and complications from tracheal placement. One complication is infection, either in the form of cellulitis at the insertion site, or a lower respiratory tract infection. The most important complication during long-term use is development of mucus balls, which form around the catheter. These balls may become large enough to cause partial tracheal obstruction. Clinically significant mucus balls occur in 10-25% of patients. Despite such complications, patients usually elect to continue transtracheal oxygen because of the treatment's benefits.

Review the efficacy of oxygen therapy every six months, or whenever there is a significant change in the patient's clinical status.

The successful use of transtracheal oxygen delivery requires a progressive program of patient support and education during a one to two month period. For patients who balk at the idea of a transtracheal catheter, the educational process might begin by having the patient talk to others who are already using transtracheal delivery, or having the patient watch a video on the subject that is available from National Jewish. The educational program should give the patient a clear understanding of the catheter system prior to its insertion, and should continue until the patient demonstrates successful independent use of the catheter.

Patient Education

All elements of oxygen therapy require thorough patient education and support if the treatment is to be successful. A physician should begin the educational process when long-term oxygen is initially prescribed, and should continue with help from the respiratory care practitioners who assist the patient with oxygen therapy at home.

It is particularly important to address the patient's concerns and attitudes about oxygen therapy. Patients often react to the news that they require oxygen therapy with questions such as: "Am I that bad?", "Can't I just use it when I feel I have to?", "Will I ever be able to get off it?", and "I could never be seen in public with that on."

The transition to routine oxygen therapy is difficult, particularly for patients who are not significantly short of breath and do not feel noticeably different when using oxygen. Physicians should stress the effect of oxygen therapy on quality of life, and avoid the mistake of emphasizing how oxygen therapy will help prolong a patient's life. Although this is a compelling medical rationale for oxygen therapy, patients may feel that they don't want to live longer if their life will be made miserable by the treatment.

Instead, emphasize that oxygen therapy will help relieve shortness of breath and help improve performance. One approach that is often successful is a tangible demonstration of the benefits of oxygen therapy. Have the patient walk in a corridor or outside for a specific length of time, such as six minutes. Then have the patient walk in a corridor or outside for a specific length of time, such as six minutes. Then have the patient walk for the same time interval while on oxygen therapy. Compare the distances walked each time, and emphasize that oxygen therapy can significantly improve the patient's ability to perform routine activities.

The most effective way to educate patients about the use of oxygen delivery equipment is a hands-on approach that centers on demonstrations with the specific equipment that the patient will use. This places a lot of educational responsibility in the hands of the therapists who help patients set up and use their equipment.

Follow-Up

No clear evidence exists on how often a patient's oxygen therapy prescription should be reviewed. This question is now being addressed by a research project at National Jewish. Despite this uncertainty, patients clearly need reevaluation as their disease progresses. For the time being, our recommendation is to review the efficacy of oxygen therapy every six months, or whenever there is a significant change in the patient's clinical status.

References

1. Corsello, PR, Make BJ. Which oxygen-conserving device is best for your patient? *J. Resp Dis* 1992, 13:27-41.

2. Couser, JT, Rassulo, J., Make BJ. Transtracheal oxygen decreases inspired minute ventilation. *Am Rev Respir Dis* 1989, 139:627-31.

3. Couser, JT, Make BJ. Respiratory tract infection complicating transtracheal oxygen therapy. *Chest* 1992, 101:273-5.

4. Lutz, M, Kraft, M., Make, B. Long-term oxygen therapy in patients with chronic obstructive pulmonary disease. *Sem Respir Med*, in press.

5. Tiep, B. Portable oxygen therapy: including oxygen conserving methodology. Futura Publishing Company, Inc., Mount Kisco, N.Y., 1991.

Chapter 73

Pulmonary Rehabilitation

What Is Pulmonary Rehabilitation?

Pulmonary rehabilitation is a program for persons with chronic lung diseases such as emphysema, chronic bronchitis, asthma, bronchiectasis, or interstitial lung disease. Most pulmonary rehabilitation programs will include medical management, education, emotional support, exercise, breathing retraining, and nutritional counseling.

The purpose of pulmonary rehabilitation is to help people lead a full, satisfying life; to restore them to their highest possible functional capacity; and to help them live a more comfortable and enjoyable life. These goal are often met by:

- decreasing respiratory symptoms and complications.

- encouraging independence through self-management and control over daily functioning.

- improving physical conditioning and exercise performance.

- improving emotional well-being.

- reducing hospitalizations.

451

The Pulmonary Rehabilitation Team

Pulmonary rehabilitation programs can be conducted while a person is a hospital inpatient, or on an outpatient basis. Many skilled professionals are part of the pulmonary rehabilitation team. In addition to physicians, the team may include:

- respiratory therapists
- dietitians
- educators
- physical therapists
- social workers
- nurses
- psychologists
- occupational therapists
- other allied health professionals

The Pulmonary Rehabilitation Program

A typical rehabilitation program includes:

- breathing exercises
- exercise reconditioning
- progressive relaxation training
- stress and panic control techniques
- smoking cessation
- educational programs to provide information on:
  medication
  diet
  exercises
  caring for and operating respiratory therapy equipment
- exercise programs that may include:
  calisthenics or stretching exercises to increase flexibility
  weight training to increase exercise endurance and conditioning
  specific exercises on stationary bicycles, treadmills, and other
  miscellaneous exercise machines

Chapter 74

National Emphysema Treatment Trial (NETT)

What Is NETT?

The National Emphysema Treatment Trial (NETT), supported by the National Heart, Lung, and Blood Institute (NHLBI), the Health Care Financing Administration (HCFA), and the Agency for Health Care Policy and Research (AHCPR), is the first multi-center clinical trial designed to determine the role, safety, and effectiveness of bilateral lung volume reduction surgery (LVRS) in the treatment of emphysema. Emphysema is a chronic lung condition that is a major cause of death and disability in the U.S. If LVRS is found to be beneficial, then a secondary objective will be to develop criteria for identifying patients who are likely to benefit from the procedure.

Why Is NETT Necessary?

In patients with emphysema, the walls between the tiny air sacs in the lungs are damaged. While healthy lungs expand with each inhalation and collapse with each exhalation, helping to move air in and out—lungs damaged by emphysema gradually lose their elasticity, becoming floppy and over-expanded like a spent rubber band. The airways, normally held open by the elastic pull of the lungs, also become floppy and collapse on exhalation. As a result, patients with

"National Emphysema Treatment Trial (NETT): Evaluation of Lung Volume Reduction Surgery for Emphysema," National Heart, Lung, and Blood Institute (NHLBI), October 8, 1998.

emphysema have increasing difficulty moving air in and out of their lungs.

In Lung Volume Reduction Surgery (LVRS), the size of the lungs is reduced. The theory underlying the surgery is that reducing the lung size will pull open the airways and allow the breathing muscles to return to a more normal and comfortable position, making breathing easier.

LVRS has been proposed as a new treatment that can improve quality of life for people with end-stage emphysema, but many questions about the procedure are unanswered—for example:

- What are the benefits and the risks compared with good medical therapy alone?

- How long do any benefits last?

- Does the surgery benefit some patients more than others?

These are questions that doctors and patients need to have answered before they can make informed, rational decisions about undertaking the surgery.

The NHLBI of the National Institutes of Health has undertaken NETT with the expectation that it will provide definitive answers to these important questions. The HCFA, which oversees the Medicare program and is cosponsoring NETT, will use the data from the study to determine whether Medicare should provide reimbursement for LVRS.

Background and Rationale for NETT

LVRS was first used to treat emphysema in the 1950s. Although some patients seemed to improve following the surgery, high mortality and morbidity associated with LVRS prevented its widespread use. In the early 1990s, some physicians began using the procedure again. Early reported successes led to the procedure's rapid spread, despite the lack of data on its long-term benefits, risks, and costs, compared with those of the current best available treatments for emphysema.

To begin to examine the issues about the safety and effectiveness of LVRS, the NHLBI convened a workshop of experts in the treatment of emphysema in 1995. The workshop participants reviewed the available data and were unanimous in their opinion that, before the surgery became widely practiced, a systematic evaluation of patient selection criteria and long-term outcomes should be undertaken.

An independent assessment of LVRS performed for HCFA concluded that the current data on the risks and benefits of LVRS were too inconclusive to justify unrestricted Medicare reimbursement for the surgery. However, because it appeared that some patients benefited from the procedure, the Center for Health Care Technology of the AHCPR, which performed the assessment, advised HCFA that a trial evaluating the effectiveness of the surgery was essential.

As a result, the NHLBI and HCFA announced in April 1996 that they would conduct a scientific study of LVRS to evaluate the safety and effectiveness of the current best available medical treatment alone and in conjunction with LVRS by excision. In late 1996, the participating clinical centers and a coordinating center were announced. Patient screening for entry into the study began in the fall of 1997.

Since the centers were selected, the NETT investigators and HCFA have continued to review data on the effectiveness of LVRS, but they have found that there is insufficient follow-up data on too many of the patients to permit them to draw conclusions. Of 1,741 LVRS cases performed at the NETT centers prior to the study, the investigators found that only 25 percent had sufficient follow-up data to determine outcome. With information missing on 75 percent of the patients, it is not possible to draw conclusions about outcomes, especially since patients who do better following surgery are more likely to return for follow-up than sicker patients.

While Medicare has complete data on 711 patients who underwent LVRS between October 1995 and January 1996, these data contrast sharply with those in the published literature, which reports successes in selected cases and low mortality. The Medicare data show that 26 percent of the patients had died by January 1997, 40 percent had been re-hospitalized (averaging 2.1 admissions and 30 hospital days), and 16 percent required long-term inpatient care. However, because there was no control group, it is not known whether these outcomes can be attributed to the surgery or to the natural history of the underlying disease.

The NETT Protocol

The trial is designed to include about 4,500 patients and to take up to 5 years to complete. The trial could be terminated early if one of the regular quarterly reviews of the data shows clear risk or benefit for one of the treatments.

People who are interested in participating in the trial should ask their physicians to send their medical history, a chest x-ray, and results of spirometry and EKG tests to the NETT center of their choice. Based on this preliminary information, the center will determine whether further screening is warranted. If so, the patient will be asked to undergo an evaluation to establish whether he or she meets all of the eligibility criteria and to provide baseline data.

Once enrolled in the study, consenting patients will complete a 6-10 week rehabilitation program in which they will receive medicines and oxygen as needed and participate in a program of exercise and breathing methods. These currently are the best known medical treatments for emphysema.

After successful completion of this rehabilitation program, consenting patients will be randomly assigned either to continue this treatment or to have lung volume reduction surgery in addition to continued medical treatment.

For this trial, surgery will be performed on both lungs, either by insertion of a tube through the chest wall (bilateral video-assisted thorascopy) or through an incision through the center of the breast bone (median sternotomy). In centers with experience in both techniques, patients assigned to surgery will be randomly assigned to one of the surgical methods.

Patients will remain under the care of their own physicians while enrolled but will be evaluated periodically for response to treatment by NETT physicians. These evaluations will be scheduled every 6 months for 2 years and every year thereafter until the conclusion of the trial. Follow-up evaluations will include tests of exercise tolerance and pulmonary and cardiovascular function, laboratory and radiologic tests, and psychosocial and quality-of-life assessments.

Eligibility Criteria

Participants in NETT must have a diagnosis of emphysema that substantially reduces their ability to function. They must meet certain pulmonary function and CT scan requirements and be approved for surgery by a cardiologist, a pulmonologist, and a thoracic surgeon.

However, they cannot participate if they:

- are smoking or have smoked tobacco within the last 4 months
- have unstable angina or cardiac arrhythmia
- have had a heart attack within the past 6 months
- have had certain, selected thoracic or cardiac surgeries or
- have another disease that is likely to interfere with participation in the trial or to reduce survival.

People who wish to participate should ask their physicians to refer them to the NETT center of their choice. For more information on the location of specific centers, please go to the list of participating centers.

Treatment Costs

Medicare recipients enrolled in NETT will receive coverage for all services integral to the study that are permitted under the Medicare law. Expenses not normally covered by Medicare, such as the costs of oral medications, will be the responsibility of the patients or, if they have additional insurance that will cover these expenses, those insurance programs. Patients may be responsible for deductibles and co-payments required by Medicare and other insurers.

Private insurers also are participating in NETT, so people interested in participating in the study should check with their insurers about coverage of services.

Chapter 75

Management of Respiratory Failure

The patient with respiratory failure cannot be adequately treated in the general care areas of the hospital. Therefore, patients in severe respiratory failure are usually treated in the intensive care unit. Current therapy for all forms of respiratory failure attempts, first, to provide support for the heart, lungs, and other affected vital organs; and second, to identify and treat the underlying cause.

Since the immediate threat to patients with respiratory failure is due to the inadequate level of oxygen delivered to the tissues, oxygenation is the basic therapy for acute respiratory failure due to lung disease. Oxygen-enriched air is usually given to the patient by nasal prongs, oxygen mask, or by placing an air tube into the trachea (windpipe).

Since prolonged high oxygen levels can be toxic, the concentration of oxygen must be carefully controlled for both short- and long-term treatment. Assisted ventilation with mechanical devices may be the first priority for neuromuscular disease patients going into respiratory failure. Additional treatments employ ventilation which helps to keep the lungs inflated at low lung volumes (positive end-expiratory pressure, PEEP), and fluid and nutritional management.

Excerpted from "Respiratory Failure," National Heart, Lung, and Blood Institute (NHLBI), NIH Publication Number 95-3531, 1995. Despite the age of this document, it still provides important information about methods commonly used to manage respiratory failure. Questions about current recommendations for treatment should be directed to a qualified health care provider.

Endotracheal Intubation. Endotracheal intubation involves insertion of a tube into the trachea. It permits delivery of precisely determined amounts of oxygen to the lungs and removal of secretions, and ensures adequate ventilation. Combined with mechanical ventilation, endotracheal intubation is the cornerstone of therapy for respiratory failure.

Mechanical Ventilation. If the patient is tiring despite ongoing therapy, a mechanical ventilator, also called a respirator, is used. The ventilator assists or controls the patient's breathing.

Positive End-Expiratory Pressure (PEEP). Positive end-expiratory pressure is used with mechanical ventilation to keep the air pressure in the trachea at a level that increases the volume of gas remaining in the lung after breathing out (expiration). This keeps the alveoli open, reduces the shunting of blood through the lungs, and improves gas exchange. Most ventilators have a PEEP adjustment.

Extracorporeal Membrane Oxygenator (ECMO). The extracorporeal membrane oxygenator (ECMO) is essentially an artificial lung. It is an appropriately cased artificial membrane which is attached to the patient externally (extracorporeally), through a vein or artery. Although the best substitute for a diseased lung that cannot handle gas exchange adequately is a healthy human lung, such substitution is often not possible. Circulating the patient's blood through the ECMO offers another approach. Gas exchange using ECMO keeps the patient alive while the damaged lungs have a chance to heal.

In 1974, the National Heart, Lung, and Blood Institute (NHLBI) organized a carefully designed clinical trial, to determine the effectiveness of ECMO for patients with acute respiratory distress syndrome. In this study, ECMO appeared to be no more useful than conventional therapy. On the other hand, ECMO seems to be an effective option in some infants with respiratory failure when treatment with mechanical ventilation fails. However ECMO is expensive, is associated with nonrespiratory complications, and is available only in a few specialized centers.

Management of Fluids and Electrolytes. Pulmonary edema, the buildup of abnormal amounts of fluid in the lung tissues, often occurs in respiratory failure. Therefore fluids are carefully managed and monitored to maintain fluid balance and avoid fluid overload which may further worsen gas exchange.

Pharmacologic Therapy. Because respiratory failure may be the end result of several different diseases, no single drug therapy is effective in all situations.

- Antibiotics help when infections (sepsis) as well as pneumonia are involved in respiratory failure.

- Bronchodilators, for example, theophylline compounds, sympathomimetic agents (albuterol, metaproterenol, isoproterenol), anticholinergics (ipratropium bromide), and corticosteroids, reverse bronchoconstriction and reduce tissue inflammation.

- Other drugs, such as digitalis, improve cardiac output, and drugs which increase blood pressure in shock can improve blood flow to the tissues.

Bronchoscopy. Patients with respiratory failure who have excessive lung secretions are sometimes helped by fiberoptic bronchoscopy, a technique for accessing the interior of the bronchi, the larger air passages of the lungs. The bronchoscope is a flexible tube with a light at the end that is passed through the nose or mouth into the trachea and bronchi. Fluid or tissue can be removed from the bronchi (aspiration), and cells for microscopic examination can be obtained by washing the interior of the larger breathing tubes (lavage).

Bronchoscopy is useful for placing or removing endotracheal tubes, removing foreign bodies from the lung, and collecting tissue samples for diagnosis.

Intravenous Nutritional Support. Nutritional supplementation is essential to maintain or restore strength when weakness and loss of muscle mass prevent patients from breathing adequately without ventilatory support. Appropriate nutrients (fats, carbohydrates, and predigested proteins) are fed intravenously for this purpose.

Physiotherapy. Physiotherapy includes chest percussion (repeated sharp blows to the chest and back to loosen secretions), suction of airways, and regular changes of body position. It helps drain secretions, maintains alveolar inflation and prevents atelectasis, incomplete expansion of the lung.

X-ray Monitoring. X-ray images of the chest help the doctor monitor the progress of lung and heart disease in respiratory failure. The portable chest radiograph taken with an x-ray machine brought to the bedside is often used for this purpose in the intensive care unit.

Lung Transplantation. Lung transplantation currently offers the only hope for certain patients with end-stage pulmonary disease. The shortage of suitable donors and the high cost of the procedure continue to be major obstacles that limit its use.

Complications of Treatment. Oxygen toxicity, pulmonary embolism (closure of the pulmonary artery or one of its branches by a blood clot or a fat globule), cardiovascular problems, barotrauma (injury to the lung tissue from excessive ventilatory pressure), pneumothorax (air in the pleural space), and gastrointestinal bleeding are some of the complications of treatment. They result from fluid overload, mechanical ventilation, PEEP, and other procedures used in the management of respiratory failure.

Weaning the Patients from Ventilators. The process of returning the patient to unassisted and spontaneous breathing is called weaning. Weaning is a complex process that requires the understanding and cooperation of the patient. It can cause great fatigue and depression in patients because of the slow- and long-term nature of the treatment procedures.

Weaning a patient too rapidly or prematurely can be dangerous. Some patients, particularly those who had severe underlying cardiac disease and prolonged episodes of acute illnesses, may require weeks to months to wean. The doctor considers weaning only when the patient is awake, has good nutrition, and is able to cough and breathe deeply.

Discontinuation of Ventilatory Support. The difficult question of whether and when to discontinue life-sustaining mechanical ventilation to the patient who is not responding to any treatment is sometimes faced by the doctor and the family. The legal, ethical, and financial implications of continuing or withholding treatment to the patient in terminal respiratory failure are important issues addressed at family, professional, and government levels.

Respecting the rights and wishes of the patient and helping the patient achieve a dignified and peaceful end while continuing to assure care and comfort is a responsibility shared by both the caregivers and the family. The family with a good understanding of respiratory failure in all its dimensions is best equipped to play its part in sharing this responsibility.

Part Five

Risks and Prevention

Chapter 76

Passive Smoke

The U.S. Environmental Protection Agency (EPA) has published a major assessment of the respiratory health risks of passive smoking (Respiratory Health Effects of Passive Smoking: Lung Cancer and Other Disorders; EPA/600/6-90/006F). The report concludes that exposure to environmental tobacco smoke (ETS)—commonly known as secondhand smoke—is responsible for approximately 3,000 lung cancer deaths each year in nonsmoking adults and impairs the respiratory health of hundreds of thousands of children.

The Environmental Protection Agency firmly maintains that the bulk of the scientific evidence demonstrates that secondhand smoke—environmental tobacco smoke, or "ETS"—causes lung cancer and other significant health threats to children and adults. EPA's report ("Respiratory Health Effects of Passive Smoking: Lung Cancer and Other Disorders," EPA/600/6-90/006F) was peer-reviewed by 18 eminent, independent scientists who unanimously endorsed the study's methodology and conclusions. Since EPA's 1993 report which estimated the risks posed by ETS, numerous independent health studies have presented an impressive accumulating body of evidence that confirms and strengthens the EPA findings. It is widely accepted in the scientific and public health communities that secondhand smoke poses significant health risks to children and adults.

A U.S. District Court decision has vacated several chapters of the EPA document "Respiratory Health Effects of Passive Smoking: Lung

"Respiratory Health Effects of Passive Smoking," U.S. Environment Protection Agency (EPA), EPA-43-F-93-003; modified February 1999.

Cancer and Other Disorders" that served as the basis for EPA's classification of secondhand smoke as a Group A carcinogen and estimates that ETS causes 3,000 lung cancer deaths in non-smokers each year. The ruling was largely based on procedural grounds. EPA is appealing this decision. None of the findings concerning the serious respiratory health effects of secondhand smoke in children were challenged.

Background

EPA studies of human exposure to air pollutants indicate that indoor levels of many pollutants often are significantly higher than outdoor levels. These levels of indoor air pollutants are of particular concern because it is estimated that most people spend approximately 90 percent of their time indoors.

In recent years, comparative risk studies performed by EPA and its Science Advisory Board have consistently ranked indoor air pollution among the top five environmental risks to public health. EPA, in close cooperation with other federal agencies and the private sector, has begun a concerted effort to better understand indoor air pollution and to reduce peoples' exposure to air pollutants in offices, homes, schools and other indoor environments where people live, work and play.

Tobacco smoking has long been recognized as a major cause of death and disease, responsible for an estimated 434,000 deaths per year in the United States. Tobacco use is known to cause lung cancer in humans, and is a major risk factor for heart disease.

In recent years, there has been concern that non-smokers may also be at risk for some of these health effects as a result of their exposure ("passive smoking") to the smoke exhaled by smokers and smoke given off by the burning end of cigarettes. As part of its effort to address all types of indoor air pollution, in 1988, EPA's Indoor Air Division (now the Indoor Environments Division) requested that EPA's Office of Research and Development (ORD) undertake an assessment of the respiratory health effects of passive smoking. The report was prepared by ORD's Office of Health and Environmental Assessment.

The document has been prepared under the authority of Title IV of Superfund (The Radon Gas and Indoor Air Quality Research Act of 1986), which directs EPA to conduct research and disseminate information on all aspects of indoor air quality.

Public and Scientific Reviews

A draft of this assessment was released for public review in June 1990. In December 1990, EPA's Science Advisory Board (SAB), a committee of independent scientists, conducted a review of the draft report and submitted its comments to the EPA Administrator in April 1991. In its comments, the SAB's Indoor Air Quality/Total Human Exposure Committee concurred with the primary findings of the report, but made a number of recommendations for strengthening it.

Incorporating these recommendations, the Agency again transmitted a new draft to the SAB in May of 1992 for a second review. Following a July 1992 meeting, the SAB panel endorsed the major conclusions of the report, including its unanimous endorsement of the classification of environmental tobacco smoke (ETS) as a Group A (known human) carcinogen.

EPA also received and reviewed more than 100 comments from the public, and integrated appropriate revisions into the final risk assessment.

Major Conclusions

Based on the weight of the available scientific evidence, EPA has concluded that the widespread exposure to environmental tobacco smoke in the U.S. presents a serious and substantial public health risk.

In Adults

ETS is a human lung carcinogen, responsible for approximately 3,000 lung cancer deaths annually in U.S. nonsmokers. ETS has been classified as a Group A carcinogen under EPA's carcinogen assessment guidelines. This classification is reserved for those compounds or mixtures which have been shown to cause cancer in humans, based on studies in human populations.

In Children

ETS exposure increases the risk of lower respiratory tract infections such as bronchitis and pneumonia. EPA estimates that between 150,000 and 300,000 of these cases annually in infants and young children up to 18 months of age are attributable to exposure to ETS. Of these, between 7,500 and 15,000 will result in hospitalization.

- ETS exposure increases the prevalence of fluid in the middle ear, a sign of chronic middle ear disease.

- ETS exposure in children irritates the upper respiratory tract and is associated with a small but significant reduction in lung function.

- ETS exposure increases the frequency of episodes and severity of symptoms in asthmatic children. The report estimates that 200,000 to 1,000,000 asthmatic children have their condition worsened by exposure to environmental tobacco smoke.

- ETS exposure is a risk factor for new cases of asthma in children who have not previously displayed symptoms.

Scope of the Report

In 1986, the National Research Council (NRC) and the U.S. Surgeon General independently assessed the health effects of exposure to ETS. Both of these reports concluded that ETS can cause lung cancer in adult non-smokers and that children of parents who smoke have increased frequency of respiratory symptoms and lower respiratory tract infections. The EPA scientific assessment builds on these reports and is based on a thorough review of all of the studies in the available literature.

Since 1986, the number of studies which examine these issues in human populations has more than doubled, resulting in a larger database with which to conduct a comprehensive assessment of the potential effects which passive smoking may have on the respiratory health of adults as well as children.

Because only a very small number of studies on the possible association between exposure to secondhand smoke and heart disease and other cancers existed in the scientific literature at the time this assessment was first undertaken, EPA has not conducted an assessment of the possible association of heart disease and passive smoking. EPA is considering whether such an assessment should be undertaken in the future, but has no plans to do so at this time.

Scientific Approach

EPA reached its conclusions concerning the potential for ETS to act as a human carcinogen based on an analysis of all of the available data, including more than 30 epidemiologic (human) studies looking specifically at passive smoking as well as information on active or direct smoking. In addition, EPA considered animal data, biological measurements of human uptake of tobacco smoke components and other available data. The conclusions were based on what is commonly known as the total weight-of-evidence" rather than on any one study or type of study.

The finding that ETS should be classified as a Group A carcinogen is based on the conclusive evidence of the dose-related lung carcinogenicity of mainstream smoke in active smokers and the similarities of mainstream and sidestream smoke given off by the burning end of the cigarette. The finding is bolstered by the statistically significant exposure-related increase in lung cancer in nonsmoking spouses of smokers which is found in an analysis of more than 30 epidemiology studies that examined the association between secondhand smoke and lung cancer.

The weight-of-evidence analysis for the noncancer respiratory effects in children is based primarily on a review of more than 100 studies, including 50 recent epidemiology studies of children whose parents smoke.

Beyond the Risk Assessment

Although EPA does not have any regulatory authority for controlling ETS, the Agency expects this report to be of value to other health professionals and policymakers in taking appropriate steps to minimize peoples' exposure to tobacco smoke in indoor environments.

In cooperation with other government agencies, EPA will continue its education and outreach program to inform the public and policy makers on what to do to reduce the health risks of ETS as well as other indoor air pollutants.

Chapter 77

Smoking Cessation

This chapter guides you from thinking about stopping smoking through actually doing it; from the day you quit to quitting for keeps. It gives tips on fighting temptation; and what to do if you give in; and on avoiding weight gain (a handy Snack Calorie Chart is included). By telling you what to expect it can help you through the day-by-day process of becoming a nonsmoker.

In this chapter, you'll find a variety of tips and helpful hints on kicking your smoking habit. Take a few moments to look at each suggestion carefully. Pick those you feel comfortable with, and decide today that you're going to use them to quit. It may take a while to find the combination that's right for you, but you can quit for good, even if you've tried to quit before.

Many smokers have successfully given up cigarettes by replacing them with new habits, without quitting "cold turkey," planning a special program, or seeking professional help.

The following approaches include many of those most popular with ex-smokers. Remember that successful methods are as different as the people who use them. What may seem silly to others may be just what you need to quit; so don't be embarrassed to try something new. These methods can make your own personal efforts a little easier.

Pick the ideas that make sense to you. And then follow through; you'll have a much better chance of success.

Text in this chapter is from an undated document produced by the National Cancer Institute (NCI), cited October 2001.

Preparing Yourself for Quitting

- Decide positively that you want to quit. Try to avoid negative thoughts about how difficult it might be.

- List all reasons you want to quit. Every night before going to bed, repeat one of those reasons 10 times.

- Develop strong personal reasons in addition to your health and obligations to others. For example, think of all the time you waste taking cigarette breaks, rushing out to buy a pack, hunting for a light, etc.

- Begin to condition yourself physically: Start a modest exercise program; drink more fluids; get plenty of rest; and avoid fatigue.

- Set a target date for quitting; perhaps a special day such as your birthday, your anniversary, or the Great American Smokeout. If you smoke heavily at work, quit during your vacation so that you're already committed to quitting when you return. Make the date sacred, and don't let anything change it. This will make it easy for you to keep track of the day you became a nonsmoker and to celebrate that date every year.

Knowing What to Expect

- Have realistic expectations; quitting isn't easy, but it's not impossible either. More than 3 million Americans quit every year.

- Understand that withdrawal symptoms are temporary. They usually last only 1-2 weeks.

- Know that most relapses occur in the first week after quitting, when withdrawal symptoms are strongest and your body is still dependent on nicotine, Be aware that this will be your hardest time, and use all your personal resources; willpower, family, friends, and the tips in this chapter; to get you through this critical period successfully.

- Know that most other relapses occur in the first week after quitting, when situational triggers, such as a particularly stressful event, occur unexpectedly. These are the times when people reach for cigarettes automatically, because they associate smoking with relaxing. This is the kind of situation that's hard to prepare yourself for until it happens, so it's especially important to recognize it if it does happen. Remember that smoking is a habit, but a habit you can break.

- Realize that most successful ex-smokers quit for good only after several attempts. You may be one of those who can quit on your first try. But if you're not, don't give up. Try again.

Involving Someone Else

- Bet a friend you can quit on your target date. Put your cigarette money aside for every day, and forfeit it if you smoke. (But if you do smoke, don't give up. Simply strengthen your resolve and try again.)

- Ask your friend or spouse to quit with you.

- Tell your family and friends that you're quitting and when. They can be an important source of support both before and after you quit.

Ways of Quitting

Switch Brands

- Switch to a brand you find distasteful.

- Change to a brand that is low in tar and nicotine a couple of weeks before your target date. This will help change your smoking behavior. However, do not smoke more cigarettes, inhale them more often or more deeply, or place your fingertips over the holes in the filters. All of these will increase your nicotine intake, and the idea is to get your body use to functioning without nicotine.

Cut Down the Number of Cigarettes You Smoke

- Smoke only half of each cigarette.

- Each day, postpone the lighting of your first cigarette 1 hour.

- Decide you'll only smoke during odd or even hours of the day.

- Decide beforehand how many cigarettes you'll smoke during the day. For each additional cigarette, give a dollar to your favorite charity.

- Change your eating habits to help you cut down. For example, drink milk, which many people consider incompatible with smoking. End meals or snacks with something that won't lead to a cigarette.

- Reach for a glass of juice instead of a cigarette for a "pick-me-up."

- Remember: Cutting down can help you quit, but it's not a substitute for quitting. If you're down to about 7 cigarettes a day, its time to set your target quit date and get ready to stick to it.

Don't Smoke "Automatically"

- Smoke only those cigarettes you really want. Catch yourself before you light up a cigarette out of pure habit.

- Don't empty your ashtrays. This will remind you of how many cigarettes you've smoked each day, and the sight and the smell of stale cigarettes butts will be very unpleasant.

- Make yourself aware of each cigarette by using the opposite hand or putting cigarettes in an unfamiliar location or a different pocket to break the automatic reach.

- If you light up many times during the day without even thinking about it, try to look in a mirror each time you put a match to your cigarette; you may decide you don't need it.

Make Smoking Inconvenient

- Stop buying cigarettes by the carton. Wait until one pack is empty before you buy another.

- Stop carrying cigarettes with you at home or at work. Make them difficult to get to.

Make Smoking Unpleasant

- Smoke only under circumstances that aren't especially pleasurable for you. If you like to smoke with others, smoke alone. Turn your chair to an empty corner and focus only on the cigarette you are smoking and all its many negative effects.

- Collect all your cigarette butts in one large glass container as a visual reminder of the filth made by smoking.

Just Before Quitting

- Practice going without cigarettes.

- Don't think of never smoking again. Think of quitting in terms of 1 day at a time.

- Tell yourself you won't smoke today, and then don't.

- Clean your clothes to rid them of the cigarette smell, which can linger a long time.

On the Day You Quit

- Throw away all your cigarettes and matches. Hide your lighters and ash trays.

- Visit the dentist and have your teeth cleaned to get rid of tobacco stains. Notice how nice they look and resolve to keep them that way.

- Make a list of things you'd like to buy for yourself or someone else. Estimate the cost in terms of packs of cigarettes, and put the money aside to buy these presents.

- Keep very busy on the big day. Go to the movies, exercise, take long walks, go bike riding.

- Remind your family and friends that this is your quit date, and ask them to help you over the rough spots of the first couple of days and weeks.

- Buy yourself a treat or do something special to celebrate.

Immediately after Quitting

- Develop a clean, fresh, nonsmoking environment around yourself; at work and at home.

- Buy yourself flowers; you may be surprised how much you can enjoy their scent now.

- The first few days after you quit, spend as much free time as possible in places where smoking isn't allowed, such as libraries. museums, theaters, department stores, and churches.

- Drink large quantities of water and fruit juice (but avoid sodas that contain caffeine).

- Try to avoid alcohol, coffee, and other beverages that you associate with cigarette smoking.

- Strike up conversation instead of a match for a cigarette.

- If you miss the sensation of having a cigarette in your hand, play with something else; a pencil, a paper clip, a marble.

- If you miss having something in your mouth, try toothpicks or a fake cigarette.

Avoid Temptation

- Instead of smoking after meals, get up from the table and brush your teeth or go for a walk.

- If you always smoke while driving, listen to a particularly interesting radio program or your favorite music, or take public transportation for a while, if you can.

- For the first 1-3 weeks, avoid situations you strongly associate with the pleasurable aspects of smoking, such as watching your favorite TV program, sitting in your favorite chair, or having a cocktail before dinner.

- Until you are confident of your ability to stay off cigarettes, limit your socializing to healthful, outdoor activities or situations where smoking is not allowed.

- If you must be in a situation where you'll be tempted to smoke (such as a cocktail or dinner party), try to associate with the nonsmokers there.

- Try to analyze cigarette ads to understand how they attempt to "sell" you on individual brands.

When You Get the Crazies

- Keep oral substitutes handy; try carrots, pickles, sunflower seeds, apples, celery, raisins, or sugarless gum instead of a cigarette.

- Take 10 deep breathes and hold the last one while lighting a match. Exhale slowly and blow out the match. Pretend it's a cigarette and crush it out in an ashtray.

- Take a shower or bath if possible.

- Learn to relax quickly and deeply. Make yourself limp, visualize a soothing, pleasing situation, and get away from it all for a moment. Concentrate on that peaceful image and nothing else.

- Light incense or a candle instead of a cigarette.

- Never allow yourself to think that "one won't hurt"; it will.

Find New Habits

- Change your habits to make smoking difficult, impossible or unnecessary, For example, it's hard to smoke while you're swimming, jogging, or playing tennis or handball. When your desire for a cigarette is intense, wash your hands or the dishes, or try new recipes.

- Do things that require you to use your hands. Try crossword puzzles, needlework, gardening, or household chores. Go bike riding or take the dog for a walk; give yourself a manicure; write letters.

- Enjoy having a clean mouth taste and maintain it by brushing your teeth frequently and using a mouthwash.

- Stretch a lot.

- Get plenty of rest.

- Pay attention to your appearance. Look and feel sharp.

- Try to find time for the activities that are the most meaningful, satisfying, and important to you.

About Gaining Weight

Many people who are considering quitting are very concerned about gaining weight. If you are concerned about weight gain, keep these points in mind:

- Quitting doesn't mean you'll automatically gain weight. When people gain it's because they often eat more once they quit.

- The benefits of giving up cigarettes far outweigh the drawbacks of adding a few pounds. You'd have to gain a very large amount of weight to offset the many substantial health benefits that a normal smoker gains by quitting. Watch what you eat, and if you are concerned about gaining weight, consider the tips that follow.

Table 77.1. Snack Calorie Chart, continued on next page.

BEVERAGES

Carbonated (per 8-ounce glass)
    Cola-type   95 calories
    Fruit flavors (10-13% sugar)   115 calories
    Ginger Ale   75 calories

Fruit drinks (per 1/2 cup)
    Apricot nectar   70 calories
    Cranberry juice   80 calories
    Grape drink   70 calories
    Lemonade (frozen)   55 calories

Fruit juices (per 1/2 cup)
    Apple juice, canned   60 calories
    Grape juice, bottled   80 calories
    Grapefruit juice, canned, unsweetened   50 calories
    Orange juice, canned, unsweetened   55 calories
    Pineapple juice, canned, unsweetened   70 calories
    Prune juice, canned   100 calories

Vegetable juices (per 1/2 cup)
    Tomato juice   25 calories
    Vegetable juice cocktail   20 calories

Coffee and tea
    Coffee, black   3-5 calories
    with 1 tsp. Sugar   18-20 calories
    with 1 tsp. Cream   3-15 calories
    Tea, plain   0-1 calories
    with 1 tsp. Sugar   15-16 calories

CANDY, CHIPS, AND PRETZELS

Candy (per ounce)
    Hard candy   110 calories
    Jelly beans   105 calories
    Marshmallows   90 calories
    Gumdrops   100 calories

Chips (per cup)
    Corn chips   230 calories
    Potato chips   115 calories

Popcorn
    (air-popped, without butter)   25 calories

Table 77.1. Snack Calorie Chart, continued from previous page.

CANDY, CHIPS, AND PRETZELS, continued

Pretzels
  Dutch, 1 twisted   60 calories
  Stick, 5 regular   10 calories

CHEESE (per ounce)

American, processed   105 calories
Cottage, creamed   30 calories
Cottage, low-fat (2%)   25 calories
Swiss, natural   105 calories

CRACKERS

Butter, 2-inch diameter   15 calories
Graham, 2 1/2 inches square, 2   55 calories
Matzoh, 6-inch diameter   80 calories
Rye   45 calories
Saltine   50 calories

FRUITS (raw)

Apple, 1 medium	80 calories	Grapefruit, ½	40 calories
Apricots, fresh, 3 medium	50 calories	Grapes, 20	30 calories
Apricots, dried, 5 halves	40 calories	Orange, 1 medium	60 calories
Banana, 1 medium	105 calories	Peach, 1 medium	35 calories
Blackberries, 1/2 cup	35 calories	Pear, 1 medium	100 calories
Blueberries, 1/2 cup	40 calories	Pineapple, 1/2 cup	40 calories
Cantaloupe, 1/4 melon	50 calories	Prunes, dried, 3	60 calories
Cherries, 10	50 calories	Raisins, 1/4 cup	110 calories
Dates, dried, 3	70 calories	Strawberries, 1 cup	45 calories
Fig, dried, 1 medium	50 calories	Watermelon, 1 cup	50 calories

NUTS (per 2 tablespoons)

Almonds	105 calories	Peanuts	105 calories
Brazil nuts	115 calories	Pecans, halves	95 calories
Cashews	100 calories		

VEGETABLES (raw)

Carrots, 1/2 cup grated   35 calories
Celery, 5-inch stalks, 3   10 calories
Pickle, 1   15-20 calories

Tips to Help You Avoid Weight Gain

- Make sure you have a well balanced diet, with the proper amounts of protein, carbohydrates and fat.

- Don't set a target date for a holiday, when the temptation of high calorie food and drinks may be too hard to resist.

- Drink a glass of water before your meals.

- Weigh yourself weekly.

- Chew sugarless gum when you want sweet foods.

- Plan menus carefully, and count calories. Don't try to lose weight; just try to maintain your prequitting weight.

Table 77.2. Withdrawal Symptoms and Activities That Might Help

Dry mouth; sore throat, gums, or tongue	Sip ice-cold water or fruit juice, or chew gum.
Headaches	Take a warm bath or shower. Try relaxation or meditation techniques.
Trouble sleeping	Don't drink coffee, tea or soda with caffeine after 6:00 p.m. Again, try relaxation or meditation techniques.
Irregularity	Add roughage to your diet, such as raw fruit, vegetables, and whole grain cereals. Drink 6-8 glasses of water a day.
Fatigue	Take a nap. Try not to push yourself during this time; don't expect too much of your body until it's had a chance to begin to heal itself over a couple of weeks.
Hunger	Drink water or low-calorie liquids. Eat low-fat, low-calorie snacks. See Snack Calorie Chart.
Tenseness, irritability	Take a walk, soak in a hot bath, try relaxation or meditation techniques.
Coughing	Sip warm herbal tea. Suck on cough drops or sugarless hard candy.

- Have low calorie foods on hand for nibbling. Use the Snack Calorie Chart to choose foods that are both nutritious and low in calories. Some good choices are fresh fruits and vegetables, fruit and vegetable juices, low-fat cottage cheese, and air-popped popcorn without butter.

- Take time for daily exercise, or join an organized exercise group.

What Happens after You Quit Smoking

Immediate Rewards

Within 12 hours after you have your last cigarette, your body will begin to heal itself. The levels of carbon monoxide and nicotine in your system will decline rapidly, and your heart and lungs will begin to repair the damage caused by cigarette smoke.

Within a few days you will probably begin to notice some remarkable changes in your body. Your sense of smell and taste may improve. You will breathe easier, and your smoker's hack will begin to disappear, although you may notice that you will continue to cough for a while. And you will be free from the mess, smell, inconvenience, expense, and dependence of cigarette smoking.

Immediate Effects

As your body begins to repair itself, instead of feeling better right away, you may feel worse for a while. It's important to understand that healing is a process; it begins immediately, but it continues over time. These "withdrawal pangs" are really symptoms of the recovery process (see Withdrawal Symptoms and Activities That Might Help).

Immediately after quitting, many ex-smokers experience "symptoms of recovery" such as temporary weight gain caused by fluid retention, irregularity, and dry, sore gums or tongue. You may feel edgy, hungry, more tired, and more short-tempered than usual and have trouble sleeping and notice that you are coughing a lot. These symptoms are the result of your body clearing itself of nicotine, a powerful addictive chemical. Most nicotine is gone from the body in 2-3 days.

Long-Range Benefits

It is important to understand that the long range after-effects of quitting are only temporary and signal the beginning of a healthier life. Now that you've quit, you've added a number of healthy productive days to each year of your life. Most important, you've greatly improved your chances for a longer life. You have significantly reduced your risk of death from heart disease, stroke, chronic bronchitis, emphysema, and several kinds of cancer; not just lung cancer. (Cigarette smoking is responsible every year for approximately 130,000 deaths from cancer, 170,000 deaths from heart disease, and 50,000 deaths from lung disease.)

Congratulations!

Now you are ready to develop a new habit; not smoking. Like any other habit, it takes time to become a part of you; unlike most other habits, though, not smoking will take some conscious effort and practice. This section of the chapter can be a big help. You will find many techniques to use for developing the nonsmoking habit and holding on to it.

By reading this section of the chapter carefully and reviewing it often, you'll become more aware of the places and situations that prompt the desire for a cigarette. You will also learn about many nonsmoking ways to deal with the urge to smoke. These are called coping skills. Finally, you will learn what to do in case you do slip and give in to the smoking urge.

Keep Your Guard Up

The key to living as a nonsmoker is to avoid letting your urges or cravings for a cigarette lead you to smoke. Don't kid yourself; even though you have made a commitment not to smoke, you will sometimes be tempted. But instead of giving in to the urge, you can use it as a learning experience.

First, remind yourself that you have quit and you are a nonsmoker. Then look closely at your urge to smoke and ask yourself:

- Where was I when I got the urge?
- What was I doing at the time?
- Whom was I with?
- What was I thinking?

The urge to smoke after you've quit often hits at predictable times. The trick is to anticipate those times and find ways to cope with them; without smoking. Naturally, it won't be easy at first. In fact, you may

482

continue to want a cigarette at times. But remember, even if you slip, it doesn't mean an end to the nonsmoking you. It does mean that you should try to identify what triggered your slip, strengthen your commitment to quitting, and try again.

Look at the following list of typical triggers. Do any of them ring a bell with you? Check off those that might trigger and urge to smoke, and add any others you can think of:

- Working under pressure
- Feeling blue
- Talking on the telephone
- Having a drink
- Watching television
- Driving your car
- Finishing a meal
- Playing cards
- Drinking coffee
- Watching someone else smoke

If you are like many new nonsmokers, the most difficult place to resist the urge to smoke is the most familiar: home. The activities most closely associated with smoking urges are eating, partying, and drinking. And, not surprisingly, most urges occur when a smoker is present.

How to Dampen That Urge

There are seven major coping skills to help you fight that urge to smoke. These tips are designed for you, the new nonsmoker, to help you nurture the nonsmoking habit.

1. Think about why you quit

Go back to your list of reasons for quitting. Look at this list several times a day; especially when you are hit with the urge to smoke. The best reasons you could have for quitting are very personally yours, and these are also the best reasons to stay a nonsmoker.

2. Know when you are rationalizing

It is easy to rationalize yourself back into smoking (see Common Rationalizations). Don't talk yourself into smoking again. A new nonsmoker in a tense situation may think, "I'll just have one cigarette to calm myself down." If thoughts like this pop into your head, stop and think again! You know better ways to relax; nonsmokers ways, such as taking a walk or doing breathing exercises.

Concern about gaining weight may also lead to rationalizations. Learn to counter thoughts such as, "I'd rather be thin, even if it means smoking." Remember that a slight weight gain is not likely to endanger your health as much as smoking would. (Cigarette smokers have about a 70-percent higher rate of premature death than nonsmokers.) And review the list of healthy, low-calorie snacks that you used when quitting.

3. Anticipate Triggers and Prepare to Avoid Them

By now you know which situations, people, and feelings are likely to tempt you to smoke. Be prepared to meet these triggers head on and counter act them. Keep using the skills that helped you cope in cutting down and quitting:

- Keep your hands busy; doodle, knit, type a letter.

- Avoid people who smoke; spend more time with nonsmoking friends.

- Find activities that make smoking difficult (gardening, washing the car, taking a shower). Exercise to help knock out that urge; it will help you to feel and look good as well.

- Put something other than a cigarette in your mouth. Chew sugarless gum or nibble on a carrot or celery stick.

- Avoid places where smoking is permitted. Sit in the nonsmoking section of restaurants, trains, and planes.

- Reduce your consumption of alcohol, which often stimulates the desire to smoke. Try to have no more than one or two drinks at a party. Better yet, have a glass of juice, soda, or mineral water.

4. Reward yourself for not smoking

Congratulations are in order each time you get through a day without smoking. After a week, give yourself a pat on the back and a reward of some kind. Buy a new record or treat yourself to a movie or concert. No matter how you do it, make sure you reward yourself in some way. It helps to remind yourself that what you are doing is important.

5. Use positive thoughts

If self-defeating thoughts start to creep in, remind yourself again that you are a nonsmoker, that you do not want to smoke, and that you have good reasons for it. Putting yourself down and trying to hold out using willpower alone are not effective coping techniques. Mobilize the power of positive thinking!

6. Use relaxation techniques

Breathing exercises help to reduce tension. Instead of having a cigarette, take a long deep breath, count to 10, and release it. Repeat this 5 times. See how much more relaxed you feel?

7. Get social support

The commitment to remain a nonsmoker can be made easier by talking about it with friends and relatives. They can congratulate you as you check off another day, week, and month as a nonsmoker. Tell the people close to you that you might be tense for a while, so they know what to expect. They'll be sympathetic when you have an urge to smoke and can be counted on to help you resist it. Remember to call on your friends when you are lonely or you feel an urge to smoke. A buddy system is a great technique.

Non Smoking Is Habit Forming

Good for you! You have made a commitment not to smoke, and by using this chapter, you know what to do if you are tempted to forget that commitment. It is difficult to stay a nonsmoker once you have had a cigarette, so do everything possible to avoid it.

If you follow the advice in this chapter and use at least one coping skill whenever you have an urge to smoke, you will have quit for keeps!

Relapse: If You Do Smoke Again

If you slip and smoke, don't be discouraged. Many former smokers tried to stop several times before they finally succeeded. Here's what you should do:

- Recognize that you have had a slip. A slip means that you have had a small setback and smoked a cigarette or two. But your first cigarette did not make you a smoker to start with, and a small setback does not make you a smoker again.

- Don't be too hard on yourself. One slip doesn't mean you're a failure or that you can't be a nonsmoker, but it is important to get yourself back on the nonsmoking track immediately.

- Identify the trigger: Exactly what was it that prompted you to smoke? Be aware of the trigger and decide now how you will cope with it when it comes up again.

- Know and Use the Coping skills described above. People who know at least one coping skill are more likely to remain non-smokers than those who do not know any.

- Sign a contract with yourself to remain a nonsmoker.

- If you think you need professional help, see your doctor. He or she can provide extra motivation for you to stop smoking. Your doctor may also prescribe nicotine gum or a nicotine patch as an alternative source of nicotine while you break the habit of smoking.

Marking Progress

- Each month, on the anniversary of your quit date, plan a special celebration.

- Periodically, write down new reasons you are glad you quit, and post these reasons where you will be sure to see them.

- Make up a calendar for the first 90 days. Cross off each day and indicate the money you saved by not smoking.

- Set other, intermediate target dates, and do something special with the money you have saved.

Common Rationalizations

Rationalization: I'm under a lot of stress, and smoking relaxes me.

Response: Your body is used to nicotine, so you naturally feel more relaxed when you give your body a substance upon which it has grown dependent. But nicotine really is a stimulant; it raises your heart rate, blood pressure, and adrenaline level. Most ex-smokers feel much less nervous just a few weeks after quitting.

Rationalization: Smoking makes me more effective in my work.

Response: Trouble concentrating can be a short-term symptom of quitting, but smoking actually deprives your brain of oxygen.

Rationalization: I've already cut down to a safe level.

Response: Cutting down is a good first step, but there's a big difference in the benefits to you between smoking a little and not smoking at all. Besides, smokers who cut back often inhale more often and more deeply, negating many of the benefits of cutting back. After you've cut back to about seven cigarettes a day, it's time to set a quit date.

Rationalization: I smoke only safe, low-tar/low-nicotine cigarettes.

Response: These cigarettes still contain harmful substances, and many smokers who use them inhale more often and more deeply to maintain their nicotine intake. Also, carbon monoxide intake often increases with a switch to low-tar cigarettes.

Rationalization: It's too hard to quit. I don't have the willpower.

Response: Quitting and staying away from cigarettes is hard, but it's not impossible. More than 3 million Americans quit every year. It's important for you to remember that many people have had to try more than once, and try more than one method, before they became ex-smokers, but they have done it, and so can you.

Rationalization: I'm worried about gaining weight.

Response: Most smokers who gain more than 5-10 pounds are eating more. Gaining weight isn't inevitable. There are certain things you can do to help keep your weight stable. (See Tips To Help You Avoid Weight Gain.)

Rationalization: I don't know what to do with my hands.

Response: That's a common complaint among ex-smokers. You can keep your hands busy in other ways; it's just a matter of getting used to the change of not holding a cigarette. Try holding something else, such as a pencil, paper clip, or marble. Practice simply keeping your hands clasped together. If you're at home, think of all the things you wish you had time to do, make a list, and consult the list for alternatives to smoking whenever your hands feel restless.

Rationalization: Sometimes I have an almost irresistible urge to have a cigarette.

Response: This is a common feeling, especially within the first 1-3 weeks. The longer you're off cigarettes, the more your urges probably will come at times when you smoked before, such as when you're drinking coffee or alcohol or are at a cocktail party where other people are smoking. These are high-risk situations, and you can help yourself by avoiding them whenever possible. If you can't avoid them, you can try to visualize in advance how you'll handle the desire for a cigarette if it arises in those situations.

Rationalization: I blew it. I smoked a cigarette.

Response: Smoking one or a few cigarettes doesn't mean you've "blown it." It does mean that you have to strengthen your determination to quit and try again; harder. Don't forget that you got through several days, perhaps even weeks or months, without a cigarette. This shows that you don't need cigarettes and that you can be a successful quitter.

Chapter 78

Smoke Inhalation Injury: Pulmonary Implications

The leading cause of death in structural fires is not thermal injury, but inhalation of smoke. Inhalation injuries occur in 10% to 20% of all hospitalized burn patients with associated mortality rates ranging from 30% to 90%. The presence of an inhalation injury has a greater effect on mortality than either patient age or surface area burned. The significance of this effect was demonstrated in an autopsy series which showed that 70% of individuals who died within 12 hours of being burned had sustained a concomitant inhalation injury.

Injury in smoke inhalation should be viewed as the result of three separate insults: exposure to heat (thermal injury), exposure to asphyxiants (asphyxiation), and pulmonary irritation (toxin-induced lung injury).

Thermal Injury to the Lung

Due to its low heat-carrying capacity, dry heat is unlikely to result in thermal damage to the lower airways. When there is thermal injury, it is usually limited to the segment of the respiratory tract above the vocal cords. This is because of the low heat-carrying capacity of dry air and the high amount of dissipation that occurs in the upper airways. It has been demonstrated that when air at 300°C was introduced into the nasopharynx, it was cooled to 50°C by the time it reached the trachea. The vocal cords provide additional protection by reflexively adducting at temperatures near 150°C. Inhalation of steam, by contrast, can cause severe thermal injury to the lower airway. Steam has 4,000 times the heat-carrying capacity of dry air and is capable of causing burns to the airway in regions distal to the respiratory bronchioles. Fortunately, steam injuries are rare.

Asphyxiants (Carbon Monoxide and Cyanide)

Two gaseous products of burning that are clinically important are carbon monoxide (CO) and hydrogen cyanide (CN). Both of these molecules can cause death by cellular asphyxia (tissue hypoxia). That is, despite adequate perfusion of the tissue by blood, there is a reduction in the oxygen supply to tissues.

Toxin-Induced Lung Injury

The thermal and asphyxiant components of an inhalation injury are apparent within a few hours of exposure. In contrast, the signs and symptoms of toxic chemical injury may take several days to manifest. During this initial "honeymoon period" the patient will appear deceptively stable with little or no pulmonary dysfunction. The severity of injury to the lung parenchyma in such cases is largely dependent on the elements of the inhaled smoke and on the duration of exposure.

Mechanism

Chemicals suspended in the smoke will react with components of the cell membrane. These interactions produce oxygen radicals which disrupt the cell membranes, damaging pulmonary endothelium and resulting in increased microvascular permeability. Furthermore, compounds such as ammonia, hydrogen chloride, and sulfur dioxide adhere to mucous membranes and form corrosive acids and alkalies. The result is death of mucosal cells, ulceration, and further edema.

Clinical Management

Any patient with a history of smoke exposure in a closed space should be considered to have an inhalation injury until proven otherwise. Burns to the face and the finding of soot in the sputum certainly are evidence that the patient was exposed to smoke, but their absence should not be used to exclude the diagnosis. Maintaining a high index of suspicion is important because symptoms and signs are frequently absent on initial evaluation. The true extent of this injury may not manifest for 24 to 72 hours following exposure. During this "calm before the storm," early symptoms may appear to be resolving; however, the peak period of mucosal sloughing has not yet occurred. The magnitude of the injury should not be underestimated based on this initial presentation.

Pulmonary function tests are not uniformly helpful in the diagnosis of smoke inhalation injury. Pulmonary function tests require the cooperation of the patient and are effort-dependent. Patients are frequently unable to comply due to concomitant thermal or traumatic injuries, the influence of narcotics, or alcohol. When dealing with a large number of patients from a mass-casualty incident, pulmonary function tests allow for the rapid evaluation and triaging of ambulatory patients.

Inhalation injuries represent the most lethal form of burn-related injury. The most deleterious component of an inhalation injury is the toxin-mediated damage to the bronchial mucosa.

Despite advances in critical care and ventilatory management, the care of the patient with inhalation injury remains mostly supportive. Appropriate fluid resuscitation combined with aggressive pulmonary care and early burn excision may reduce the mortality rate from the accepted 30% to 70%.

Chapter 79

Air Pollution and
Lung Function

Even in a mountain wilderness, periods of moderate levels of ozone—the main ingredient of urban smog—can decrease active people's lung function, a study led by researchers at Brigham and Women's Hospital and the Harvard School of Public Health has found.

The researchers said their two-year study showed ozone levels common to non-urban parts of the United States were associated with decreases in lung function in adult hikers on Mt. Washington in the White Mountain National Forest in New Hampshire. These declines were more pronounced in hikers with a history of asthma or wheezing.

Their study results are published today in the *Environmental Health Perspectives*, the monthly journal of the National Institute of Environmental Health Sciences.

The study evaluated the effects of ozone and other air pollutants, including fine particulate matter and suspended acid droplets, on the lung function of 530 nonsmokers hiking on New Hampshire's Mount Washington during two summers. When ozone went up slightly, lung function decreased, the researchers said.

The hikers ranged from 18 to 64 years of age and hiked an average of eight hours each. During this time, they were exposed to average ozone concentrations from 21 to 74 parts per billion (ppb) per hour. The overall average exposure was 40 ppb, which the researchers called "a relatively low level characteristic of much of the continental United States."

NIEHS PR#1-98, National Institute of Environmental Health Sciences (NIEHS), 1998.

Researchers measured the hikers' forced expiratory volume—the volume of air they could expel from their lungs in one second—and forced vital capacity—the total volume of air expelled from the lungs—before and after their hikes. They found that a 50 ppb increase in ozone concentration was associated with decreased lung function over the course of the hike—an average 2.6 percent decline in forced expiratory volume, and a 2.2 percent decline in forced vital capacity.

The investigators found that hikers with a history of asthma or wheezing had an even greater decline: Their ozone-related changes were approximately four times greater than those of the remaining subjects. The researchers say these effects are important because they occurred among hikers exposed to relatively low ozone concentrations when compared to the recently revised National Ambient Air Quality Standard of 80 ppb over eight hours.

"Physicians, public health officials and the general public should be aware of the potentially negative health impact of relatively low levels of air pollutants, not only among residents of urban and industrial regions, but also among individuals engaged in outdoor recreation in wilderness areas," said lead author Susan Korrick, MD, MPH, an environmental epidemiologist at the Channing Laboratory at Brigham and Women's Hospital, which is in Boston.

The research was funded in part by the National Institute of Environmental Health Sciences, which is a part of the National Institutes of Health; the U.S. Environmental Protection Agency; the Appalachian Mountain Club, and the White Mountain National Forest.

Chapter 80

Asbestos in Your Home

This chapter will help you understand asbestos: what it is, its health effects, where it is in your home, and what to do about it.

Even if asbestos is in your home, this is usually NOT a serious problem. The mere presence of asbestos in a home or a building is not hazardous. The danger is that asbestos materials may become damaged over time. Damaged asbestos may release asbestos fibers and become a health hazard.

THE BEST THING TO DO WITH ASBESTOS MATERIAL IN GOOD CONDITION IS TO LEAVE IT ALONE! Disturbing it may create a health hazard where none existed before. Read this chapter before you have any asbestos material inspected, removed, or repaired.

Where Asbestos Hazards May Be Found in the Home

1. Some roofing and siding shingles are made of asbestos cement.

2. Houses built between 1930 and 1950 may have asbestos as insulation.

3. Asbestos may be present in textured paint and in patching compounds used on wall and ceiling joints. Their use was banned in 1977.

"Asbestos in Your Home," U.S. Environmental Protection Agency (EPA), available online at http://www.epa.gov/iaq/pubs/asbestos.html, April 1997, modified March 1998.

4. Artificial ashes and embers sold for use in gas-fired fireplaces may contain asbestos.

5. Older products such as stove-top pads may have some asbestos compounds.

6. Walls and floors around woodburning stoves may be protected with asbestos paper, millboard, or cement sheets.

7. Asbestos is found in some vinyl floor tiles and the backing on vinyl sheet flooring and adhesives.

8. Hot water and steam pipes in older houses may be coated with an asbestos material or covered with an asbestos blanket or tape.

9. Oil and coal furnaces and door gaskets may have asbestos insulation.

What Is Asbestos?

Asbestos is a mineral fiber. It can be positively identified only with a special type of microscope. There are several types of asbestos fibers. In the past, asbestos was added to a variety of products to strengthen them and to provide heat insulation and fire resistance.

How Can Asbestos Affect My Health?

From studies of people who were exposed to asbestos in factories and shipyards, we know that breathing high levels of asbestos fibers can lead to an increased risk of: lung cancer; mesothelioma, a cancer of the lining of the chest and the abdominal cavity; and asbestosis, in which the lungs become scarred with fibrous tissue.

The risk of lung cancer and mesothelioma increases with the number of fibers inhaled. The risk of lung cancer from inhaling asbestos fibers is also greater if you smoke. People who get asbestosis have usually been exposed to high levels of asbestos for a long time. The symptoms of these diseases do not usually appear until about 20 to 30 years after the first exposure to asbestos.

Most people exposed to small amounts of asbestos, as we all are in our daily lives, do not develop these health problems. However, if disturbed, asbestos material may release asbestos fibers, which can be inhaled into the lungs. The fibers can remain there for a long time, increasing the risk of disease. Asbestos material that would crumble easily if handled, or that has been sawed, scraped, or sanded into a powder, is more likely to create a health hazard.

Where Can I Find Asbestos and When Can it Be a Problem?

Most products made today do not contain asbestos. Those few products made which still contain asbestos that could be inhaled are required to be labeled as such. However, until the 1970s, many types of building products and insulation materials used in homes contained asbestos. Common products that might have contained asbestos in the past, and conditions which may release fibers, include:

- STEAM PIPES, BOILERS, and FURNACE DUCTS insulated with an asbestos blanket or asbestos paper tape. These materials may release asbestos fibers if damaged, repaired, or removed improperly.

- RESILIENT FLOOR TILES (vinyl asbestos, asphalt, and rubber), the backing on VINYL SHEET FLOORING, and ADHESIVES used for installing floor tile. Sanding tiles can release fibers. So may scraping or sanding the backing of sheet flooring during removal.

- CEMENT SHEET, MILLBOARD, and PAPER used as insulation around furnaces and woodburning stoves. Repairing or removing appliances may release asbestos fibers. So may cutting, tearing, sanding, drilling, or sawing insulation.

- DOOR GASKETS in furnaces, wood stoves, and coal stoves. Worn seals can release asbestos fibers during use.

- SOUNDPROOFING OR DECORATIVE MATERIAL sprayed on walls and ceilings. Loose, crumbly, or water-damaged material may release fibers. So will sanding, drilling, or scraping the material.

- PATCHING AND JOINT COMPOUNDS for walls and ceilings, and TEXTURED PAINTS. Sanding, scraping, or drilling these surfaces may release asbestos.

- ASBESTOS CEMENT ROOFING, SHINGLES, and SIDING. These products are not likely to release asbestos fibers unless sawed, dilled, or cut.

- ARTIFICIAL ASHES AND EMBERS sold for use in gas-fired fireplaces. Also, other older household products such as FIRE-PROOF GLOVES, STOVE-TOP PADS, IRONING BOARD COVERS, and certain HAIRDRYERS.

- AUTOMOBILE BRAKE PADS AND LININGS, CLUTCH FACINGS, and GASKETS.

What Should Be Done about Asbestos in the Home?

If you think asbestos may be in your home, don't panic! Usually the best thing is to LEAVE asbestos material that is in good condition ALONE.

Generally, material in good condition will not release asbestos fibers. THERE IS NO DANGER unless fibers are released and inhaled into the lungs.

Check material regularly if you suspect it may contain asbestos. Don't touch it, but look for signs of wear or damage such as tears, abrasions, or water damage. Damaged material may release asbestos fibers. This is particularly true if you often disturb it by hitting, rubbing, or handling it, or if it is exposed to extreme vibration or air flow.

Sometimes, the best way to deal with slightly damaged material is to limit access to the area and not touch or disturb it. Discard damaged or worn asbestos gloves, stove-top pads, or ironing board covers. Check with local health, environmental, or other appropriate officials to find out proper handling and disposal procedures.

If asbestos material is more than slightly damaged, or if you are going to make changes in your home that might disturb it, repair or removal by a professional is needed. Before you have your house remodeled, find out whether asbestos materials are present.

How to Identify Materials That Contain Asbestos

You can't tell whether a material contains asbestos simply by looking at it, unless it is labeled. If in doubt, treat the material as if it contains asbestos or have it sampled and analyzed by a qualified professional. A professional should take samples for analysis, since a professional knows what to look for, and because there may be an increased health risk if fibers are released. In fact, if done incorrectly, sampling can be more hazardous than leaving the material alone. Taking samples yourself is not recommended. If you nevertheless choose to take the samples yourself, take care not to release asbestos fibers into the air or onto yourself. Material that is in good condition and will not be disturbed (by remodeling, for example) should be left alone. Only material that is damaged or will be disturbed should be sampled. Anyone who samples asbestos-containing materials should have as much information as possible on the handling of asbestos before sampling, and at a minimum, should observe the following procedures:

- Make sure no one else is in the room when sampling is done.

- Wear disposable gloves or wash hands after sampling.

- Shut down any heating or cooling systems to minimize the spread of any released fibers.

- Do not disturb the material any more than is needed to take a small sample.

- Place a plastic sheet on the floor below the area to be sampled.

- Wet the material using a fine mist of water containing a few drops of detergent before taking the sample. The water/detergent mist will reduce the release of asbestos fibers.

- Carefully cut a piece from the entire depth of the material using, for example, a small knife, corer, or other sharp object. Place the small piece into a clean container (for example, a 35 mm film canister, small glass or plastic vial, or high quality resealable plastic bag).

- Tightly seal the container after the sample is in it.

- Carefully dispose of the plastic sheet. Use a damp paper towel to clean up any material on the outside of the container or around the area sampled. Dispose of asbestos materials according to state and local procedures.

- Label the container with an identification number and clearly state when and where the sample was taken.

- Patch the sampled area with the smallest possible piece of duct tape to prevent fiber release.

- Send the sample to an EPA-approved laboratory for analysis.

How to Manage an Asbestos Problem

If the asbestos material is in good shape and will not be disturbed, do nothing! If it is a problem, there are two types of corrections: repair and removal.

REPAIR usually involves either sealing or covering asbestos material.

Sealing (encapsulation) involves treating the material with a sealant that either binds the asbestos fibers together or coats the material so fibers are not released. Pipe, furnace, and boiler insulation can sometimes be repaired this way. This should be done only by a professional trained to handle asbestos safely.

Covering(enclosure) involves placing something over or around the material that contains asbestos to prevent release of fibers. Exposed insulated piping may be covered with a protective wrap or jacket.

With any type of repair, the asbestos remains in place. Repair is usually cheaper than removal, but it may make later removal of asbestos, if necessary, more difficult and costly. Repairs can either be major or minor.

Asbestos Do's And Don'ts for the Homeowner

- **Do** keep activities to a minimum in any areas having damaged material that may contain asbestos.
- **Do** take every precaution to avoid damaging asbestos material.
- **Do** have removal and major repair done by people trained and qualified in handling asbestos. It is highly recommended that sampling and minor repair also be done by asbestos professionals.

- **Don't** dust, sweep, or vacuum debris that may contain asbestos.
- **Don't** saw, sand, scrape, or drill holes in asbestos materials.
- **Don't** use abrasive pads or brushes on power strippers to strip wax from asbestos flooring. Never use a power stripper on a dry floor.
- **Don't** sand or try to level asbestos flooring or its backing. When asbestos flooring needs replacing, install new floorcovering over it, if possible.
- **Don't** track material that could contain asbestos through the house. If you cannot avoid walking through the area, have it cleaned with a wet mop. If the material is from a damaged area, or if a large area must be cleaned, call an asbestos professional.

Major repairs must be done only by a professional trained in methods for safely handling asbestos.

Minor repairs should also be done by professionals since there is always a risk of exposure to fibers when asbestos is disturbed.

Doing minor repairs yourself is not recommended since improper handling of asbestos materials can create a hazard where none existed. If you nevertheless choose to do minor repairs, you should have as much information as possible on the handling of asbestos before doing anything. Contact your state or local health department or regional EPA office for information about asbestos training programs in your area. Your local school district may also have information about asbestos professionals and training programs for school buildings. Even if you have completed a training program, do not try anything more than minor repairs. Before undertaking minor repairs, carefully examine the area around the damage to make sure it is stable. As a general matter, any damaged area which is bigger than the size of your hand is not a minor repair.

Before undertaking minor repairs, be sure to follow all the precautions described earlier for sampling asbestos material. Always wet the asbestos material using a fine mist of water containing a few drops of detergent. Commercial products designed to fill holes and seal damaged areas are available. Small areas of material such as pipe insulation can be covered by wrapping a special fabric, such as rewettable glass cloth, around it. These products are available from stores which specialize in asbestos materials and safety items.

Removal is usually the most expensive method and, unless required by state or local regulations, should be the last option considered in most situations. This is because removal poses the greatest risk of fiber release. However, removal may be required when remodeling or making major changes to your home that will disturb asbestos material. Also, removal may be called for if asbestos material is damaged extensively and cannot be otherwise repaired. Removal is complex and must be done only by a contractor with special training. Improper removal may actually increase the health risks to you and your family.

Asbestos Professionals:
Who Are They and What Can They Do?

Asbestos professionals are trained in handling asbestos material. The type of professional will depend on the type of product and what needs to be done to correct the problem. You may hire a general asbestos contractor or, in some cases, a professional trained to handle specific products containing asbestos.

Asbestos professionals can conduct home inspections, take samples of suspected material, assess its condition, and advise about what corrections are needed and who is qualified to make these corrections.

501

Once again, material in good condition need not be sampled unless it is likely to be disturbed. Professional correction or abatement contractors repair or remove asbestos materials. Some firms offer combinations of testing, assessment, and correction. A professional hired to assess the need for corrective action should not be connected with an asbestos-correction firm. It is better to use two different firms so there is no conflict of interest. Services vary from one area to another around the country.

The federal government has training courses for asbestos professionals around the country. Some state and local governments also have or require training or certification courses. Ask asbestos professionals to document their completion of federal or state-approved training. Each person performing work in your home should provide proof of training and licensing in asbestos work, such as completion of EPA-approved training. State and local health departments or EPA regional offices may have listings of licensed professionals in your area.

If you have a problem that requires the services of asbestos professionals, check their credentials carefully. Hire professionals who are trained, experienced, reputable, and accredited—especially if accreditation is required by state or local laws. Before hiring a professional, ask for references from previous clients. Find out if they were satisfied. Ask whether the professional has handled similar situations. Get cost estimates from several professionals, as the charges for these services can vary.

Though private homes are usually not covered by the asbestos regulations that apply to schools and public buildings, professionals should still use procedures described during federal or state-approved training. Homeowners should be alert to the chance of misleading claims by asbestos consultants and contractors. There have been reports of firms incorrectly claiming that asbestos materials in homes must be replaced. In other cases, firms have encouraged unnecessary removals or performed them improperly. Unnecessary removals are a waste of money. Improper removals may actually increase the health risks to you and your family. To guard against this, know what services are available and what procedures and precautions are needed to do the job properly.

In addition to general asbestos contractors, you may select a roofing, flooring, or plumbing contractor trained to handle asbestos when it is necessary to remove and replace roofing, flooring, siding, or asbestos-cement pipe that is part of a water system. Normally, roofing and flooring contractors are exempt from state and local licensing requirements because they do not perform any other asbestos-correction work.

Asbestos-containing automobile brake pads and linings, clutch facings, and gaskets should be repaired and replaced only by a professional using special protective equipment. Many of these products are now available without asbestos. For more information, read "Guidance for Preventing Asbestos Disease Among Auto Mechanics," available from regional EPA offices.

If You Hire a Professional Asbestos Inspector

- Make sure that the inspection will include a complete visual examination and the careful collection and lab analysis of samples. If asbestos is present, the inspector should provide a written evaluation describing its location and extent of damage, and give recommendations for correction or prevention.

- Make sure an inspecting firm makes frequent site visits if it is hired to assure that a contractor follows proper procedures and requirements. The inspector may recommend and perform checks after the correction to assure the area has been properly cleaned.

If You Hire a Corrective-Action Contractor

- Check with your local air pollution control board, the local agency responsible for worker safety, and the Better Business Bureau. Ask if the firm has had any safety violations. Find out if there are legal actions filed against it.

- Insist that the contractor use the proper equipment to do the job. The workers must wear approved respirators, gloves, and other protective clothing.

- Before work begins, get a written contract specifying the work plan, cleanup, and the applicable federal, state, and local regulations which the contractor must follow (such as notification requirements and asbestos disposal procedures). Contact your state and local health departments, EPA's regional office, and the Occupational Safety and Health Administration's regional office to find out what the regulations are. Be sure the contractor follows local asbestos removal and disposal laws. At the end of the job, get written assurance from the contractor that all procedures have been followed.

- Assure that the contractor avoids spreading or tracking asbestos dust into other areas of your home. They should seal the work area from the rest of the house using plastic sheeting and duct tape, and also turn off the heating and air conditioning system. For some repairs, such as pipe insulation removal, plastic glove bags may be adequate. They must be sealed with tape and properly disposed of when the job is complete.

- Make sure the work site is clearly marked as a hazard area. Do not allow household members and pets into the area until work is completed.

- Insist that the contractor apply a wetting agent to the asbestos material with a hand sprayer that creates a fine mist before removal. Wet fibers do not float in the air as easily as dry fibers and will be easier to clean up.

- Make sure the contractor does not break removed material into small pieces. This could release asbestos fibers into the air. Pipe insulation was usually installed in preformed blocks and should be removed in complete pieces.

- Upon completion, assure that the contractor cleans the area well with wet mops, wet rags, sponges, or HEPA (high efficiency particulate air) vacuum cleaners. A regular vacuum cleaner must never be used. Wetting helps reduce the chance of spreading asbestos fibers in the air. All asbestos materials and disposable equipment and clothing used in the job must be placed in sealed, leakproof, and labeled plastic bags. The work site should be visually free of dust and debris. Air monitoring (to make sure there is no increase of asbestos fibers in the air) may be necessary to assure that the contractor's job is done properly. This should be done by someone not connected with the contractor.

Caution!

Do not dust, sweep, or vacuum debris that may contain asbestos. These steps will disturb tiny asbestos fibers and may release them into the air. Remove dust by wet mopping or with a special HEPA vacuum cleaner used by trained asbestos contractors.

Chapter 81

Asbestos in the Workplace

What Is Asbestos?

Asbestos is a widely used, mineral-based material that is resistant to heat and corrosive chemicals. Typically, asbestos appears as a whitish, fibrous material which may release fibers that range in texture from coarse to silky; however, airborne fibers that can cause health damage may be too small to see with the naked eye.

Who Is Exposed?

An estimated 1.3 million employees in construction and general industry face significant asbestos exposure on the job. Heaviest exposures occur in the construction industry, particularly during the removal of asbestos during renovation or demolition. Employees are also likely to be exposed during the manufacture of asbestos products (such as textiles, friction products, insulation, and other building materials) and during automotive brake and clutch repair work.

What Are the Dangers of Asbestos Exposure?

Exposure to asbestos can cause asbestosis (scarring of the lungs resulting in loss of lung function that often progresses to disability and to death); mesothelioma (cancer affecting the membranes lining

Occupational Safety and Health Association (OSHA), Fact Sheet Number 93-06, 1993. Despite the date of this document, it provides general information about a U.S. Department of Labor program that may be of help to the reader.

the lungs and abdomen); lung cancer; and cancers of the esophagus, stomach, colon, and rectum.

What Protections Are Mandatory?

The U.S. Occupational Safety and Health Administration (OSHA) has issued revised regulations covering asbestos exposure in general industry and construction. Both standards set a maximum exposure limit and include provisions for engineering controls and respirators, protective clothing, exposure monitoring, hygiene facilities and practices, warning signs, labeling, record keeping, and medical exams.

Nonasbestiform tremolite, anthophyllite, and actinolite were excluded from coverage under the asbestos standard in May 1992.

Here are some of the highlights of the revised rules, published in the Federal Register June 20, 1986; and on Sept. 14, 1988:

- *Permissible Exposure Limit:* In both general industry and construction, workplace exposure must be limited to 0.2 fibers per cubic centimeter of air (0.2 f/cc), averaged over an eight-hour work shift. The excursion or short-term limit is one fiber per cubic centimeter of air (1 f/cc) averaged over a sampling period of 30 minutes.

- *Exposure Monitoring:* In general industry, employers must do initial monitoring for workers who may be exposed above the "action level" of 0.1 f/cc. Subsequent monitoring must be conducted at reasonable intervals, in no case longer than six months for employees exposed above the action level.

  In construction, daily monitoring must be continued until exposure drops below the action level (0.1 f/cc). Daily monitoring is not required where employees are using supplied-air respirators operated in the positive pressure mode.

- *Methods of Compliance:* In both general industry and construction, employers must control exposures using engineering controls, to the extent feasible. Where engineering controls are not feasible to meet the exposure limit, they must be used to reduce employee exposures to the lowest levels attainable and must be supplemented by the use of respiratory protection.

- *Respirators:* In general industry and construction, the level of exposure determines what type of respirator is required; the standards specify the respirator to be used.

- *Regulated Areas:* In general industry and construction, regulated areas must be established where the 8-hour TWA or 30-minute excursion values for airborne asbestos exceed the prescribed permissible exposure limits. Only authorized persons wearing appropriate respirators can enter a regulated area. In regulated areas, eating, smoking, drinking, chewing tobacco or gum, and applying cosmetics are prohibited.

  Warning signs must be displayed at each regulated area and must be posted at all approaches to regulated areas.

- *Labels:* Caution labels must be placed on all raw materials, mixtures, scrap, waste, debris, and other products containing asbestos fibers.

- *Recordkeeping:* The employer must keep an accurate record of all measurements taken to monitor employee exposure to asbestos. This record is to include: the date of measurement, operation involving exposure, sampling and analytical methods used, and evidence of their accuracy; number, duration, and results of samples taken; type of respiratory protective devices worn; name, social security number, and the results of all employee exposure measurements. This record must be kept for 30 years.

- *Protective Clothing:* For any employee exposed to airborne concentrations of asbestos that exceed the PEL, the employer must provide and require the use of protective clothing such as coveralls or similar full-body clothing, head coverings, gloves, and foot covering. Wherever the possibility of eye irritation exists, face shields, vented goggles, or other appropriate protective equipment must be provided and worn.

  In construction, there are special regulated-area requirements for asbestos removal, renovation, and demolition operations. These provisions include a negative pressure area, decontamination procedures for workers, and a "competent person" with the authority to identify and control asbestos hazards. The standard includes an exemption from the negative pressure enclosure requirements for certain small scale, short duration operations provided special work practices prescribed in an appendix to the standard are followed.

507

- *Hygiene Facilities and Practices:* Clean change rooms must be furnished by employers for employees who work in areas where exposure is above the TWA and/or excursion limit. Two lockers or storage facilities must be furnished and separated to prevent contamination of the employee's street clothes from protective work clothing and equipment. Showers must be furnished so that employees may shower at the end of the work shift. Employees must enter and exit the regulated area through the decontamination area.

  The equipment room must be supplied with impermeable, labeled bags and containers for the containment and disposal of contaminated protective clothing and equipment.

  Lunchroom facilities for those employees must have a positive pressure, filtered air supply and be readily accessible to employees. Employees must wash their hands and face prior to eating, drinking or smoking. The employer must ensure that employees do not enter lunchroom facilities with protective work clothing or equipment unless surface fibers have been removed from the clothing or equipment.

  Employees may not smoke in work areas where they are occupationally exposed to asbestos.

- *Medical Exams:* In general industry, exposed employees must have a preplacement physical examination before being assigned to an occupation exposed to airborne concentrations of asbestos at or above the action level or the excursion level. The physical examination must include chest X-ray, medical and work history, and pulmonary function tests. Subsequent exams must be given annually and upon termination of employment, though chest X-rays are required annually only for older workers whose first asbestos exposure occurred more than 10 years ago.

  In construction, examinations must be made available annually for workers exposed above the action level or excursion limit for 30 or more days per year or who are required to wear negative pressure respirators; chest X-rays are at the discretion of the physician.

Chapter 82

Radon

EPA Recommends

- Test your home for radon—it's easy and inexpensive.
- Fix your home if your radon level is 4 picocuries per liter (pCi/L) or higher.
- Radon levels less than 4 pCi/L still pose a risk, and in many cases may be reduced.

Radon is estimated to cause about 14,000 deaths per year. However, this number could range from 7,000 to 30,000 deaths per year The numbers of deaths from other causes are taken from 1990 National Safety Council reports.

Radon Is a Cancer-Causing, Radioactive Gas

You can't see radon. And you can't smell it or taste it. But it may be a problem in your home. Radon is estimated to cause many thousands of deaths each year. That's because when you breathe air containing radon, you can get lung cancer. In fact, the Surgeon General has warned that radon is the second leading cause of lung cancer in the United States today. Only smoking causes more lung cancer deaths. If you smoke and your home has high radon levels, your risk of lung cancer is especially high.

U.S. Environmental Protection Agency (EPA), EPA Document Number 402-K92-001, modified March 1999.

Radon Can Be Found All Over the U.S.

Radon comes from the natural (radioactive) breakdown of uranium in soil, rock and water and gets into the air you breathe. Radon can be found all over the U.S. It can get into any type of building—homes, offices, and schools—and build up to high levels. But you and your family are most likely to get your greatest exposure at home. That's where you spend most of your time.

You Should Test for Radon

Testing is the only way to know if you and your family are at risk from radon. EPA and the Surgeon General recommend testing all homes below the third floor for radon. EPA also recommends testing in schools.

Testing is inexpensive and easy—it should only take a few minutes of your time. Millions of Americans have already tested their homes for radon.

You Can Fix a Radon Problem

There are simple ways to fix a radon problem that aren't too costly. Even very high levels can be reduced to acceptable levels.

How Does Radon Get into Your Home?

Radon is a radioactive gas. It comes from the natural decay of uranium that is found in nearly all soils. It typically moves up through the ground to the air above and into your home through cracks and other holes in the foundation. Your home traps radon inside, where it can build up. Any home may have a radon problem. This means new and old homes, well-sealed and drafty homes, and homes with or without basements.

Radon from soil gas is the main cause of radon problems. Sometimes radon enters the home through well water. In a small number of homes, the building materials can give off radon, too. However, building materials rarely cause radon problems by themselves.

Radon gets in through:

- Cracks in solid floors
- Construction joints
- Cracks in walls
- Gaps in suspended floors

- Gaps around service pipes
- Cavities inside walls
- The water supply

Nearly 1 out of every 15 homes in the U.S. is estimated to have elevated radon levels. Elevated levels of radon gas have been found in homes in your state. Contact your state radon office for general information about radon in your area. While radon problems may be more common in some areas, any home may have a problem. The only way to know about your home is to test. Radon can be a problem in schools and workplaces, too. Ask your state radon office about radon problems in schools and workplaces in your area.

How to Test Your Home

You can't see radon, but it's not hard to find out if you have a radon problem in your home. All you need to do is test for radon. Testing is easy and should only take a few minutes of your time. The amount of radon in the air is measured in "picocuries per liter of air," or "pCi/L." Sometimes test results are expressed in Working Levels (WL) rather than picocuries per liter (pCi/L). There are many kinds of low-cost "do-it-yourself" radon test kits you can get through the mail and in hardware stores and other retail outlets. Make sure you buy a test kit that has passed EPA's testing program or is state-certified. These kits will usually display the phrase "Meets EPA Requirements." If you prefer, or if you are buying or selling a home, you can hire a trained contractor to do the testing for you. Make certain you hire an EPA-qualified or state-certified radon tester. Call your state radon office for a list of these testers.

There are Two General Ways to Test for Radon:

- SHORT-TERM TESTING: The quickest way to test is with short-term tests. Short-term tests remain in your home for two days to 90 days, depending on the device. "Charcoal canisters," "alpha track," "electret ion chamber," "continuous monitors," and "charcoal liquid scintillation" detectors are most commonly used for short-term testing. Because radon levels tend to vary from day to day and season to season, a short-term test is less likely than a long-term test to tell you your year-round average radon level. If you need results quickly, however, a short-term test followed by a second short-term test may be used to decide whether to fix your home.

- LONG-TERM TESTING: Long-term tests remain in your home for more than 90 days. "Alpha track" and "electret" detectors are commonly used for this type of testing. A long-term test will give you a reading that is more likely to tell you your home's year-round average radon level than a short-term test.

How to Use a Test Kit

Follow the instructions that come with your test kit. If you are doing a short-term test, close your windows and outside doors and keep them closed as much as possible during the test. (If you are doing a short-term test lasting just 2 or 3 days, be sure to close your windows and outside doors at least 12 hours before beginning the test, too. You should not conduct short-term tests lasting just 2 or 3 days during unusually severe storms or periods of unusually high winds.) The test kit should be placed in the lowest lived-in level of the home (for example, the basement if it is frequently used, otherwise the first floor). It should be put in a room that is used regularly (like a living room, playroom, den or bedroom) but not your kitchen or bathroom. Place the kit at least 20 inches above the floor in a location where it won't be disturbed—away from drafts, high heat, high humidity, and exterior walls. Leave the kit in place for as long as the package says. Once you've finished the test, reseal the package and send it to the lab specified on the package right away for study. You should receive your test results within a few weeks.

Testing is easy and should only take a few minutes of your time.

EPA recommends the following testing steps:

1. Take a short-term test. If your result is 4 pCi/L or higher (0.02 Working Levels [WL] or higher) take a follow-up test (Step 2) to be sure.

2. Follow up with either a long-term test or a second short-term test. For a better understanding of your year-round average radon level, take a long-term test. If you need results quickly, take a second short-term test. The higher your initial short-term test result, the more certain you can be that you should take a short-term rather than a long-term follow up test. If your first short-term test result is several times the action level—for example, about 10 pCi/L or higher—you should take a second short-term test immediately.

3. If you followed up with a long-term test: Fix your home if your long-term test result is 4 pCi/L or more (0.02 Working Levels

[WL] or higher). If you followed up with a seconds short-term test: The higher your short-term results, the more certain you can be that you should fix your home. Consider fixing your home if the average of your first and second test is 4 pCi/L or higher (0.02 Working Levels [WL] or higher).

What Your Test Results Mean

The average indoor radon level is estimated to be about 1.3 pCi/L, and about 0.4 pCi/L of radon is normally found in the outside air. The U.S. Congress has set a long-term goal that indoor radon levels be no more than outdoor levels. While this goal is not yet technologically achievable in all cases, most homes today can be reduced to 2 pCi/L or below.

Sometimes short-term tests are less definitive about whether or not your home is above 4 pCi/L. This can happen when your results are close to 4 pCi/L. For example, if the average of your two short-term test results is 4.1 pCi/L, there is about a 50% chance that your year-round average is somewhat below 4 pCi/L. However, EPA believes that any radon exposure carries some risk—no level of radon is safe. Even radon levels below 4 pCi/L pose some risk, and you can reduce your risk of lung cancer by lowering your radon level.

If your living patterns change and you begin occupying a lower level of your home (such as a basement) you should retest your home on that level.

Even if your test result is below 4 pCi/L, you may want to test again sometime in the future.

Radon and Home Sales

More and more, home buyers and renters are asking about radon levels before they buy or rent a home. Because real estate sales happen quickly, there is often little time to deal with radon and other issues. The best thing to do is to test for radon NOW and save the results in case the buyer is interested in them. Fix a problem if it exists so it won't complicate your home sale. If you are planning to move, call your state radon office for EPA's pamphlet "Home Buyer's and Seller's Guide to Radon," which addresses some common questions. During home sales:

- Buyers often ask if a home has been tested, and if elevated levels were reduced.

513

- Buyers frequently want tests made by someone who is not involved in the home sale. Your state office (see below) has a list of qualified testers.

- Buyers might want to know the radon levels in areas of the home (like a basement they plan to finish) that the seller might not otherwise test.

Today many homes are built to prevent radon from coming in. Your state or local area may require these radon-resistant construction features. Radon-resistant construction features usually keep radon levels in new homes below 2 pCi/L. If you are buying or renting a new home, ask the owner or builder if it has radon-resistant features.

Test your home now and save your results. If you find high radon levels, fix your home before you decide to sell it.

Radon in Water

Compared with radon entering the home through soil, radon entering the home through water will in most cases be a small source of risk. Radon gas can enter the home through well water. It can be released into the air you breathe when water is used for showering and other household uses. Research suggests that swallowing water with high radon levels may pose risks, too, although risks from swallowing water containing radon are believed to be much lower than those from breathing air containing radon.

While radon in water is not a problem in homes served by most public water supplies, it has been found in well water. If you've tested the air in your home and found a radon problem, and your water comes from a well, contact a lab certified to measure radiation in water to have your water tested. If you're on a public water supply and are concerned that radon may be entering your home through the water, call your public water supplier.

Radon problems in water can be readily fixed. The most effective treatment is to remove radon from the water before it enters the home. This is called point-of-entry treatment. Treatment at your water tap is called point-of-use treatment. Unfortunately, point-of-use treatment will not reduce most of the inhalation risk from radon.

If you've tested the air in your home and found a radon problem, and your water comes from a well, have your water tested.

If high radon levels are found and the home has a well, you can find publications and documents developed by EPA's Office of Ground

Water and Drinking Water relating to radon in drinking water and the radon in drinking water rule at http://www.epa.gov/safewater/radon.html.

How to Lower the Radon Level in Your Home

Since there is no known safe level of radon, there can always be some risk. But the risk can be reduced by lowering the radon level in your home.

A variety of methods are used to reduce radon in your home. In some cases, sealing cracks in floors and walls may help to reduce radon. In other cases, simple systems using pipes and fans may be used to reduce radon. Such systems are called "sub-slab depressurization," and do not require major changes to your home. These systems remove radon gas from below the concrete floor and the foundation before it can enter the home. Similar systems can also be installed in houses with crawl spaces. Radon contractors use other methods that may also work in your home. The right system depends on the design of your home and other factors.

Ways to reduce radon in your home are discussed in EPA's "Consumer's Guide to Radon Reduction." You can get a copy from your state radon office.

The cost of making repairs to reduce radon depends on how your home was built and the extent of the radon problem. Most homes can be fixed for about the same cost as other common home repairs like painting or having a new hot water heater installed. The average house costs about $1,200 for a contractor to fix, although this can range from about $500 to about $2,500. Lowering high radon levels requires technical knowledge and special skills. You should use a contractor who is trained to fix radon problems. The EPA Radon Contractor Proficiency (RCP) Program [Now the National Radon Proficiency Program (RPP)] tests these contractors. EPA provides a list of RCP contractors (now referred to as "Mitigation Service Providers") on the world wide web and to state radon offices. A mitigation contractor who has passed the EPA test will carry a special RPP identification card. A trained mitigation contractor can study the radon problem in your home and help you pick the right treatment method.

Check our proficiency internet site or contact your state radon office for names of qualified or state certified radon mitigation contractors in your area. Picking someone to fix your radon problem is much like choosing a contractor for other home repairs—you may want to get references and more than one estimate.

If you plan to fix the problem in your home yourself, you should first contact your state radon office for EPA's technical guide, "Radon Reduction Techniques for Detached Houses." You should also test your home again after it is fixed to be sure that radon levels have been reduced. Most radon reduction systems include a monitor that will alert you if the system needs servicing. In addition, it's a good idea to retest your home sometime in the future to be sure radon levels remain low.

Most homes can be fixed for about the same cost as other common home repairs.

Radon and Home Renovations

If you are planning any major structural renovation, such as converting an unfinished basement area into living space, it is especially important to test the area for radon before you begin the renovation. If your test results indicate a radon problem radon-resistant techniques can be inexpensively included as part of the renovation. Because major renovations can change the level of radon in any home, always test again after work is completed. Most homes can be fixed for about the same cost as other common home repairs.

The Risk of Living with Radon

Radon gas decays into radioactive particles that can get trapped in your lungs when you breathe. As they break down further, these particles release small bursts of energy. This can damage lung tissue and lead to lung cancer over the course of your lifetime. Not everyone exposed to elevated levels of radon will develop lung cancer. And the amount of time between exposure and the onset of the disease may be many years.

Like other environmental pollutants, there is some uncertainty about the magnitude of radon health risks. However, we know more about radon risks than risks from most other cancer-causing substances. This is because estimates of radon risks are based on studies of cancer in humans (underground miners). Additional studies on more typical populations are under way.

Smoking combined with radon is an especially serious health risk. Stop smoking and lower your radon level to reduce your lung cancer risk.

Children have been reported to have greater risk than adults of certain types of cancer from radiation, but there are currently no conclusive data on whether children are at greater risk than adults from radon.

Your chances of getting lung cancer from radon depend mostly on:

- How much radon is in your home
- The amount of time you spend in your home
- Whether you are a smoker or have ever smoked

Scientists are more certain about radon risks than risks from most other cancer-causing substances.

It's never too late to reduce your risk of lung cancer. Don't wait to test and fix a radon problem. If you are a smoker, stop smoking.

Table 82.1. Radon Risk if You Smoke

Radon Level	If 1,000 people who smoked were exposed to this level over a lifetime...	The risk of cancer from radon exposure compares to...	WHAT TO DO: Stop smoking and...
20 pCi/L	About 135 people could get lung cancer	100 times the risk of drowning	Fix your home
10 pCi/L	About 71 people could get lung cancer	100 times the risk of dying in a home fire	Fix your home
8 pCi/L	About 57 people could get lung cancer		Fix your home
4 pCi/L	About 29 people could get lung cancer	100 times the risk of dying in an airplane crash	Fix your home
2 pCi/L	About 15 people could get lung cancer	2 times the risk of dying in a car crash	Consider fixing between 2 and 4 pCi/L
1.3 pCi/L	About 9 people could get lung cancer	(Average indoor radon level)	(Reducing radon levels below 2 pCi/L is difficult.)
0.4 pCi/L	About 3 people could get lung cancer	(Average outdoor radon level)	(Reducing radon levels below 2 pCi/L is difficult.)

Note: If you are a former smoker, your risk may be lower.

Some Common Myths about Radon

MYTH: Scientists are not sure that radon really is a problem.

FACT: Although some scientists dispute the precise number of deaths due to radon, all the major health organizations (like the Centers for Disease Control and Prevention, the American Lung Association and the American Medical Association) agree with estimates that radon causes thousands of preventable lung cancer deaths every year. This is especially true among smokers, since the risk to smokers is much greater than to non-smokers.

MYTH: Radon testing devices are not reliable and are difficult to find.

FACT: Radon testing can be conducted by a professionally trained EPA-listed or state-certified radon tester.

Active radon devices can continuously gather and periodically record radon levels to reveal any unusual swings in the radon level during the test.

Reliable testing devices are also available through the mail, in hardware stores and other retail outlets. Call your state radon office for a list of radon device companies that have met EPA requirements for reliability or are state-certified.

MYTH: Radon testing is difficult and time-consuming.

FACT: Radon testing is easy. You can test your own home or you can hire an EPA-listed or state-certified radon tester. Either approach takes only a small amount of the homeowner's time or effort.

MYTH: Homes with radon problems cannot be fixed.

FACT: There are solutions to radon problems in homes. Thousands of home owners have already lowered elevated radon levels in their homes. Radon levels can be readily lowered for $500 to $2,500. Call your state radon office for a list of contractors that have met EPA requirements or are state-certified.

MYTH: Radon affects only certain types of homes.

FACT: Radon can be a problem in all types of homes such as old homes, new homes, drafty homes, insulated homes, homes with basements and homes without basements. Construction materials and the way the home has been built may also affect radon levels.

MYTH: Radon is only a problem in certain parts of the country.

FACT: High radon levels have been found in every state. Radon problems do vary from area to area, but the only way to know the home's radon level is to test.

MYTH: A neighbor's test result is a good indication of whether your home has a radon problem.

FACT: It is not. Radon levels vary from home to home. The only way to know if your home has a radon problem is to test it.

Table 82.2. Radon Risk if You Have Never Smoked

Radon Level	If 1,000 people who never smoked were exposed to this level over a lifetime...	The risk of cancer from radon exposure compares to...	WHAT TO DO:
20 pCi/L	About 8 people could get lung cancer	The risk of being killed in a violent crime	Fix your home
10 pCi/L	About 4 people could get lung cancer		Fix your home
8 pCi/L	About 3 people could get lung cancer	10 times the risk of dying in an airplane crash	Fix your home
4 pCi/L	About 2 people could get lung cancer	The risk of drowning	Fix your home
2 pCi/L	About 1 person could get lung cancer	The risk of dying in a home fire	Consider fixing between 2 and 4 pCi/L
1.3 pCi/L	Less than 1 person could get lung cancer	(Average indoor radon level)	(Reducing radon levels below 2 pCi/L is difficult.)
0.4 pCi/L	Less than 1 person could get lung cancer	(Average outdoor radon level)	(Reducing radon levels below 2 pCi/L is difficult.)

Note: If you are a former smoker, your risk may be higher.

MYTH: Everyone should test his or her water for radon.

FACT: While radon gets into some homes through the water, it is important to first test the air in the home for radon. If high radon levels are found and the home has a well, call the Safe Drinking Water Hotline at 1 800-426-4791, or your state radon office for more information.

MYTH: It is difficult to sell a home where radon problems have been discovered.

FACT: Where radon problems have been fixed, home sales have not been blocked. The added protection could be a good selling point.

MYTH: I have lived in my home for so long, it does not make sense to take action now.

FACT: You will reduce your risk of lung cancer when you reduce radon levels, even if you have lived with a radon problem for a long time.

MYTH: Short-term tests cannot be used for making a decision about whether to reduce the home's high radon levels.

FACT: Short-term tests may be used to decide whether to reduce the home's high radon levels. However, the closer the short-term testing result is to 4 pCi/L, the less certainty there is about whether the home's year-round average is above or below that level. Keep in mind that radon levels below 4 pCi/L still pose some risk and that radon levels can be reduced in some homes to 2 pCi/L or below.

National Radon Hotline

1-800-767-7236

Chapter 83

Formaldehyde

What Is Formaldehyde?

Formaldehyde is an important industrial chemical used to make other chemicals, building materials, and household products. It is one of the large family of chemical compounds called volatile organic compounds or 'VOCs'. The term volatile means that the compounds vaporize, that is, become a gas, at normal room temperatures. Formaldehyde serves many purposes in products. It is used as a part of:

- the glue or adhesive in pressed wood products (particleboard, hardwood plywood, and fiberboard);
- preservatives in some paints, coatings, and cosmetics;
- the coating that provides permanent press quality to fabrics and draperies;
- the finish used to coat paper products; and
- certain insulation materials (ureaformaldehyde foam insulation).

Formaldehyde is released into the air by burning wood, kerosene or natural gas, by automobiles, and by cigarettes. Formaldehyde can off-gas from materials made with it. It is also a naturally occurring substance.

"An Update on Formaldehyde," U.S. Consumer Product Safety Commission and U.S. Environmental Protection Agency (EPA), modified April 1998.

This chapter tells you where you may come in contact with formaldehyde, how it may affect your health, and how you might reduce your exposure to it.

Why Should You Be Concerned?

Formaldehyde is a colorless, strong-smelling gas. When present in the air at levels above 0.1 ppm (parts in a million parts of air), it can cause watery eyes, burning sensations in the eyes, nose and throat, nausea, coughing, chest tightness, wheezing, skin rashes, and allergic reactions. It also causes cancer in laboratory animals and may cause cancer in humans.

Formaldehyde can affect people differently. Some people are very sensitive to formaldehyde while others may not have any noticeable reaction to the same level.

Persons have developed allergic reactions (allergic skin disease and hives) to formaldehyde through skin contact with solutions of formaldehyde or durable-press clothing containing formaldehyde. Others have developed asthmatic reactions and skin rashes from exposure to formaldehyde.

You should understand that formaldehyde is just one of several gases present indoors that may cause illnesses. Many of these gases, as well as colds and flu, cause similar symptoms.

What Levels of Formaldehyde Are Normal?

Formaldehyde is normally present at low levels, usually less than 0.03 ppm, in both out door and indoor air. The outdoor air in rural areas has lower concentrations while urban areas have higher concentrations. Residences or offices that contain products that release formaldehyde to the air can have formaldehyde levels of greater than 0.03 ppm. Products that may add formaldehyde to the air include particleboard used as sub-flooring or shelving, fiberboard in cabinets and furniture, plywood wall panels, and urea-formaldehyde as insulation. As formaldehyde levels increase, illness or discomfort is more likely to occur and may be more serious.

Efforts have been made by both the government and industry to reduce exposure to formaldehyde. CPSC voted to ban urea-formaldehyde foam insulation. That ban was overturned in the courts, but these actions greatly reduced the residential use of the product. CPSC, the Department of Housing and Urban Development (HUD), and other federal agencies are working with the pressed wood industry to further reduce the release of the chemical from their products. However, it would be unrealistic to expect to completely remove formaldehyde from the air. Some persons who are extremely sensitive to formaldehyde may need to reduce or stop using these products.

What Affects Formaldehyde Levels?

Formaldehyde levels in the indoor air depend mainly on what is releasing the formaldehyde (the source), the temperature, the humidity, and the air exchange rate (the amount of outdoor air entering or leaving the indoor area). Increasing the flow of outdoor air to the inside decreases the formaldehyde levels. Decreasing this flow of outdoor air by sealing the residence or office increases the formaldehyde level in the in door air.

As the temperature rises, more formaldehyde comes off from the product. The reverse is also true; less formaldehyde comes off at lower temperature. Humidity also affects the release of formaldehyde from the product. As humidity rises more formaldehyde is released.

The formaldehyde levels in a residence change with the season and from day-to-day and day-to-night. Levels may be high on a hot and humid day and low on a cool, dry day. Understanding these factors is important when you consider measuring the levels of formaldehyde.

Some sources—such as pressed wood products containing urea-formaldehyde glues, urea-formaldehyde foam insulation, durable press fabrics, and draperies—release more formaldehyde when new. As they age, the formaldehyde release decreases.

What Are the Major Sources?

- *Urea-formaldehyde foam insulation:* During the 1970s, many home owners installed this insulation to save energy. Many of these homes had high levels of formaldehyde soon afterwards. Sale of urea formaldehyde foam insulation has largely stopped. Formaldehyde release from this product decreases rapidly after the first few months and reaches background levels in a few years. Therefore, urea-formaldehyde foam insulation installed 5 to 10 years ago is unlikely to still release formaldehyde.

- *Durable-press fabrics, draperies, and coated paper products:* In the early 1960s, there were several reports of allergic reactions to formaldehyde from durable press fabrics and coated paper products. Such reports have declined in recent years as industry has taken steps to reduce formaldehyde levels. Draperies made of formaldehyde treated durable press fabrics may add slightly to indoor formaldehyde levels.

- *Cosmetics, paints, coatings, and some wet-strength paper products:* The amount of formaldehyde present in these products is small and is of slight concern. However, persons sensitive to formaldehyde may have allergic reactions.

- *Pressed Wood Products:* Pressed wood products, especially those containing ureaformaldehyde glues, are a source of formaldehyde. These products include particleboard used in subfloors, shelves, cabinets, and furniture; plywood wall panels, and medium-density fiberboard used in drawers, cabinets, and furniture. Medium-density fiberboard, which contains a higher glue content, has the potential to release the most formaldehyde.

- *Combustion Sources:* Burning materials such as wood, kerosene, cigarettes, and natural gas, and operating internal combustion engines (e.g. automobiles), produces small quantities of formaldehyde. Combustion sources add small amounts of formaldehyde to indoor air.

Products such as carpets or gypsum board do not contain formaldehyde when new. They may trap formaldehyde emitted from other sources and later release the formaldehyde into the indoor air when the temperature and humidity change.

Do You Have Formaldehyde-Related Symptoms?

There are several formaldehyde-related symptoms, such as watery eyes, runny nose, burning sensation in eyes, nose, and throat, headaches, and fatigue. These symptoms may also occur because of the common cold, the flu or other pollutants that may be present in the indoor air. If these symptoms lessen when you are away from home or office but reappear upon your return, they may be caused by indoor pollutants, including formaldehyde. Examine your environment. Have you recently moved into a new or different home or office? Have you recently remodeled or installed new cabinets, or furniture? Symptoms may be due to formaldehyde exposure. You should contact your physician and/or state or local health department for help. Your physician can help to determine if the cause of your symptoms is formaldehyde or other pollutants.

Should You Measure Formaldehyde?

Only trained professionals should measure formaldehyde because they know how to interpret the results. If you become ill, and the illness persists following the purchase of furniture or remodeling with pressed wood products, you might not need to measure formaldehyde. Since these are likely sources, you can take action. You may become ill after painting, sealing, making repairs, and/or applying pest control treatment in your home or office. In such cases, indoor air pollutants other than formaldehyde may be the cause. If the source is not obvious, you should consult an physician to determine whether or not your symptoms might relate to indoor air quality problems.

If your physician believes that you may be sensitive to formaldehyde, you may want to make some measurements. As discussed earlier, many factors can affect the level of formaldehyde on a given day in an office or residence. This is why a professional is best suited to make an accurate measurement of the levels.

Do-it-yourself formaldehyde measuring devices are available. These devices can only provide a "ball park" figure for the formaldehyde level in the area. If you use such a device, you must carefully follow the instructions.

How Do You Reduce Formaldehyde Exposure?

Every day you probably use many products that contain formaldehyde. You may not be able to avoid coming in contact with some formaldehyde in your normal daily routine. If you are sensitive to formaldehyde, you will need to avoid many everyday items to reduce symptoms. For most people, a low-level exposure to formaldehyde (up to 0.1 ppm) does not produce symptoms. People who suspect they are sensitive to formaldehyde should work closely with a knowledgeable physician to make sure that formaldehyde is causing their symptoms.

You can avoid exposure to higher levels by:

• Purchasing low formaldehyde-releasing pressed wood products for use in construction or remodeling of homes, and for furniture, cabinets etc. These could include oriented strand board and softwood plywood for construction, low formaldehyde-emitting pressed wood products or solid wood for furniture and cabinets. Some products are labeled as low-emitting, or ask for help in identifying low-emitting products.

• Using alternative products such as lumber or metal.

- Avoiding the use of foamed-in-place insulation containing form-aldehyde, especially urea-formaldehyde foam insulation.

- Washing durable-press fabrics before use.

How Do You Reduce Existing Formaldehyde Levels?

The choice of methods to reduce formaldehyde is unique to your situation. People who can help you select appropriate methods are your state or local health department, physician, or professional expert in indoor air problems. Here are some of the methods to reduce indoor levels of formaldehyde.

- Bring large amounts of fresh air into the home. Increase ventilation by opening doors and windows and installing an exhaust fan(s).

- Reduce the humidity level in your home.

- Seal the surfaces of the formaldehyde-containing product. You may use a vapor barrier such as some paints, varnishes, or a layer of vinyl or polyurethane-like materials. Be sure to seal completely, with a material that does not itself contain formaldehyde.

- Remove from your home the product that is releasing formaldehyde in the indoor air. When other materials in the area such as carpets, gypsum boards, etc., have absorbed formaldehyde, these products may also start releasing it into the air. Overall levels of formaldehyde can be lower if you increase the ventilation over an extended period.

One method NOT recommended by CPSC is a chemical treatment with strong ammonia (28-29% ammonia in water) which results in a temporary decrease in formaldehyde levels. We strongly discourage such treatment since ammonia in this strength is extremely dangerous to handle. Ammonia may damage the brass fittings of a natural gas system, adding a fire and explosion danger.

Chapter 84

Combustion Appliances and Indoor Air Pollution

Hazards may be associated with almost all types of appliances. The purpose of this chapter is to answer some common questions you may have about the potential for one specific type of hazard—indoor air pollution—associated with one class of appliances—combustion appliances.

Combustion appliances are those which burn fuels for warmth, cooking, or decorative purposes. Typical fuels are gas, both natural and liquefied petroleum (LP); kerosene; oil; coal; and wood. Examples of the appliances are space heaters, ranges, ovens, stoves, furnaces, fireplaces, water heaters, and clothes dryers. These appliances are usually safe. However, under certain conditions, these appliances can produce combustion pollutants that can damage your health, or even kill you.

Possible health effects range from headaches, dizziness, sleepiness, and watery eyes to breathing difficulties or even death. Similar effects may also occur because of common medical problems or other indoor air pollutants.

Should I be concerned about indoor air pollution?

YES. Studies have shown that the air in our homes can be even more polluted than the outdoor air in big cities. Because people spend a lot of time indoors, the quality of the air indoors can affect their

"What You Should Know about Combustion Appliances and Indoor Air Pollution," U.S. Environmental Protection Agency (EPA), March 1997, revised March 1999.

health. Infants, young children and the elderly are a group shown to be more susceptible to pollutants. People with chronic respiratory or cardiovascular illness or immune system diseases are also more susceptible than others to pollutants.

Many factors determine whether pollutants in your home will affect your health. They include the presence, use, and condition of pollutant sources, the level of pollutants both indoors and out, the amount of ventilation in your home, and your overall health.

Most homes have more than one source of indoor air pollution. For example, pollutants come from tobacco smoke, building materials, decorating products, home furnishings, and activities such as cooking, heating, cooling, and cleaning. Living in areas with high outdoor levels of pollutants usually results in high indoor levels. Combustion pollutants are one category of indoor air pollutants.

What are combustion pollutants?

Combustion pollutants are gases or particles that come from burning materials. The combustion pollutants discussed in this chapter come from burning fuels in appliances. The common fuels burned in these appliances are natural or LP gas, fuel oil, kerosene, wood, or coal. The types and amounts of pollutants produced depend upon the type of appliance, how well the appliance is installed, maintained, and vented, and the kind of fuel it uses. Some of the common pollutants produced from burning these fuels are carbon monoxide, nitrogen dioxide, particles, and sulfur dioxide. Particles can have hazardous chemicals attached to them. Other pollutants that can be produced by some appliances are unburned hydrocarbons and aldehydes.

Combustion always produces water vapor. Water vapor is not usually considered a pollutant, but it can act as one. It can result in high humidity and wet surfaces. These conditions encourage the growth of biological pollutants such as house dust mites, molds, and bacteria.

Where do combustion pollutants come from?

Combustion pollutants found indoors include: outdoor air, tobacco smoke, exhaust from car and lawn mower internal combustion engines, and some hobby activities such as welding, woodburning, and soldering. Combustion pollutants can also come from vented or unvented combustion appliances. These appliances include space heaters, gas ranges and ovens, furnaces, gas water heaters, gas clothes dryers, wood or coal-burning stoves, and fireplaces. As a group these are called "combustion appliances."

What are vented and unvented appliances?

Vented appliances are appliances designed to be used with a duct, chimney, pipe, or other device that carry the combustion pollutants outside the home. These appliances can release large amounts of pollutants directly into your home, if a vent is not properly installed, or is blocked or leaking.

Unvented appliances do not vent to the outside, so they release combustion pollutants directly into the home.

Table 84.1 shows typical appliance problems that cause the release of pollutants in your home. Many of these problems are hard for a homeowner to identify. A professional is needed.

Can I use charcoal grills or charcoal hibachis indoors?

No. Never use these appliances inside homes, trailers, truck-caps, or tents. Carbon monoxide from burning and smoldering charcoal can kill you if you use it indoors for cooking or heating. There are about 25 deaths each year from the use of charcoal grills and hibachis indoors.

NEVER burn charcoal inside homes, trailers, tents, or other enclosures. The carbon monoxide can kill you.

What are the health effects of combustion pollutants?

The health effects of combustion pollutants range from headaches and breathing difficulties to death. The health effects may show up immediately after exposure or occur after being exposed to the pollutants for a long time. The effects depend upon the type and amount of pollutants and the length of time of exposure to them. They also depend upon several factors related to the exposed person. These include the age and any existing health problems. There are still some questions about the level of pollutants or the period of exposure needed to produce specific health effects. Further studies to better define the release of pollutants from combustion appliances and their health effects are needed.

Health Problems Associated with Some Common Combustion Pollutants

These pollutants include carbon monoxide, nitrogen dioxide, particles, and sulfur dioxide. Even if you are healthy, high levels of carbon monoxide can kill you within a short time. The health effects of the other pollutants are generally more subtle and are more likely to

Table 84.1. Combustion Appliances and Potential Problems

Appliances	Fuel	Typical Potential Problems
Central Furnaces; Room Heaters;	Natural or Liquefied Petroleum Gas Fireplaces	Cracked heat exchanger; Not enough air to burn fuel properly; Defective/ blocked flue; Maladjusted burner
Central Furnaces	Oil	Cracked heat exchanger; Not enough air to burn fuel properly; Defective/blocked flue; Maladjusted burner
Central Heaters; Room Heaters	Wood	Cracked heat exchanger; Not enough air to burn fuel properly; Defective/blocked flue; Green or treated wood
Central Furnaces; Stoves	Coal	Cracked heat exchanger; Not enough air to burn fuel properly; Defective grate
Room Heaters; Central Heaters	Kerosene	Improper adjustment; Wrong fuel (not-K-1); Wrong wick or wick height; Not enough air to burn fuel properly
Water Heaters	Natural or Liquefied Petroleum Gas	Not enough air to burn fuel properly; Defective/blocked flue; Maladjusted burner
Ranges; Ovens	Natural or Liquefied Petroleum Gas	Not enough air to burn fuel properly; Maladjusted burner; Misuse as a room heater
Stoves; Fireplaces	Wood; Coal	Not enough air to burn fuel properly; Defective/blocked flue; Green or treated wood; Cracked heat exchanger or firebox

affect susceptible people. It is always a good idea to reduce exposure to combustion pollutants by using and maintaining combustion appliances properly.

Carbon Monoxide

Each year, according to CPSC, there are more than 200 carbon monoxide deaths related to the use of all types of combustion appliances in the home. Exposure to carbon monoxide reduces the blood's ability to carry oxygen. Often a person or an entire family may not recognize that carbon monoxide is poisoning them. The chemical is odorless and some of the symptoms are similar to common illnesses. This is particularly dangerous because carbon monoxide's deadly effects will not be recognized until it is too late to take action against them.

Carbon monoxide exposures especially affect unborn babies, infants, and people with anemia or a history of heart disease. Breathing low levels of the chemical can cause fatigue and increase chest pain in people with chronic heart disease. Breathing higher levels of carbon monoxide causes symptoms such as headaches, dizziness, and weakness in healthy people. Carbon monoxide also causes sleepiness, nausea, vomiting, confusion, and disorientation. At very high levels it causes loss of consciousness and death.

Nitrogen Dioxide

Breathing high levels of nitrogen dioxide causes irritation of the respiratory tract and causes shortness of breath. Compared to healthy people, children, and individuals with respiratory illnesses such as asthma, may be more susceptible to the effects of nitrogen dioxide.

Some studies have shown that children may have more colds and flu when exposed to low levels of nitrogen dioxide. When people with asthma inhale low levels of nitrogen dioxide while exercising, their lung airways can narrow and react more to inhaled materials.

Particles

Particles suspended in the air can cause eye, nose, throat, and lung irritation. They can increase respiratory symptoms, especially in people with chronic lung disease or heart problems. Certain chemicals attached to particles may cause lung cancer, if they are inhaled. The risk of lung cancer increases with the amount and length of exposure. The health effects from inhaling particles depend upon many factors, including the size of the particle and its chemical make-up.

Sulfur Dioxide

Sulfur dioxide at low levels of exposure can cause eye, nose, and respiratory tract irritation. At high exposure levels, it causes the lung airways to narrow. This causes wheezing, chest tightness, or breathing problems. People with asthma are particularly susceptible to the effects of sulfur dioxide. They may have symptoms at levels that are much lower than the rest of the population.

Other Pollutants

Combustion may release other pollutants. They include unburned hydrocarbons and aldehydes. Little is known about the levels of these pollutants in indoor air and the resulting health effects.

What do I do if I suspect that combustion pollutants are affecting my health?

If you suspect you are being subjected to carbon monoxide poisoning get fresh air immediately. Open windows and doors for more ventilation, turn off any combustion appliances, and leave the house. You could lose consciousness and die from carbon monoxide poisoning if you do nothing. It is also important to contact a doctor IMMEDIATELY for a proper diagnosis. Remember to tell your doctor that you suspect carbon monoxide poisoning is causing your problems. Prompt medical attention is important.

Remember that some symptoms from combustion pollutants—headaches, dizziness, sleepiness, coughing, and watery eyes—may also occur because of common medical problems. These medical problems include colds, the flu, or allergies. Similar symptoms may also occur because of other indoor air pollutants. Contact your doctor for a proper diagnosis.

To help your doctor make the correct diagnosis, try to have answers to the following questions:

- Do your symptoms occur only in the home? Do they disappear or decrease when you leave home, and reappear when you return?

- Is anyone else in your household complaining of similar symptoms, such as headaches, dizziness, or sleepiness? Are they complaining of nausea, watery eyes, coughing, or nose and throat irritation?

- Do you always have symptoms?

- Are your symptoms getting worse?

- Do you often catch colds or get the flu?

- Are you using any combustion appliances in your home?

- Has anyone inspected your appliances lately? Are you certain they are working properly?

Your doctor may take a blood sample to measure the level of carbon monoxide in your blood if he or she suspects carbon monoxide poisoning. This sample will help determine whether carbon monoxide is affecting your health.

Contact qualified appliance service people to have your appliances inspected and adjusted if needed. You should be able to find a qualified person by asking your appliance distributor or your fuel supplier. In some areas, the local fuel company may be able to inspect and adjust the appliance.

How can I reduce my exposure to combustion pollutants?

Proper selection, installation, inspection and maintenance of your appliances are extremely important in reducing your exposure to these pollutants. Providing good ventilation in your home and correctly using your appliance can also reduce your exposure to these pollutants.

Additionally, there are several different residential carbon monoxide detectors for sale. The CPSC is encouraging the development of detectors that will provide maximum protection. These detectors would warn consumers of harmful carbon monoxide levels in the home. They may soon be widely available to reduce deaths from carbon monoxide poisoning.

Appliance Selection

- Choose vented appliances whenever possible.

- Only buy combustion appliances that have been tested and certified to meet current safety standards. Examples of certifying organizations are Underwriters Laboratories (UL) and the American Gas Association (AGA) Laboratories. Look for a label that clearly shows the certification.

- All currently manufactured vented gas heaters are required by industry safety standards to have a safety shut-off device. This device helps protect you from carbon monoxide poisoning by shutting off an improperly vented heater.

- Check your local and state building codes and fire ordinances to see if you can use an unvented space heater, if you consider purchasing one. They are not allowed to be used in some communities, dwellings, or certain rooms in the house.

- If you must replace an unvented gas space heater with another, make it a new one. Heaters made after 1982 have a pilot light safety system called an oxygen depletion sensor (ODS). This system shuts off the heater when there is not enough fresh air, before the heater begins producing large amounts of carbon monoxide. Look for the label that tells you that the appliance has this safety system. Older heaters will not have this protection system.

- Consider buying gas appliances that have electronic ignitions rather than pilot lights. These appliances are usually more energy efficient and eliminate the continuous low-level pollutants from pilot lights.

- Buy appliances that are the correct size for the area you want to heat. Using the wrong size heater may produce more pollutants in your home and is not an efficient use of energy.

- Talk to your dealer to determine the type and size of appliance you will need. You may wish to write to the appliance manufacturer or association for more information on the appliance. Some addresses are in the back of this chapter.

- All new woodstoves are EPA-certified to limit the amounts of pollutants released into the outdoor air. For more information on selecting, installing, operating, and maintaining woodburning stoves, write to the EPA Wood Heater Program. Their address is at the bottom of this chapter. Before buying a woodstove check your local laws about the installation and use of woodstoves.

Proper Installation

You should have your appliances professionally installed. Professionals should follow the installation directions and applicable building codes. Improperly installed appliances can release dangerous pollutants in your home and may create a fire hazard. Be sure that the installer checks for backdrafting on all vented appliances. A qualified installer knows how to do this.

Ventilation

- To reduce indoor air pollution, a good supply of fresh outdoor air is needed. The movement of air into and out of your home is very important. Normally, air comes through cracks around doors and windows. This air helps reduce the level of pollutants indoors. This supply of fresh air is also important to help carry pollutants up the chimney, stovepipe, or flue to the outside.

- Keep doors open to the rest of the house from the room where you are using an unvented gas space heater or kerosene heater, and crack open a window. This allows enough air for proper combustion and reduces the level of pollutants, especially carbon monoxide.

- Use a hood fan, if you are using a range. They reduce the level of pollutants you breath, if they exhaust to the outside. Make sure that enough air is coming into the house when you use an exhaust fan. If needed, slightly open a door or window, especially if other appliances are in use. For proper operation of most combustion appliances and their venting system, the air pressure in the house should be greater than that outside. If not, the vented appliances could release combustion pollutants into the house rather than outdoors. If you suspect that you have this problem you may need the help of a qualified person to solve it.

- Make sure that your vented appliance has the vent connected and that nothing is blocking it. Make sure there are no holes or cracks in the vent. Do not vent gas clothes dryers or water heaters into the house for heating. This is unsafe.

- Open the stove's damper when adding wood. This allows more air into the stove. More air helps the wood burn properly and prevents pollutants from being drawn back into the house instead of going up the chimney. Visible smoke or a constant smoky odor inside the home when using a woodburning stove is a sign that the stove is not working properly. Soot on furniture in the rooms where you are using the stove also tells this. Smoke and soot are signs that the stove is releasing pollutants into the indoor air.

Correct Use

- Read and follow the instructions for all appliances so you understand how they work. Keep the owner's manual in a convenient place to refer to when needed. Also, read and follow the warning labels because they tell you important safety information that you need to know. Reading and following the instructions and warning labels could save your life.

- Always use the correct fuel for the appliance.

- Only use water-clear ASTM 1-K kerosene for kerosene heaters. The use of kerosene other than 1-K could lead to a release of more pollutants in your home. Never use gasoline in a kerosene heater because it can cause a fire or an explosion. Using even small amounts of gasoline could cause a fire.

- Use seasoned hardwoods (elm, maple, oak) instead of softwoods (cedar, fir, pine) in woodburning stoves and fireplaces. Hardwoods are better because they burn hotter and form less creosote, an oily, black tar that sticks to chimneys and stove pipes. Do not use green or wet woods as the primary wood because they make more creosote and smoke. Never burn painted scrap wood or wood treated with preservatives, because they could release highly toxic pollutants, such as arsenic or lead. Plastics, charcoal, and colored paper such as comics, also produce pollutants. Never burn anything that the stove or fireplace manufacturer does not recommend.

- Never use a range, oven, or dryer to heat your home. When you misuse gas appliances in this way, they can produce fatal amounts of carbon monoxide. They can produce high levels of nitrogen dioxide, too.

- Never use an unvented combustion heater overnight or in a room where you are sleeping. Carbon monoxide from combustion heaters can reach dangerous levels.

- Never ignore a safety device when it shuts off an appliance. It means that something is wrong. Read your appliance instructions to find out what you should do or have a professional check out the problem.

- Never ignore the smell of fuel. This usually indicates that the appliance is not operating properly or is leaking fuel. Leaking fuel will not always be detectible by smell. If you suspect that you have a fuel leak have it fixed as soon as possible. In most cases you should shut off the appliance, extinguish any other flames or pilot lights, shut off other appliances in the area, open windows and doors, call for help, and leave the area.

Inspection and Maintenance

• Have your combustion appliance regularly inspected and maintained to reduce your exposure to pollutants. Appliances that are not working properly can release harmful and even fatal amounts of pollutants, especially carbon monoxide.

• Have chimneys and vents inspected when installing or changing vented heating appliances. Some modifications may be required. For example, if a change was made in your heating system from oil to natural gas, the flue gas produced by the gas system could be hot enough to melt accumulated oil combustion debris in the chimney or vent. This debris could block the vent forcing pollutants into the house. It is important to clean your chimney and vents especially when changing heating systems.

What are the inspection and maintenance procedures?

The best advice is to follow the recommendations of the manufacturer. The same combustion appliance may have different inspection and maintenance requirements, depending upon where you live.

In general, check the flame in the furnace combustion chamber at the beginning of the heating season. Natural gas furnaces should have a blue flame with perhaps only a slight yellow tip. Call your appliance service representative to adjust the burner if there is a lot of yellow in the flame, or call your local utility company for this service. LP units should have a flame with a bright blue center that may have a light yellow tip. Pilot lights on gas water heaters and gas cooking appliances should also have a blue flame. Have a trained service representative adjust the pilot light if it is yellow or orange.

Before each heating season, have flues and chimneys inspected and cleaned before each heating season for leakage and for blockage by creosote or debris. Creosote buildup or leakage could cause black stains on the outside of the chimney or flue. These stains can mean that pollutants are leaking into the house.

Table 84.2 (on the next page) shows how and when to take care of your appliance.

Table 84.2. Inspection and Maintenance Schedules

Appliance	Inspection/ Frequency	Maintenance/ Frequency
Gas Hot Air Heating System	Air Filters—Clean /change filter— Monthly As needed; Look at flues for rust and soot—Yearly	Qualified person check/ clean chimney, clean/adjust burners, check heat exchanger and operation— Yearly (at start of heating season)
Gas/Oil Water/ Steam Heating Systems and Water Heaters	Look at flues for rust and soot—Yearly	Qualified person check/ clean chimney, clean combustion chamber, adjust burners, check operation— Yearly (at start of heating season)
Kerosene Space Heaters	Look to see that mantle is properly seated— daily when in use; Look to see that fuel tank is free of water and other contaminants— daily or before refueling	Check and replace wick— Yearly (at start of heating season); Clean Combustion chamber—Yearly (at start of heating season); Drain fuel tank—Yearly (at end of heating season)
Wood/Coal Stoves	Look at flues for rust and soot—Yearly	Qualified person check/ clean chimney, check seams and gaskets, check operation—Yearly (at start of heating season)

Chapter 85

Indoor Environmental Quality (IEQ)

During the last 20 years, concerns associated with the quality of the indoor office environment have escalated in the American workplace. The National Institute for Occupational Safety and Health (NIOSH) has seen the number of request for the Institute's assistance rise dramatically, as public concern about this problem continues to increase.

What is Indoor Environmental Quality (IEQ)?

The public is probably more familiar with the terms "Indoor Air Quality" and "Sick Building Syndrome." "Indoor Air Quality," as the name implies, simply refers to the quality of the air in an office environment. "Sick Building Syndrome" is a term many people use to convey a wide range of symptoms they believe can be attributed to the building itself. Workers typically implicate the workplace environment because their symptoms are alleviated when they leave the office.

NIOSH prefers to use the term "Indoor Environmental Quality" (or IEQ) to describe the problems occurring in office buildings and schools throughout the nation. The Institute, through its Health Hazard Evaluation (HHE) Program, evaluates potential health hazards in workplaces in response to requests from employers, employees, employee representatives, state and local government agencies, and Federal agencies. NIOSH investigators have found that concerns

---

Document #705002, National Institute for Occupational Safety and Health (NIOSH), June 1997, updated August 1997.

about air quality may be caused by a number of factors, encompassing much more than air contamination.

Other factors such as comfort, noise, lighting, ergonomic stressors (poorly designed work stations and tasks) and job related psychosocial stressors can individually and in combination contribute to complaints. Hence, IEQ more accurately describes the scope of the problem.

What are the typical symptoms associated with IEQ?

The symptoms reported to NIOSH have been diverse and usually not suggestive of any particular medical diagnosis. A typical spectrum of symptoms includes headaches, unusual fatigue, varying degrees of itching or burning eyes, skin irritation, nasal congestion, dry or irritated throats, and nausea.

How big is the IEQ problem?

During the last decade, there has been a significant increase in public concern about IEQ. NIOSH scientists have completed approximately 1300 evaluations related to the indoor office environment since the late 1970's, and the number of these requests as a percentage of the total has risen dramatically.

In 1980, requests to evaluate office environments made up only 8% of the total requests for NIOSH investigations. In 1990, the Institute received 150 IEQ requests, which accounted for 38% of the total. Since 1990, IEQ requests have made up 52% all requests.

Why are IEQ problems increasing?

During the 1970's, ventilation requirements were changed to conserve fossil fuels, and virtually air-tight buildings emerged. At the same time, a revolution occurred in office work throughout the country. Computers and other new work technologies forced a change in office procedures and productivity, and ergonomic and organizational stress problems may have increased. Coupled with the conservation measures and changing technology was a dramatic increase in the number of workers in white collar jobs. Greater awareness of the potential for IEQ problems may also be contributing to a rise in reporting of suspected problems. All of these factors may have contributed to the increase.

Media coverage of IEQ has profoundly influenced the number of IEQ requests the Institute receives. Following a network television report on the subject in October 1992, NIOSH received over 6,000 phone calls and nearly 800 requests for investigations.

What types of IEQ problems has NIOSH found in the workplace?

NIOSH investigators have found IEQ problems caused by ventilation system deficiencies, overcrowding, off gassing from materials in the office and mechanical equipment, tobacco smoke, microbiological contamination, and outside air pollutants. NIOSH has also found comfort problems due to improper temperature and relative humidity conditions, poor lighting, and unacceptable noise levels, as well as adverse ergonomic conditions, and job related psychosocial stressors.

What is typically involved in an investigation?

Evaluation of a potential hazard can involve various methods of investigation. These include: direct observation of production processes and work practices, measurement of contamination levels and extent of employee exposure, medical testing or physical examinations, confidential interviews, and review of employer's records of injuries and illnesses, medical tests, and job histories.

What do investigators look for during an IEQ evaluation?

NIOSH investigators typically look at four elements to determine if there is an IEQ problem.

1. *Pollutant sources:* Is there a source of contamination or discomfort indoors, outdoors, or within the mechanical systems in the building?

2. *The Heating, Ventilating, and Air Conditioning System (HVAC) system:* Can the HVAC system control existing contaminants and ensure thermal comfort? Is it properly maintained and operated?

3. *Pollutant pathways and driving forces:* The HVAC system is the primary pathway. Are the pressure relationships maintained between areas of the building so that the flow of the air goes from cleaner areas to dirtier areas?

4. *Occupants:* Do the building occupants understand that their activities affect the air quality?

NIOSH investigators then look at factors beyond air quality including physical factors, such as lighting, vibration, noise, ergonomic factors, and psychosocial aspects of the workplace.

What help is available in solving IEQ problems?

Many IEQ problems can be solved with inhouse expertise. NIOSH, in conjunction with the Environmental Protection Agency (EPA), has published a guide to provide help in solving these problems. This publication, *Building Air Quality: A Guide for Building Owners and Managers*, provides practical advice for evaluating IEQ problems. Furthermore, NIOSH through its Health Hazard Evaluation (HHE) Program, evaluates potential health hazards in workplaces in response to requests from employers, employees, employee representatives, state and local government agencies and Federal agencies.

However, because of the extraordinary number of IEQ requests, NIOSH is not able to conduct a site visit in response to every request. NIOSH will evaluate each request and respond within the constraints of available resources.

Chapter 86

Home Air Ducts

What is Air Duct Cleaning?

Most people are now aware that indoor air pollution is an issue of growing concern and increased visibility. Many companies are marketing products and services intended to improve the quality of your indoor air. You have probably seen an advertisement, received a coupon in the mail, or been approached directly by a company offering to clean your air ducts as a means of improving your home's indoor air quality. These services typically—but not always—range in cost from $450 to $1,000 per heating and cooling system, depending on the services offered, the size of the system to be cleaned, system accessibility, climatic region, and level of contamination.

Duct cleaning generally refers to the cleaning of various heating and cooling system components of forced air systems, including the supply and return air ducts and registers, grilles and diffusers, heat exchangers heating and cooling coils, condensate drain pans (drip pans), fan motor and fan housing, and the air handling unit housing.

If not properly installed, maintained, and operated, these components may become contaminated with particles of dust, pollen or other debris. If moisture is present, the potential for microbiological growth (e.g., mold) is increased and spores from such growth may be released into the home's living space. Some of these contaminants may cause

"Should You Have the Air Ducts in Your Home Cleaned?" U.S. Environmental Protection Agency (EPA), Publication Number EPA-402-K-97-002, October 1997, revised February 17, 1998.

allergic reactions or other symptoms in people if they are exposed to them. If you decide to have your heating and cooling system cleaned, it is important to make sure the service provider agrees to clean all components of the system and is qualified to do so. Failure to clean a component of a contaminated system can result in re-contamination of the entire system, thus negating any potential benefits. Methods of duct cleaning vary, although standards have been established by industry associations concerned with air duct cleaning. Typically, a service provider will use specialized tools to dislodge dirt and other debris in ducts, then vacuum them out with a high-powered vacuum cleaner.

In addition, the service provider may propose applying chemical biocides, designed to kill microbiological contaminants, to the inside of the duct work and to other system components. Some service providers may also suggest applying chemical treatments (sealants or other encapsulants) to seal or cover the inside surfaces of the air ducts and equipment housings because they believe the sealant will control mold growth or prevent the release of dirt particles or fibers from ducts. These practices have yet to be fully researched and you should be fully informed before deciding to permit the use of biocides or sealants in your air ducts. They should only be applied, if at all, after the system has been properly cleaned of all visible dust or debris.

Deciding Whether or Not to Have Your Air Ducts Cleaned

Knowledge about the potential benefits and possible problems of air duct cleaning is limited. Since conditions in every home are different, it is impossible to generalize about whether or not air duct cleaning in your home would be beneficial.

If no one in your household suffers from allergies or unexplained symptoms or illnesses and if, after a visual inspection of the inside of the ducts, you see no indication that your air ducts are contaminated with large deposits of dust or mold (no musty odor or visible mold growth), having your air ducts cleaned is probably unnecessary. It is normal for the return registers to get dusty as dust-laden air is pulled through the grate. This does not indicate that your air ducts are contaminated with heavy deposits of dust or debris; the registers can be easily vacuumed or removed and cleaned.

On the other hand, if family members are experiencing unusual or unexplained symptoms or illnesses that you think might be related to your home environment, you should discuss the situation with your doctor.

You may consider having your air ducts cleaned simply because it seems logical that air ducts will get dirty over time and should occasionally be cleaned. While the debate about the value of periodic duct cleaning continues, no evidence suggests that such cleaning would be detrimental, provided that it is done properly.

On the other hand, if a service provider fails to follow proper duct cleaning procedures, duct cleaning can cause indoor air problems. For example, an inadequate vacuum collection system can release more dust, dirt, and other contaminants than if you had left the ducts alone. A careless or inadequately trained service provider can damage your ducts or heating and cooling system, possibly increasing your heating and air conditioning costs or forcing you to undertake difficult and costly repairs or replacements.

You should consider having the air ducts in your home cleaned if:

- There is substantial visible mold growth inside hard surface (e.g., sheet metal) ducts or on other components of your heating and cooling system. There are several important points to understand concerning mold detection in heating and cooling systems:

  Many sections of your heating and cooling system may not be accessible for a visible inspection, so ask the service provider to show you any mold they say exists.

  You should be aware that although a substance may look like mold, a positive determination of whether it is mold or not can be made only by an expert and may require laboratory analysis for final confirmation. For about $50, some microbiology laboratories can tell you whether a sample sent to them on a clear strip of sticky household tape is mold or simply a substance that resembles it.

  If you have insulated air ducts and the insulation gets wet or moldy it cannot be effectively cleaned and should be removed and replaced.

  If the conditions causing the mold growth in the first place are not corrected, mold growth will recur.

- Ducts are infested with vermin, e.g. (rodents or insects); or

- Ducts are clogged with excessive amounts of dust and debris and/or particles are actually released into the home from your supply registers.

Other Important Considerations

Duct cleaning has never been shown to actually prevent health problems. Neither do studies conclusively demonstrate that particle (e.g., dust) levels in homes increase because of dirty air ducts or go down after cleaning. This is because much of the dirt that may accumulate inside air ducts adheres to duct surfaces and does not necessarily enter the living space. It is important to keep in mind that dirty air ducts are only one of many possible sources of particles that are present in homes. Pollutants that enter the home both from outdoors and indoor activities such as cooking, cleaning, smoking, or just moving around can cause greater exposure to contaminants than dirty air ducts. Moreover, there is no evidence that a light amount of household dust or other particulate matter in air ducts poses any risk to health.

EPA does not recommend that air ducts be cleaned except on an as-needed basis because of the continuing uncertainty about the benefits of duct cleaning under most circumstances. If a service provider or advertiser asserts that EPA recommends routine duct cleaning or makes claims about its health benefits, you should notify EPA by writing to the address listed at the end of this guidance. EPA does, however, recommend that if you have a fuel burning furnace, stove, or fireplace, they be inspected for proper functioning and serviced before each heating season to protect against carbon monoxide poisoning. Some research also suggests that cleaning dirty cooling coils, fans and heat exchangers can improve the efficiency of heating and cooling systems. However, little evidence exists to indicate that simply cleaning the duct system will increase your system's efficiency.

If you think duct cleaning might be a good idea for your home, but you are not sure, talk to a professional. The company that services your heating and cooling system may be a good source of advice. You may also want to contact professional duct cleaning service providers and ask them about the services they provide. Remember, they are trying to sell you a service, so ask questions and insist on complete and knowledgeable answers.

Suggestions for Choosing a Duct Cleaning Service Provider

To find companies that provide duct cleaning services, check your Yellow Pages under "duct cleaning" or contact the National Air Duct Cleaners Association (NADCA). Do not assume that all duct cleaning service providers are equally knowledgeable and responsible. Talk to at least three different service providers and get written estimates before deciding whether to have your ducts cleaned. When the service providers come to your home, ask them to show you the contamination that would justify having your ducts cleaned.

Do not hire duct cleaners who make sweeping claims about the health benefits of duct cleaning—such claims are unsubstantiated. Do not hire duct cleaners who recommend duct cleaning as a routine part of your heating and cooling system maintenance. You should also be wary of duct cleaners who claim to be certified by EPA. EPA neither establishes duct cleaning standards nor certifies, endorses, or approves duct cleaning companies.

Do not allow the use of chemical biocides or sealants unless you fully understand the pros and the cons.

Check references to be sure other customers were satisfied and did not experience any problems with their heating and cooling system after cleaning.

Contact your county or city office of consumer affairs or local Better Business Bureau to determine if complaints have been lodged against any of the companies you are considering.

Interview potential service providers to ensure:

- they are experienced in duct cleaning and have worked on systems like yours;

- they will use procedures to protect you, your pets, and your home from contamination; and

- they comply with NADCA's air duct cleaning standards and, if your ducts are constructed of fiber glass duct board or insulated internally with fiber glass duct liner, with the North American Insulation Manufacturers Association's (NAIMA) recommendations.

Ask the service provider whether they hold any relevant state licenses. As of 1996, the following states require air duct cleaners to hold special licenses: Arizona, Arkansas, California, Florida, Georgia, Michigan and Texas. Other states may require them as well.

If the service provider charges by the hour, request an estimate of the number of hours or days the job will take, and find out whether there will be interruptions in the work. Make sure the duct cleaner you choose will provide a written agreement outlining the total cost and scope of the job before work begins.

What to Expect From an Air Duct Cleaning Service Provider

If you choose to have your ducts cleaned, the service provider should:

- Open access ports or doors to allow the entire system to be cleaned and inspected.

- Inspect the system before cleaning to be sure that there are no asbestos-containing materials (e.g., insulation, register boots, etc.) in the heating and cooling system. Asbestos-containing materials require specialized procedures and should not be disturbed or removed except by specially trained and equipped contractors.

- Use vacuum equipment that exhausts particles outside of the home or use only high-efficiency particle air (HEPA) vacuuming equipment if the vacuum exhausts inside the home.

- Protect carpet and household furnishings during cleaning.

- Use well-controlled brushing of duct surfaces in conjunction with contact vacuum cleaning to dislodge dust and other particles.

- Use only soft-bristled brushes for fiberglass duct board and sheet metal ducts internally lined with fiberglass. (Although flex duct can also be cleaned using soft-bristled brushes, it can be more economical to simply replace accessible flex duct.)

- Take care to protect the duct work, including sealing and re-insulating any access holes the service provider may have made or used so they are airtight.

- Follow NADCA's standards for air duct cleaning and NAIMA's recommended practice for ducts containing fiber glass lining or constructed of fiber glass duct board.

How to Determine if the Duct Cleaner Did A Thorough Job

A thorough visual inspection is the best way to verify the cleanliness of your heating and cooling system. Some service providers use remote photography to document conditions inside ducts. All portions of the system should be visibly clean; you should not be able to detect any debris with the naked eye. Show the Post-Cleaning Consumer Checklist to the service provider before the work begins. After completing the job, ask the service provider to show you each component of your system to verify that the job was performed satisfactorily.

If you answer "No" to any of the questions on the checklist, this may indicate a problem with the job. Ask your service provider to correct any deficiencies until you can answer "yes" to all the questions on the checklist. (Checklist is provided in Table 86.1)

How to Prevent Duct Contamination

Whether or not you decide to have the air ducts in your home cleaned, committing to a good preventive maintenance program is essential to minimize duct contamination.

To prevent dirt from entering the system:

- Use the highest efficiency air filter recommended by the manufacturer of your heating and cooling system.

- Change filters regularly.

- If your filters become clogged, change them more frequently.

- Be sure you do not have any missing filters and that air cannot bypass filters through gaps around the filter holder.

- When having your heating and cooling system maintained or checked for other reasons, be sure to ask the service provider to clean cooling coils and drain pans.

- During construction or renovation work that produces dust in your home, seal off supply and return registers and do not operate the heating and cooling system until after cleaning up the dust.

- Remove dust and vacuum your home regularly. (Use a high efficiency vacuum (HEPA) cleaner or the highest efficiency filter bags your vacuum cleaner can take. Vacuuming can increase the amount of dust in the air during and after vacuuming as well as in your ducts).

- If your heating system includes in-duct humidification equipment, be sure to operate and maintain the humidifier strictly as recommended by the manufacturer.

To prevent ducts from becoming wet:

- Moisture should not be present in ducts. Controlling moisture is the most effective way to prevent biological growth in air ducts.

Moisture can enter the duct system through leaks or if the system has been improperly installed or serviced. Research suggests that condensation (which occurs when a surface temperature is lower than the dew point temperature of the surrounding air) on or near cooling coils of air conditioning units is a major factor in moisture contamination of the system. The presence of condensation or high relative humidity is an important indicator of the potential for mold growth on any type of duct. Controlling moisture can often be difficult, but here are some steps you can take:

- Promptly and properly repair any leaks or water damage.

- Pay particular attention to cooling coils, which are designed to remove water from the air and can be a major source of moisture contamination of the system that can lead to mold growth.

- Make sure the condensate pan drains properly. The presence of substantial standing water and/or debris indicates a problem requiring immediate attention.

- Check any insulation near cooling coils for wet spots.

- Make sure ducts are properly sealed and insulated in all non-air-conditioned spaces (e.g., attics and crawl spaces). This will help to prevent moisture due to condensation from entering the system and is important to make the system work as intended. To prevent water condensation, the heating and cooling system must be properly insulated.

Table 86.1. Post-Cleaning Consumer Checklist

General

- Did the service provider obtain access to and clean the entire heating and cooling system, including ductwork and all components (drain pans, humidifiers, coils, and fans)?

- Has the service provider adequately demonstrated that duct work and plenums are clean? (Plenum is a space in which supply or return air is mixed or moves; can be duct, joist space, attic and crawl spaces, or wall cavity.)

Heating

- Is the heat exchanger surface visibly clean?

Table 86.1. Post-Cleaning Consumer Checklist, continued

Cooling Components
- Are both sides of the cooling coil visibly clean?
- If you point a flashlight into the cooling coil, does light shine through the other side? It should if the coil is clean.
- Are the coil fins straight and evenly spaced (as opposed to being bent over and smashed together)?
- Is the coil drain pan completely clean and draining properly?

Blower
- Are the blower blades clean and free of oil and debris?
- Is the blower compartment free of visible dust or debris?

Plenums
- Is the return air plenum free of visible dust or debris?
- Do filters fit properly and are they the proper efficiency as recommended by HVAC system manufacturer?
- Is the supply air plenum (directly downstream of the air handling unit) free of moisture stains and contaminants?

Metal Ducts
- Are interior ductwork surfaces free of visible debris? (Select several sites at random in both the return and supply sides of the system.)

Fiber Glass
- Is all fiber glass material in good condition (i.e., free of tears and abrasions; well adhered to underlying materials)?

Access Doors
- Are newly installed access doors in sheet metal ducts attached with more than just duct tape (e.g., screws, rivets, mastic, etc.)?
- With the system running, is air leakage through access doors or covers very slight or non-existent?

Air Vents
- Have all registers, grilles, and diffusers been firmly reattached to the walls, floors, and/or ceilings?
- Are the registers, grilles, and diffusers visibly clean?

System Operation
- Does the system function properly in both the heating and cooling modes after cleaning?

Unresolved Issues of Duct Cleaning

Does duct cleaning prevent health problems?

The bottom line is: no one knows. There are examples of ducts that have become badly contaminated with a variety of materials that may pose risks to your health. The duct system can serve as a means to distribute these contaminants throughout a home. In these cases, duct cleaning may make sense. However, a light amount of household dust in your air ducts is normal. Duct cleaning is not considered to be a necessary part of yearly maintenance of your heating and cooling system, which consists of regular cleaning of drain pans and heating and cooling coils, regular filter changes and yearly inspections of heating equipment. Research continues in an effort to evaluate the potential benefits of air duct cleaning.

In the meantime educate yourself about duct cleaning by contacting some or all of the sources of information listed at the end of this publication and asking questions of potential service providers.

Are duct materials other than bare sheet metal ducts more likely to be contaminated with mold and other biological contaminants?

You may be familiar with air ducts that are constructed of sheet metal. However, many modern residential air duct systems are constructed of fiber glass duct board or sheet metal ducts that are lined on the inside with fiber glass duct liner. Since the early 1970's, a significant increase in the use of flexible duct, which generally is internally lined with plastic or some other type of material, has occurred. The use of insulated duct material has increased due to improved temperature control, energy conservation, and reduced condensation. Internal insulation provides better acoustical (noise) control. Flexible duct is very low cost. These products are engineered specifically for use in ducts or as ducts themselves, and are tested in accordance with standards established by Underwriters Laboratories (UL), the American Society for Testing and Materials (ASTM), and the National Fire Protection Association (NFPA).

Many insulated duct systems have operated for years without supporting significant mold growth. Keeping them reasonably clean and dry is generally adequate. However, there is substantial debate about whether porous insulation materials (e.g., fiber glass) are more prone to microbial contamination than bare sheet metal ducts. If enough dirt and moisture are permitted to enter the duct system, there may be no significant difference in the rate or extent of microbial growth in internally lined or bare sheet metal ducts. However, treatment of mold contamination on bare sheet metal is much easier. Cleaning and treatment with an EPA-registered biocide are possible. Once fiberglass duct liner is contaminated with mold, cleaning is not sufficient to prevent regrowth and there are no EPA-registered biocides for the treatment of porous duct materials. EPA, NADCA, and NAIMA all recommend the replacement of wet or moldy fiber glass duct material.

In the meantime experts do agree that moisture should not be present in ducts and if moisture and dirt are present, the potential exists for biological contaminants to grow and be distributed throughout the home. Controlling moisture is the most effective way to prevent biological growth in all types of air ducts.

- Correct any water leaks or standing water.

- Remove standing water under cooling coils of air handling units by making sure that drain pans slope toward the drain.

- If humidifiers are used, they must be properly maintained.

- Air handling units should be constructed so that maintenance personnel have easy, direct access to heat exchange components and drain pans for proper cleaning and maintenance.

- Fiber glass, or any other insulation material that is wet or visibly moldy (or if an unacceptable odor is present) should be removed and replaced by a qualified heating and cooling system contractor.

- Steam cleaning and other methods involving moisture should not be used on any kind of duct work.

Should chemical biocides be applied to the inside of air ducts?

Air duct cleaning service providers may tell you that they need to apply a chemical biocide to the inside of your ducts to kill bacteria (germs), and fungi (mold) and prevent future biological growth. Some duct cleaning service providers may propose to introduce ozone to kill biological contaminants. Ozone is a highly reactive gas that is regulated in the outside air as a lung irritant. However, there remains considerable controversy over the necessity and wisdom of introducing chemical biocides or ozone into the duct work.

553

Among the possible problems with biocide and ozone application in air ducts:

- Little research has been conducted to demonstrate the effectiveness of most biocides and ozone when used inside ducts. Simply spraying or otherwise introducing these materials into the operating duct system may cause much of the material to be transported through the system and released into other areas of your home.

- Some people may react negatively to the biocide or ozone, causing adverse health reactions.

Chemical biocides are regulated by EPA under Federal pesticide law. A product must be registered by EPA for a specific use before it can be legally used for that purpose. The specific use(s) must appear on the pesticide (e.g., biocide) label, along with other important information. It is a violation of federal law to use a pesticide product in any manner inconsistent with the label directions.

A small number of products are currently registered by EPA specifically for use on the inside of bare sheet metal air ducts. A number of products are also registered for use as sanitizers on hard surfaces, which could include the interior of bare sheet metal ducts. While many such products may be used legally inside of unlined ducts if all label directions are followed, some of the directions on the label may be inappropriate for use in ducts. For example, if the directions indicate "rinse with water", the added moisture could stimulate mold growth.

All of the products discussed above are registered solely for the purpose of sanitizing the smooth surfaces of unlined (bare) sheet metal ducts. No products are currently registered as biocides for use on fiber glass duct board or fiber glass lined ducts, so it is important to determine if sections of your system contain these materials before permitting the application of any biocide.

In the meantime before allowing a service provider to use a chemical biocide in your duct work, the service provider should:

- Demonstrate visible evidence of microbial growth in your duct work. Some service providers may attempt to convince you that your air ducts are contaminated by demonstrating that the microorganisms found in your home grow on a settling plate (i.e., petri dish). This is inappropriate. Some microorganisms are always present in the air, and some growth on a settling plate is normal. As noted earlier, only an expert can positively identify a substance as biological growth and lab analysis may be required for final confirmation. Other testing methods are not reliable.

• Explain why biological growth cannot be removed by physical means, such as brushing, and further growth prevented by controlling moisture.

If you decide to permit the use of a biocide, the service provider should:

• Show you the biocide label, which will describe its range of approved uses.

• Apply the biocide only to un-insulated areas of the duct system after proper cleaning, if necessary to reduce the chances for regrowth of mold.

• Always use the product strictly according to its label instructions.

While some low toxicity products may be legally applied while occupants of the home are present, you may wish to consider leaving the premises while the biocide is being applied as an added precaution.

Do sealants prevent the release of dust and dirt particles into the air?

Manufacturers of products marketed to coat and seal duct surfaces claim that these sealants prevent dust and dirt particles inside air ducts from being released into the air. As with biocides, a sealant is often applied by spraying it into the operating duct system. Laboratory tests indicate that materials introduced in this manner tend not to completely coat the duct surface. Application of sealants may also affect the acoustical (noise) and fire retarding characteristics of fiber glass lined or constructed ducts and may invalidate the manufacturer's warranty.

Questions about the safety, effectiveness and overall desirability of sealants remain. For example, little is known about the potential toxicity of these products under typical use conditions or in the event they catch fire.

In addition, sealants have yet to be evaluated for their resistance to deterioration over time which could add particles to the duct air.

In the meantime most organizations concerned with duct cleaning, including EPA, NADCA, NAIMA, and the Sheet Metal and Air

Conditioning Contractors' National Association (SMACNA) do not currently recommend the routine use of sealants in any type of duct. Instances when the use of sealants may be appropriate include the repair of damaged fiber glass insulation or when combating fire damage within ducts. Sealants should never be used on wet duct liner, to cover actively growing mold, or to cover debris in the ducts, and should only be applied after cleaning according to NADCA or other appropriate guidelines or standards.

To Learn More About Indoor Air Quality

U.S. Environmental Protection Agency
Office of Radiation and Indoor Air
Indoor Environments Division (6604J)
401 M St., S.W.
Washington, DC 20460
Tel: 202- 564-9370; Fax: 202-565-2038
Internet: http://www.epa.gov
E-Mail: webmaster.oria@epamail.epa.gov

Indoor Air Quality InformationClearinghouse (IAQ INFO)
P.O. Box 37133
Washington, DC 20013-7133
Toll Free: 800-438-4318
Tel: 703-356-4020; Fax: 703-356-5386
E-Mail: IAQINFO@aol.com

To Learn More About Air Duct Cleaning

National Air Duct Cleaners Association (NADCA)
1518 K Street, NW Suite 503
Washington, DC 20005
Tel: 202-737-2926
Internet: http://www.nadca.com

North American Insulation Manufacturers Association (NAIMA)
44 Canal Center Plaza, Suite 310
Alexandria, VA 22314
Tel: 703-684-0084; Fax: 703-684-0427
Internet: http://www.naima.org

Consumer Checklist

- Learn as much as possible about air duct cleaning before you decide to have your ducts cleaned by reading this guidance and contacting the sources of information provided.

- Consider other possible sources of indoor air pollution first if you suspect an indoor air quality problem exists in your home.

- Have your air ducts cleaned if they are visibly contaminated with substantial mold growth, pests or vermin, or are clogged with substantial deposits of dust or debris.

- Ask the service provider to show you any mold or other biological contamination they say exists. Get laboratory confirmation of mold growth or decide to rely on your own judgment and common sense in evaluating apparent mold growth.

- Get estimates from at least three service providers.

- Check references.

- Ask the service provider whether he/she holds any relevant state licenses. As of 1996, the following states require air duct cleaners to hold special licenses: Arizona, Arkansas, California, Florida, Georgia, Michigan and Texas. Other states may also require licenses.

- Insist that the service provider give you knowledgeable and complete answers to your questions.

- Find out whether your ducts are made of sheet metal, flex duct, or constructed of fiber glass duct board or lined with fiber glass since the methods of cleaning vary depending on duct type. Remember, a combination of these elements may be present.

- Permit the application of biocides in your ducts only if necessary to control mold growth and only after assuring yourself that the product will be applied strictly according to label directions. As a precaution, you and your pets should leave the premises during application.

- Do not permit the use of sealants except under unusual circumstances where other alternatives are not feasible.

- Make sure the service provider follows the National Air Duct Cleaning Association's (NADCA) standards and, if the ducts are constructed of flex duct, duct board, or lined with fiber glass, the guidelines of the North American Insulation Manufacturers Association (NAIMA).

• Commit to a preventive maintenance program of yearly inspections of your heating and cooling system, regular filter changes, and steps to prevent moisture contamination.

Chapter 87

Residential Air Cleaners

Air Cleaning

Air cleaning is one of three methods of reducing pollutants in indoor air. In order of effectiveness, the three methods are:

1. removal of the source or control of its emissions,

2. ventilation,

3. air cleaning.

Air cleaning can be used as an adjunct to source control and ventilation. However, air cleaning alone cannot adequately remove all of the pollutants typically found in indoor air.

Should You Use an Air Cleaner?

Many factors need to be considered in determining whether use of an air cleaner is appropriate in a particular setting. Therefore, the decision whether or not to use an air cleaner is left to the individual. EPA has not taken a position either for or against the use of these devices in the home.

"Indoor Air Facts No. 7," Environment Protection Agency (EPA), EPA Document Number 20A-4001, March 1997, modified July 1998.

Will Air Cleaning Reduce Health Effects?

Air cleaners may reduce the health effects from some particles—small solid or liquid substances suspended in air, such as dust or light spray mists.

Some air cleaners, under the right conditions, can effectively remove certain respirable-size particles (for example, tobacco smoke particles). These invisible particles are of concern because they can be inhaled deeply into the lungs. Removing such particles may reduce associated health effects in exposed people. These effects may range from eye and lung irritation to more serious effects such as cancer and decreased lung function.

Some controversy exists about whether air cleaners can reduce the allergic reactions produced by larger particles such as pollen, house dust allergens, some molds, and animal dander. Most of these particles are found where they settle on surfaces in the home, rather than in the air. They cannot be removed by an air cleaner unless disturbed and resuspended in the air.

Air cleaners that do not contain special media, such as activated carbon or alumina, will not remove gaseous pollutants, including radon, or reduce their associated health effects. Whether air cleaners that contain these media are effective in reducing health risks from gaseous pollutants cannot be adequately assessed at this time. In addition, the effectiveness of air cleaners in reducing the health risks from radon progeny (decay products) cannot be adequately evaluated at present.

The removal of gaseous pollutants and radon and its progeny is not addressed further in this fact sheet. Health effects from these pollutants may be serious, however, and they are of concern in indoor air.

Types of Air Cleaners

Some air cleaners may be installed in the ducts which are part of central heating or air-conditioning systems in homes. Portable air cleaners stand alone in a room.

Types of air cleaners include:

- Mechanical filters, similar to, and including, the typical furnace filter.

- Electronic air cleaners (for example, electrostatic precipitators) which trap charged particles using an electrical field.

- Ion generators which act by charging the particles in a room. The charged particles are then attracted to walls, floors, draperies, etc. or a charged collector.

- "Hybrid" devices, which contain two or more of the particle removal devices discussed above.

Assessing Potential Performance

At a minimum, you should consider the following major factors affecting the performance of the air cleaner:

- The percentage of the particles removed as they go through the device (that is, the efficiency).

- The amount of air handled by the device. For example, an air cleaner may have a high efficiency filter, but it may process only 10 cubic feet of air each minute. Suppose that the air cleaner is put in a room of typical size, containing 1000 cubic feet of air. In this room, it will take a long time for all the air to be processed. In some cases, pollutants may be generated more quickly than they are removed.

- The effective volume of the air to be cleaned. A single portable unit used in a room within a large building in which the air flows between several apartments or offices would be of little or no value.

- The decrease in performance which may occur between maintenance periods and if periodic maintenance is not performed on schedule.

Additional Factors to Consider

- Ion generators and electronic air cleaners may produce ozone, particularly if they are not properly installed and maintained.

- Ozone can be a lung irritant.

- Gases and odors from particles collected by the devices may be redispersed into the air. The odor of tobacco smoke is largely due to gases in the smoke, rather than particles. Thus, you may smell a tobacco odor even when the smoke particles have been removed.

- Some devices scent the air to mask odors, which may lead you to believe that the odor-causing pollutants have been removed.

- Ion generators, especially those that do not contain a collector, may cause soiling of walls and other surfaces.

- You may be bothered by noise from portable air cleaners, even at low speeds.

- Maintenance costs, such as costs for the replacement of filters, may be significant. You should consider these costs in addition to the initial cost of purchase. In general, the most effective units are also the most costly.

Obtaining Adequate Performance

Proper installation, use, and care. Follow the manufacturer's directions to assure that the air cleaner works properly. To avoid any electrical or mechanical hazards, be sure the unit is listed with Underwriters Laboratories (UL) or another recognized independent safety testing laboratory. Perform routine maintenance, as required. Generally speaking, air cleaners rigor frequent cleaning and filter replacement to function properly.

Proper placement. Place portable air cleaners so:

- They are near a specific pollutant source, if one exists.

- They force the cleaned air into occupied areas.

- The inlet and outlet are not blocked by walls, furniture, or other obstructions.

- For in-duct devices, assure that the inlets and outlets of the heating or cooling system are not blocked by furniture and other obstructions.

Comparing Air Cleaners

One common method of rating high efficiency filters uses a procedure in Military Standard 282. This procedure measures how well small particles of a specific chemical are removed by the filter.

The Federal government has not published guidelines or standards that can be used to determine how well low to medium efficiency air cleaners work. However, standards have been developed by private standard-setting trade associations. These standards may be useful in comparing air cleaners.

For further information on standards for in-duct air cleaners, contact your local heating or air-conditioning contractor or:

Air-Conditioning & Refrigeration Institute (ARI)
4100 North Fairfax Drive, Suite 200
Arlington, VA 22203
Tel: 703-524-8800
Fax: 703-528-3816
Internet: http://www.ari.org
E-Mail: ari@ari.org

For further information on standards for portable air cleaners:

Association of Home Appliance Manufacturers (AHAM)
1111 18th Street, N.W.
Suite 402
Washington, D.C. 20036
Tel: 202-872-5955
Fax: 202-872-9354
Internet: http://www.aham.org

Chapter 88

Indoor Environmental Air Quality in Schools

Why IAQ Is Important to Your School?

Most people are aware that outdoor air pollution can damage their health, but many do not know that indoor air pollution can also cause harm. Environmental Protection Agency (EPA) studies of human exposure to air pollutants indicate that indoor levels of pollutants may be 2-5 times, and occasionally more than 100 times, higher than outdoor levels. These levels of indoor air pollutants are of particular concern because it is estimated that most people spend about 90% of their time indoors. Comparative risk studies performed by EPA and its Science Advisory Board have consistently ranked indoor air pollution among the top four environmental risks to the public.

Failure to prevent indoor air problems, or failure to act promptly, can have consequences such as:

- increasing the chances for long-term and short-term health problems for students and staff

- impacting the student learning environment, comfort, and attendance

- reducing productivity of teachers and staff due to discomfort, sickness, or absenteeism

---

"IAQ Tools for Schools," U.S. Environmental Protection Agency (EPA), December 1996, modified January 2000.

- faster deterioration and reduced efficiency of the school physical plant and equipment

- increasing the chance that schools will have to be closed, or occupants temporarily moved

- straining relationships among school administration and parents and staff

- creating negative publicity that could damage a school's or administration's image and effectiveness

- creating potential liability problems

Indoor air problems can be subtle and do not always produce easily recognized impacts on health, well-being, or the physical plant. Children are especially susceptible to air pollution. For this and the reasons noted above, air quality in schools is of particular concern. Proper maintenance of indoor air is more than a "quality" issue, it includes safety and good management of our investment in the students, staff, and facilities.

Good indoor air quality contributes to a favorable learning environment for students, productivity for teachers and staff, and a sense of comfort, health, and well-being for school occupants. These combine to assist a school in its core mission—educating children.

Understanding IAQ Problems and Solutions

Over the past forty or fifty years, exposure to indoor air pollutants has increased due to a variety of factors, including the construction of more tightly sealed buildings, reduced ventilation rates to save energy, the use of synthetic building materials and furnishings, and the use of chemically-formulated personal care products, pesticides, and housekeeping supplies. In addition, our activities and decisions, such as delaying maintenance to "save" money, can lead to problems from sources and ventilation. Four basic factors affect IAQ: sources of indoor air pollutants, the heating, ventilation, and air-conditioning (HVAC) system, pollutant pathways, and occupants.

Sources of Indoor Air Pollutants

Indoor air contaminants can begin within the building or be drawn in from outdoors. If pollutant sources are not controlled, IAQ problems can occur, even if the HVAC system is working properly. Air pollutants consist of numerous particles, fibers, mists, molds, bacteria, and gases. It may be helpful to think of air pollutant sources as fitting into one of the categories in the table shown below.

In addition to the number of potential pollutants, indoor air pollutant levels can vary within the school building, or even a single classroom. Pollutants can also vary with time, such as only once each week when floor stripping is done, or continuously such as when fungi is growing in the HVAC system.

HVAC System Design and Operation

The heating, ventilation, and air-conditioning (HVAC) system includes all heating, cooling, and ventilating equipment serving a school. A properly designed and functioning HVAC system:

- controls temperature and humidity to provide thermal comfort

- distributes adequate amounts of outdoor air to meet ventilation needs of school occupants

- isolates and removes odors and pollutants through pressure control, filtration, and exhaust fans

Not all HVAC systems are designed to do all of these things. Some buildings rely only on natural ventilation. Others lack cooling, and many have little or no humidity control.

Pollutant Pathways and Driving Forces

Airflow patterns in buildings are caused by mechanical ventilation systems, human activity, and natural effects such as wind. Air pressure differences created by these forces move airborne pollutants from areas of higher pressure to areas of lower pressure through any available openings in building walls, ceilings, floors, doors, windows, and HVAC system. An inflated balloon is an example of this driving force. As long as the opening to the balloon is kept shut, no air will flow, but when open, air will move from inside (area of higher pressure) to the outside (area of lower pressure). Even if the opening is small, air will move until the pressures inside and outside are equal.

Building Occupants and Health

Building occupants in schools include the staff, students, and other people who spend extended periods of time in the school. The effects of IAQ problems on occupants are often vague symptoms rather than clearly defined illnesses. Symptoms commonly attributed to IAQ problems include:

- headache, fatigue, and shortness of breath
- sinus congestion, cough, and sneezing
- eye, nose, throat, and skin irritation
- dizziness and nausea

All of these symptoms, however, may also be caused by other factors, and are not necessarily due to air quality problems. Environmental stressors such as improper lighting, noise, vibration, overcrowding, and psychosocial problems (such as job or home stress) can produce symptoms that are similar to those associated with poor air quality, but require different solutions.

Because people are different, one individual may react to a particular IAQ problem while surrounding occupants have no noticeable ill effects. In other cases, complaints may be widespread. In addition to different degrees of reaction, an indoor air pollutant or problem can trigger different types of reactions in different people. Some groups that may be particularly susceptible to effects of indoor air contaminants include:

- allergic or asthmatic individuals, or people with sensitivity to chemicals
- people with respiratory disease
- people whose immune systems are suppressed due to radiation or chemotherapy, or disease
- contact lens wearers

Six Basic Control Strategies

There are six basic methods for lowering concentrations of indoor air pollutants.

Source Management includes source removal, source substitution, and source encapsulation. Source management is the most effective control method when it can be practically applied. The best prevention method is never to bring unnecessary pollutants into the school building. Examples of source removal include not allowing buses to idle near outdoor air intakes, not placing garbage in rooms where HVAC equipment is located, and banning smoking within the school. Source substitution includes actions such as selecting less toxic art material or interior paint than the products which are currently in use. Source encapsulation involves placing a barrier around the source so that it releases fewer pollutants into the indoor air.

Local Exhaust is very effective in removing sources of pollutants before they can be dispersed into the indoor air, exhausting the contaminated air outside. Well known examples include restrooms, kitchens, and science lab fume hoods. Other examples of pollutants that originate at specific points and that can be easily exhausted include science lab and housekeeping storage rooms, printing and duplicating rooms, and vocational/industrial areas such as welding booths.

Ventilation uses cleaner (i.e., outdoor) air to dilute the contaminated (i.e., indoor) air that people are breathing. Generally, local building codes specify the amount of outdoor air that must be continuously supplied to an occupied area. For situations such as painting, pesticide application, or chemical spills, temporarily increasing the ventilation can be useful in diluting the concentration of fumes in the air.

Exposure Control includes the principles of time of use and location of use. An example of time of use would be to strip and wax floors on Friday after school is dismissed, so that the floor products have a chance to release gases over the weekend, reducing the level of odors or contaminants in the air when the school is occupied. An example of location of use involves moving the contaminating source as far as possible from occupants, or relocating susceptible occupants.

Air Cleaning primarily involves the filtration of particles from the air as the air passes through the ventilation equipment. Gaseous contaminants can also be removed, but usually this type of system should be engineered on a case-by-case basis.

Education of the school occupants is critical. If school staff are provided information about the sources and effects of contaminants under their control, and about the proper operation of the ventilation system, they will better understand their indoor environment and can act to reduce their personal exposure.

How Do I Know if There Is an IAQ Problem

Diagnosing symptoms that relate to IAQ can be tricky. Acute (short-term) symptoms of IAQ problems typically are similar to those from colds, allergies, fatigue, or the flu. There are clues, however, that can serve as indicators of potential indoor air problems:

- the symptoms are widespread within a class or within the school, potentially indicating a ventilation problem

- the symptoms disappear when the students or staff leave the school building for the day

- the onset is sudden after some change at school, such as painting or pesticide application

- persons with allergies, asthma, or chemical sensitivities have reactions indoors but not outdoors

- a doctor has diagnosed a student or staff member as having an indoor air-related illness

However, a lack of symptoms does not mean that the quality of the air within the school is acceptable. Symptoms from long-term health effects (such as lung cancer due to radon) often do not become evident for many years. For this reason, schools should establish a preventive indoor air program to minimize exposure of students and staff to indoor air pollutants.

What Should I Do if I Think a School has an IAQ Problem

If your child, or someone else you know, is experiencing symptoms that you believe may be related to their school environment, contact a school official immediately, such as the school IAQ Coordinator, or the health and safety coordinator. Whether or not the school has a known problem, encourage the school to obtain and use the Indoor Air Quality Tools for Schools Kit. This easy-to-use Kit shows schools how to carry out a practical plan of action at little or no cost, using in-house staff.

The Kit includes simple checklists for all school employees, a flexible step-by-step guide for using the checklists, an Indoor Air Quality Problem Solving Wheel, a fact sheet on indoor air pollution sources and solutions, sample memos to help school personnel respond to inquiries, and sample policies.

The Kit is co-sponsored by the National PTA, National Education Association, Council for American Private Education, Association of School Business Officials, American Federation of Teachers, and the American Lung Association.

The Federal government, as well as most State and local governments, do not have regulations or enforcement capabilities regarding indoor air quality in schools. For some schools, assistance may be available from the local or State departments of health or environment. The Federal or State occupational safety and health office (OSHA) may also provide some help.

What You Can Do

1. Ensure that your school gets the Indoor Air Quality Tools for Schools Kit

2. Ensure that your school uses the Kit

How to Order the Kit

IAQ Tools for Schools Action Kit (Kit) shows schools how to carry out a practical plan of action to improve indoor air quality at little or no cost using common-sense activities and in-house staff. The Kit provides simple-to-follow checklists, background information, sample memos and policies, a recommended IAQ Management Plan, and a unique IAQ Problem Solving Wheel. Ten appendices include information on topics such as hiring outside assistance, and mold and moisture control.

The IAQ Tools for Schools—Taking Action and Ventilation Basics Videos are available free of charge and can be obtained by calling the IAQ INFO Clearinghouse at 1-800-438-4318.

Schools and school districts may obtain a free copy of the IAQ Tools for Schools and video by faxing a request on official school/school district letterhead to EPA's Indoor Air Quality Clearinghouse at 703-356-5386 or you may write to:

EPA Kit
P.O. Box 37133
Washington, DC 20013-7133
http://www.epa.gov/iaq/schools/scholkit.html

Chapter 89

Occupational Respiratory Diseases

Who is at risk for work-related lung disease?

If the air you breathe at work contains an excessive amount of dust, fumes, smoke, gases, vapors or mists, you may be at risk for a lung disease that can cause a breathing problem. Workers who smoke are at a much greater risk of lung disease if they are exposed to substances in the workplace that cause lung disease. Poor ventilation, closed-in working areas and heat increase the danger. Outside air pollution can also increase the risk of lung disease in people who work in jobs that expose them to substances that can cause lung disease.

What substances in the workplace can hurt my lungs?

Many substances found in the workplace can cause breathing problems. Some of them are as follows:

- Dusts from such things as wood, cotton, coal, asbestos, silica and talc. Dust from cereal grains, coffee, pesticides, drug or enzyme powders, metals and fiberglass can also hurt your lungs.

- Fumes such as from metals that are heated and cooled quickly. This process results in fine, solid particles being carried in the air. Examples of jobs that involve exposure to fumes from metals and other substances that are heated and cooled quickly include welding, smelting, furnace work, pottery making, plastics manufacture and rubber operations.

- Smoke from burning organic materials. Smoke can contain a variety of dusts, gases and vapors, depending on what is burning. Firefighters are at special risk.

- Gases such as formaldehyde, ammonia, chlorine, sulfur dioxide, ozone and nitrogen oxides. These gases can be found in jobs where chemical reactions occur and in jobs with high heat operations, such as welding, brazing, smelting, oven drying and furnace work.

- Vapors, which are a form of gas given off by all liquids. Vapors, such as those given off by solvents, usually irritate the nose and throat first, before they affect the lungs.

- Mists or sprays from paints, lacquers (for example, varnishes), hair spray, pesticides, cleaning products, acids, oils and solvents (such as turpentine).

What kinds of breathing problems can occur following exposure to such substances?

Some substances can cause you to have upper respiratory irritation, or irritation of your nose and/or throat and cold-like symptoms, such as a runny nose and scratchy throat. Viral infections and allergies produce similar symptoms. You should become suspicious of a work-related illness if you often feel like your nose and throat are irritated and breathing problems seem to occur when you are at work.

Breathing in substances at work can also cause you to have bronchitis, a flu-like illness, asthma and emphysema. A person with bronchitis has a persistent cough that produces mucus or sputum and lasts at least three months a year. Cigarette smoking is the most common cause of bronchitis, but workplace toxins can also play a role.

Frequent episodes of flu-like illness may be caused by a substances you breathe in your workplace. If you notice that you often have what seems to be the flu, your illness may be caused by something you are exposed to at work.

There are different work-related lung diseases that can make you feel as though you have the flu. One of them is allergic alveolitis (also known as "farmer's lung"), which can occur after excessive exposure to moldy hay. Metal fume fever is another occupational lung disease that can produce flu-like symptoms. It occurs from inhalation of metal vapors, such as in welding and other metallic operations. Polymer fume fever, from breathing the fumes of polymers such as Teflon, also may make you feel like you have the flu. A worker with one of these conditions develops breathing problems, cough, fever, muscle aches and general malaise (a feeling of being tired and having no energy) four to six hours after exposure to the substance. If such symptoms occur again and again when you are at work, this pattern is a clue that your illness may be related to your work.

If you develop asthma for the first time as an adult, the illness could be related to something you are exposed to at work. Asthma symptoms include wheezing, a persistent dry cough or trouble breathing.

Emphysema usually occurs in older people who smoke. However, people who have worked with coal, asbestos or silica dust for 20 years or more can develop emphysema. They may have a cough, fatigue, chest tightness and difficulty breathing.

What should I do if I think something in the air at work is making me sick?

You will want to see your family doctor. Before doing so, you need to gather some information to help your doctor make a diagnosis. One way you can do this is to keep a written record about your illness. Try to write down the following information:

- When you first started to experience your symptoms

- How often you experience symptoms

- The time of day that the symptoms are worse

- Whether you feel better on some days

- How you feel your symptoms relate to work

Even if the pattern of your symptoms does not seem to be clearly related to your work, it is important to record the timing of your symptoms accurately.

Also, make a note of your shift or work hours, and the days of the week you work and are off work. Try to recall previous jobs, hobbies and smoking habits—anything that might have affected your lungs. If your doctor has sent you an occupational health history form, fill it out as completely as possible.

Write down the list of all of the ingredients listed on the containers of materials you are using in the workplace. Also write down any descriptions of handling precautions and first-aid measures that are printed on the label. If possible, try to get the chemical name, instead of the brand name, to show your doctor.

Ask to see the material safety data sheets (MSDSs) at your workplace. These are information sheets about the products that you use in the workplace. All employers are required by law to complete these forms, and you have a right to see them. Obtain copies of the MSDSs and bring them with you to your doctor's appointment.

How can I keep from having my lungs damaged by something I'm exposed to at work?

If you smoke, stop. This is the most important thing you can do for your overall health, regardless of your workplace risks. Cigarette smoking irritates the lungs and impairs their self-cleaning ability, so smokers are at greater risk of developing some work-related lung diseases than are nonsmokers. For example, asbestos workers who smoke more than a pack of cigarettes a day greatly increase their risk of lung cancer. Such workers have up to 90 times the chance of dying of lung cancer, compared with workers who neither smoke nor work with asbestos.

If you are exposed to a substance at work that can cause lung disease, a respirator should be used at work as a temporary measure until changes are made in the workplace that prevent exposure to the substance. You must be properly fitted and trained in the use of the respirator. Over time you should be periodically refitted and retrained in how to use this equipment. The respirator must be carefully cleaned after each use, and it should be checked and maintained to ensure that it works properly.

If you are exposed to damaging substances at work, talk to your supervisor about the need for adequate ventilation and new procedures to eliminate your exposure. A change in ingredients, work practices or machinery can reduce hazards in the air. Ventilation systems can remove pollutants and toxins from the air to reduce exposure and prevent buildup. Local exhaust ventilation can be used to remove polluted air at the point where it is generated by a hazardous process or machine. At some jobs, people can be separated from the hazards.

This information provides a general overview on occupational respiratory disorders and may not apply to everyone. Talk to your family doctor to find out if this information applies to you and to get more information on this subject.

Chapter 90

Farm Respiratory Hazards

Do Farmer-Set Fires Endanger Health?

Fall is burning season in the wheat fields of eastern Washington State. To prepare for planting in 1998, farmers burned about 229,000 acres of wheat stubble, an increase over recent years. Although a tighter state permitting system substantially reduced the acreage burned in 1999, clean air activitists are concerned that the state has not tightened up enough.

A hot issue. Farmers argue that agricultural burning is a necessary tool, but neighbors worry that the smoke may lead to health problems such as asthma, particularly in children.

The fires are used to help control crop diseases and to clear fields before using a relatively new farming technique called minimum tillage, which reduces soil erosion but requires machinery that can get clogged by heavy stubble. Nationally, fires are also used to clear stubble from grass seed fields in Idaho, rice fields in California, and sugarcane fields in Florida. In eastern Washington, grass growers stopped burning their fields in 1998 in accordance with an agreement with the state's Department of Ecology, which regulates agricultural burning in Washington. But the emphasis on minimum tillage, among other factors, has caused a larger number of wheat fires to take grass's place.

"Do Farmer-Set Fires Endanger Health?" U.S. Environmental Protection Agency (EPA), 2000.

Burning is a major source of air pollution in Spokane and surrounding areas. "It's a unique pollution, different from auto exhaust," says Patricia Hoffman, a veterinarian who heads Save Our Summers, a citizens group that opposes agricultural burning. "It's a high-concentration, high-intensity exposure for a short period. It's very dangerous for people with asthma or heart or lung problems."

Of Spokane County's approximately 500,000 residents, she says, about 40,000 have asthma and 3,000 have emphysema. These asthma rates are around twice the national average. Timothy Krautkraemer, age 10, is a Spokane asthma patient who stays indoors during the burning season. "He can't participate in activities that others participate in," says his father, Jeffrey. "It's pretty rough on a 10-year-old."

The family has joined a federal lawsuit with another family and Save Our Summers against the Washington Department of Ecology. They argue that the burning constitutes discrimination against asthma sufferers, violating the Americans with Disabilities Act.

Michael McCarthy, a Spokane pulmonary pediatric specialist, says he's "totally convinced [the burning is] an extremely important public health problem." McCarthy believes the increased asthma rates are due to the smoke and a dry, dusty climate where frequent air inversions can cause smoke to linger for days.

While McCarthy admits he cannot prove that any particular patient has been injured by the smoke, he says his medical experience is persuasive. For example, he says, patients who travel during the burning season tell him, "As soon as I get out of Spokane, I feel better, and as soon as I get back, I feel worse." The evidence may be anecdotal, McCarthy adds, but "so many have told me this, it's become a reality for me."

Roe Roberts, an associate professor of health administration at Eastern Washington University in Spokane, studied the effects of grass-fire smoke in eastern Washington during the mid-1990s. Her research, published in the June 1998 issue of the Journal of Environmental Health, found that concentrations of smoke particles smaller than 2.5 microns in diameter correlated with weekend purchases of bronchodilators, which are used to open bronchial airways. Roberts says that because weekend purchases often represent emergency purchases, they provide an indirect measure of the effects of smoke on lung-disease patients.

Even some wheat growers recognize the problem. In the July 1999 issue of the trade journal Wheat Life, David Roseberry, past president of the Washington Association of Wheat Growers, wrote, "Evidence affirming the negative consequences of inhaling smoke—all smoke, not just cigarette smoke—has been continuously building to a surprising extent."

Department of Ecology spokesman Larry Altose says the department recognizes that "smoke from agricultural fires is causing serious health problems and people are very interested in addressing this issue to bring it under control." The Washington Association of Wheat Growers signed an agreement with the Department of Ecology in February 1999 specifying a 50% decline in burning over seven years. Altose says permits are issued to farmers who show that burning is "necessary according to best management practices."

Hoffman says the 50% overall reduction mandated by the agreement will not protect public health because it was based on 1998 figures, when a record amount of acreage was burned. But Altose says the Department of Ecology believes the 50% reduction will make a big difference, especially when coupled with new "best management" practices used by farmers, which discourage the use of fire. "We've already seen burning decrease by 50% this fall," he says.

Chapter 91

Respiratory Safety and Health in Mines

Mining the earth—underground and on the surface—for coal, ore, and stone, remains one of the most dangerous industries in the United States.

Approximately 400,000 miners are employed in over 11,000 surface and underground mines in the U.S.

Each year, an estimated 2,000 miners die from lung diseases caused by exposure to coal mine dust. The Federal Black Lung Program paid over $18 billion to beneficiaries in the 1980s.

Mining has the highest rate for fatal injuries of all U.S. industries. More than 80 miners die from fatal work injuries each year.

In 1993, one in eight underground coal miners was injured on the job, nearly twice the average of U.S. industry.

The primary focus of NIOSH mining research is to prevent lung diseases, the most prevalent health problem among miners. Recently, Congress and the Administration transferred the management of the mine safety research functions of the former Bureau of Mines (BoM) to NIOSH, consolidating into one program all federal occupational health and safety research. Workplace hazards, and ways to control them, cut across many industries. Mining research activities provide new opportunities for improving safety and health research for all workers.

"NIOSH Facts: Mine Safety and Health," National Institute for Occupational Safety and Health (NIOSH), 1996, updated August 1997.

NIOSH Makes a Difference in the Health of Miners

While significant progress has been made to reduce mine worker respiratory disease since the enactment of the Federal Coal Mine Health and Safety Act of 1969, serious problems remain. Some dust samples collected in underground and surface mines exceed Federal dust standards. Even miners with lifetime exposures to coal mine dust at the current federal standard have an elevated risk of developing occupational respiratory diseases. NIOSH assesses mine dust health effects and develops exposure controls and other prevention strategies.

Preventing Silicosis in Mine Drillers

Silicosis, a preventable and often fatal lung disease, is caused by inhaling fine particles of silica. Silicosis persists, even with knowledge of how it can be prevented. Each year, thousands of coal workers are afflicted with silicosis.

NIOSH field investigations identified numerous examples of high silica exposures and tragic cases of silicosis deaths in mine drillers. NIOSH and its partners developed a national program to promote the health of surface coal miners. To reduce silicosis among miners, NIOSH:

- Disseminates information to inspectors, miners, and employers throughout the surface mining industry describing steps to prevent silicosis.

- Produced a video for the surface mining community.

- Provides technical assistance to establish a program providing health screening and follow up care for surface miners in Pennsylvania.

Unpredictable geological conditions, confined work spaces, poor visibility and the use of large, powerful equipment are hazards in mining. Coal and metal miners who suffer injuries tend to lose twice as many days of work as workers in other industries. With the incorporation of the former BoM into NIOSH, NIOSH has increased capacity to improve mine safety through training, prevention strategies, and technologies.

Chapter 92

Personal Respiratory Protection

Preventing Inhalation of Airborne Hazards

The human body has marvelous defense mechanisms against air pollutants which ensure effective functioning of the lungs. However, when exposed to specific hazards in the workplace including certain chemical vapors, bioaerosols, mineral dusts or agricultural dusts, we require additional protection to prevent the development of disease. Some of these occupational lung diseases include asbestosis, lung cancer, beryllium disease, silicosis, asthma and tuberculosis. Often, inhaled agents do not target the lungs themselves, but rather use the respiratory tract as an organ of uptake. Therefore, protecting the lungs from these noxious materials will prevent not just respiratory disease but other forms of disease as well.

The concept of respiratory protection is not new—as early as the first century A.D., Roman mine workers, wearing masks made from dried animal bladders, shielded their lungs from the toxic red oxide of lead. Today, technological advances continue to create thousands of new chemicals and new occupational hazards. These advances, ironically, have also meant the development of more sophisticated methods for protecting workers. While the challenges may be new, the principles remain the same.

Principles of Respiratory Protection

In general, a respirator is any device designed to protect the wearer from hazardous air. More specifically, a respirator is a face piece, hood or helmet that is equipped with a filter or connected to a breathable air source. (A surgical mask, designed to protect a sterile environment from the wearer, is not a respirator) It is important to note that engineering and administrative strategies (e.g., using less hazardous materials) should be the primary factors in preventing worker exposure. When these measures are not adequate, not feasible or not yet implemented, a respirator may be required to protect the employee and mitigate the hazard.

The Occupational Safety and Health Administration (OSHA), a division of the Department of Labor, determines and enforces the regulations for the use of respirators.

Under current OSHA standards, the employer is responsible for implementing a respirator program and assuring that regulatory requirements are met. A complete program, detailed in written guidelines, is necessary to instruct workers on the fit, care, use and limitations of a particular respirator so that protection is optimized. Without such a program, a respirator may not be used in the workplace.

An initial medical evaluation is required to determine whether or not a worker is able to use a respirator. A "high-risk" worker with cardiac disease, for instance, would not be able to support a heavier respirator like a self-contained breathing apparatus, which could weigh as much as 30 pounds. The medical screening may involve a specially designed questionnaire, or, if necessary, a more thorough physical exam conducted by a physician. Finally, the program administrator, who is trained in respiratory protection, considers the kind of exposure, the demands of the job and the physical characteristics of the worker to select which type of respirator is most appropriate.

A successful respiratory program encompasses three basic principles: obtaining information about a hazard; following an employer's written program; and, using a respirator properly. This last concept sounds simple—but respirator protection can be rendered ineffective when not given the careful attention it requires.

Types of Respirators

There are two major categories of respirators: air-supplied respirators and air-purifying respirators. With air-supplied respirators, air travels to the mask or suit through a hose from an independent source outside the environment or from a compressed air cylinder worn on the back.

Air-supplied set-ups offer the greatest amount of protection, but can be heavy or cumbersome. Air-purifying respirators, however, remove hazardous agents from the air that is present in the work environment. This is accomplished through filtration, adsorption or chemical reaction. Within this category are negative-pressure respirators, which work when a user sucks in air through a filter. A second type, powered air-purifying respirators (PAPRs), use a fan unit to blow air through a filter to a mask, helmet or hood. The motorized air pump, battery and filter usually are worn on a waist belt.

Negative-pressure respirators are frequently used because of their versatility, light weight and low cost. The N95 disposable particulate respirator, named for its classification and filter efficiency, looks similar to a surgical mask and is often found in health care environments. The elastomeric respirator, available in half-face or full-face designs, is similar to the disposable particulate respirator but is reusable and made from flexible materials that create a more effective face-mask seal. A tight-fitting face piece—though essential for protection—can become uncomfortably hot and can hinder the ability to communicate. Also, any obstruction on or around the face such as hair, eye glasses or even deep creases in the skin can interfere with a tight face-mask seal.

All respirators are tested and certified by the National Institute for Occupational Safety and Health (NIOSH). It is this data that OSHA uses when formulating health standards. An assigned protection factor (APF) represents the protection expected for a particular type of respirator when it is worn by workers who have been fitted and trained in its use. The protection factor is the ratio of the contaminant concentration outside the respirator to the contaminant concentration inside the face piece (i.e., a protection factor of 10 means that the concentration inside the mask is one-tenth that outside).

Occupation: Farmer

Problems

- He performs multiple duties around the farm. His exposures include grain dust, hog confinement houses, pesticides and diesel fumes.

- He is unable to wear a negative-pressure respirator due to the following:

  he has a beard

  he has discomfort during hot weather

  he has claustrophobia

  some of his work requires a hard hat and eye protection

  he has mild asthma

  he wears glasses

Solution

He was fit with a loose-fitting helmet of a PABR Air Hat that would accommodate his beard, while delivering a constant flow of cool air for comfort during a long summer work day. He received literature on the product as well as information on where to purchase the respirator set-up.

Occupation: Welder

Problems

- He needed a half-face negative-pressure respirator that would fit under a welding mask and not restrict his movement.

- He forwarded his Material Safety Data Sheets containing information on the treated metals he works with.

Solution

The PRPP was able to consult on the proper filters to wear on his mask. He had a quantitative fit test for a backpack set-up with a harness system to keep away the filters from the exposure. This arrangement allows a welding shield to be placed over the mask and keeps the filters tight to the body and away from the immediate exposure area.

Occupation: Respiratory Therapist

Problems

- She has a latex allergy

- She works on a medical/surgical floor, occasionally caring for patients with TB

- She needs personal respiratory protection against TB because she occasionally assists with bronchoscopies and intubations.

Solution

The PRPP conducted a fit test for a latex-free N95 duck bill respirator for the therapist to wear in TB isolation rooms. In addition, she received training on a powered air-purifying respirator (PAPR) with a hood to provide a higher level of protection during bronchoscopies.

Healthcare Workers and the Prevention of Tuberculosis

Healthcare workers are in a unique position—they work in close proximity to infectious diseases like tuberculosis and need adequate protection, yet do not want to isolate or frighten a patient by using a respirator that hinders communication or looks intimidating. There must be a balance between this need for protection and the need for comfort, communication, practicality and efficient patient care. The bottom line is that only certain types of respirators protect a healthcare worker from TB.

Since the resurgence of tuberculosis in the late 1980's, there has been an increased interest in the prevention of occupational tuberculosis (i.e., transmission of tuberculosis from patients to healthcare workers). This outbreak, attributed to a new multidrug-resistant TB bacteria, spurred the research for better preventative actions. In 1990, the Centers for Disease Control first recommended the use of disposable particulate respirators for the prevention of occupational TB.

Data showed that the surgical masks being used leaked and did not prevent transmission of TB. In 1993, this recommendation was changed to the use of disposable respirators with high efficiency particulate (HEPA) air filters. In 1995, NIOSH updated and modernized the process for certifying non-powered, air-purifying, particulate-filter respirators. These "Part 84" respirators have passed more demanding testing criteria than used previously. OSHA now mandates the use of this N95 class (N=not resistant to oil; 95=95% efficient) of respirators, at minimum, for protecting against tuberculosis. A final TB standard for respiratory protection is pending.

Most respirators recommended for protection against TB are air-purifying respirators like the disposable N95, a negative-pressure particulate respirator that is most commonly used in healthcare settings because of its unintimidating appearance, low cost, and practicality. A major disadvantage, however, of the N95 is the difficulty in assuring a reliable face-mask seal with each use.

It is important to note that a respirator with an exhalation or exhaust valve should never be provided to patients with infectious TB: exhaust valves allow droplets and particles exhaled by the patient to escape, potentially releasing infectious aerosol.

Another commonly used respirator for TB protection is the elastomeric negative-pressure respirator that is reusable. The body is made of flexible materials that provide a tight face-mask seal. Though it comes in both half-face and full-face designs, the former is more frequently used in healthcare settings. The masks have a head-strap and neck-strap that that allow the respirator to be removed and replaced quickly and easily.

The importance of using a respirator properly can't be emphasized enough. Understanding how to fit, care for and use a respirator is the only means to ensure protection. Adhering to regulations seems that much more challenging for healthcare workers treating and caring for patients infected with tuberculosis. But respiratory protection, when not give the careful attention it requires, is ineffective.

Chapter 93

Selection and Use of Particulate Respirators

How effective are the Part 84 filter respirators against particles smaller than 0.3 micrometer in diameter?

The 0.3-micrometer diameter used in the certification testing is approximately the most penetrating particle size for particulate filters. Although it seems contrary to expectation, smaller particles do not penetrate as readily as 0.3-micrometer particles. Therefore, these respirators will filter all other particle sizes at least as well as the certified efficiency level.

How effective are the Part 84 filter respirators against asbestos fibers or other rod-shaped particles?

Although fibers or rod-shaped particles may have very small cross-sectional diameters relative to their lengths, the Part 84 particulate filter respirators will be at least as efficient against this particle shape as the certified efficiency level.

How do I tell a new Part 84 particulate filter from the Part 11 predecessors?

There are several labeling changes for Part 84 filter respirators

From "NIOSH Guide to the Selection and Use of Particulate Respirators," National Institute for Occupational Safety and Health (NIOSH), NIOSH Publication Number 96-101, January 1996. Available online at http://www.cdc.gov/niosh/userguid.html; cited April 2000.

that should enable users to distinguish between the Part 11 and Part 84 respirators. These are as follows:

- NIOSH and DHHS emblems on Part 84 labels replace NIOSH and MSHA logos on Part 11 labels.

- The approval number will be in the format of TC-84A-xxxx for Part 84 devices rather than TC-21C-xxxx or TC-23C-xxxx for Part 11 devices (except for particulate PAPRs, which will continue to be numbered with the sequence TC-21C-xxxx or TC-23C-xxxx).

- The certification filter series and efficiency levels (e.g., N95, P100, etc.) are included on the Part 84 filter approval label.

How long can I use my particulate respirator for TB exposures before I discard it?

In the health care setting, the filter material used in respirators may remain functional for weeks to months [CDC 1994]. As long as there is no oil mist, reuse is limited only by considerations of hygiene, damage, and breathing resistance. Respirators with replaceable filters are designed for reuse, and a respirator classified as disposable may be reused by the same health care worker as long as it remains functional.

Before each use, the filter material should be inspected. If the filter material is physically damaged or soiled, the filter should be changed (in the case of respirators with replaceable filters) or the respirator should be discarded (in the case of disposable respirators). Your employer should develop standard operating procedures for storing, reusing, and disposing of respirators designated as disposable and for disposing of replaceable filters.

Is it always necessary to fit-check a respirator before each use?

Fit-checking your respirator before each use is important to minimize contaminant leakage into the face piece. Your respirator manufacturer has recommended fit-checking procedures that should be followed by the user each time the respirator is worn.

Chapter 94

Ozone Generators

There is a large body of written material on ozone and the use of ozone indoors. However, much of this material makes claims or draws conclusions without substantiation and sound science. In developing "Ozone Generators that are Sold as Air Cleaners," the EPA reviewed a wide assortment of this literature, including information provided by a leading manufacturer of ozone generating devices. In keeping with EPA's policy of insuring that the information it provides is based on sound science, only peer reviewed, scientifically supported findings and conclusions were relied upon in developing this document.

Ozone generators that are sold as air cleaners intentionally produce the gas ozone. Often the vendors of ozone generators make statements and distribute material that lead the public to believe that these devices are always safe and effective in controlling indoor air pollution. For almost a century, health professionals have refuted these claims. The purpose of this chapter is to provide accurate information regarding the use of ozone-generating devices in indoor occupied spaces. This information is based on the most credible scientific evidence currently available.

Some vendors suggest that these devices have been approved by the federal government for use in occupied spaces. To the contrary, NO agency of the federal government has approved these devices for use in occupied spaces. Because of these claims, and because ozone

"Ozone Generators That Are Sold as Air Cleaners: An Assessment of Effectiveness and Health Consequences," U.S. Environmental Protection Agency (EPA), April 1998, modified March 1999.

can cause health problems at high concentrations, several federal government agencies have worked in consultation with the U.S. Environmental Protection Agency to produce this public information document.

What Is Ozone?

Ozone is a molecule composed of three atoms of oxygen. Two atoms of oxygen form the basic oxygen molecule—the oxygen we breathe that is essential to life. The third oxygen atom can detach from the ozone molecule, and re-attach to molecules of other substances, thereby altering their chemical composition. It is this ability to react with other substances that forms the basis of manufacturers' claims.

How Is Ozone Harmful?

The same chemical properties that allow high concentrations of ozone to react with organic material outside the body give it the ability to react with similar organic material that makes up the body, and potentially cause harmful health consequences. When inhaled, ozone can damage the lungs. Relatively low amounts can cause chest pain, coughing, shortness of breath, and, throat irritation. Ozone may also worsen chronic respiratory diseases such as asthma and compromise the ability of the body to fight respiratory infections. People vary widely in their susceptibility to ozone. Healthy people, as well as those with respiratory difficulty, can experience breathing problems when exposed to ozone. Exercise during exposure to ozone causes a greater amount of ozone to be inhaled, and increases the risk of harmful respiratory effects. Recovery from the harmful effects can occur following short-term exposure to low levels of ozone, but health effects may become more damaging and recovery less certain at higher levels or from longer exposures.

Manufacturers and vendors of ozone devices often use misleading terms to describe ozone. Terms such as "energized oxygen" or "pure air" suggest that ozone is a healthy kind of oxygen. Ozone is a toxic gas with vastly different chemical and toxicological properties from oxygen. Several federal agencies have established health standards or recommendations to limit human exposure to ozone.

Is There Such a Thing as "Good Ozone" and "Bad Ozone"?

The phrase "good up high—bad nearby" has been used by the U.S. Environmental Protection Agency (EPA) to make the distinction between ozone in the upper and lower atmosphere. Ozone in the upper atmosphere—referred to as "stratospheric ozone"—helps filter out damaging ultraviolet radiation from the sun. Though ozone in the stratosphere is protective, ozone in the atmosphere—which is the air we breathe—can be harmful to the respiratory system. Harmful levels of ozone can be produced by the interaction of sunlight with certain chemicals emitted to the environment (e.g., automobile emissions and chemical emissions of industrial plants). These harmful concentrations of ozone in the atmosphere are often accompanied by high concentrations of other pollutants, including nitrogen dioxide, fine particles, and hydrocarbons. Whether pure or mixed with other chemicals, ozone can be harmful to health.

Are Ozone Generators Effective?

Available scientific evidence shows that at concentrations that do not exceed public health standards, ozone has little potential to remove indoor air contaminants. Some manufacturers or vendors suggest that ozone will render almost every chemical contaminant harmless by producing a chemical reaction whose only by-products are carbon dioxide, oxygen and water. This is misleading.

First, a review of scientific research shows that, for many of the chemicals commonly found in indoor environments, the reaction process with ozone may take months or years. For all practical purposes, ozone does not react at all with such chemicals. And contrary to specific claims by some vendors, ozone generators are not effective in removing carbon monoxide or formaldehyde.

Second, for many of the chemicals with which ozone does readily react, the reaction can form a variety of harmful or irritating by-products. For example, in a laboratory experiment that mixed ozone with chemicals from new carpet, ozone reduced many of these chemicals, including those which can produce new carpet odor. However, in the process, the reaction produced a variety of aldehydes, and the total concentration of organic chemicals in the air increased rather than decreased after the introduction of ozone. In addition to aldehydes, ozone may also increase indoor concentrations of formic acid, both of which can irritate the lungs if produced in sufficient amounts. Some of the potential by-products produced by ozone's reactions with other chemicals are themselves very reactive and capable of producing irritating and corrosive by-products. Given the complexity of the chemical reactions that occur, additional research is needed to more completely understand the complex interactions of indoor chemicals in the presence of ozone.

Third, ozone does not remove particles (e.g., dust and pollen) from the air, including the particles that cause most allergies. However, some ozone generators are manufactured with an "ion generator" or "ionizer" in the same unit. An ionizer is a device that disperses negatively (and/or positively) charged ions into the air. These ions attach to particles in the air giving them a negative (or positive) charge so that the particles may attach to nearby surfaces such as walls or furniture, or attach to one another and settle out of the air. In recent experiments, ionizers were found to be less effective in removing particles of dust, tobacco smoke, pollen or fungal spores than either high efficiency particle filters or electrostatic precipitators. However, it is apparent from other experiments that the effectiveness of particle air cleaners, including electrostatic precipitators, ion generators, or pleated filters varies widely.

There is evidence to show that at concentrations that do not exceed public health standards, ozone is not effective at removing many odor-causing chemicals.

In an experiment designed to produce formaldehyde concentrations representative of an embalming studio, where formaldehyde is the main odor producer, ozone showed no effect in reducing formaldehyde concentration. Other experiments suggest that body odor may be masked by the smell of ozone but is not removed by ozone. Ozone is not considered useful for odor removal in building ventilation systems.

While there are few scientific studies to support the claim that ozone effectively removes odors, it is plausible that some odorous chemicals will react with ozone. For example, in some experiments, ozone appeared to react readily with certain chemicals, including some chemicals that contribute to the smell of new carpet. Ozone is also believed to react with acrolein, one of the many odorous and irritating chemicals found in secondhand tobacco smoke.

If used at concentrations that do not exceed public health standards, ozone applied to indoor air does not effectively remove viruses, bacteria, mold, or other biological pollutants.

Some data suggest that low levels of ozone may reduce airborne concentrations and inhibit the growth of some biological organisms while ozone is present, but ozone concentrations would have to be 5-10 times higher than public health standards allow before the ozone could decontaminate the air sufficiently to prevent survival and regeneration of the organisms once the ozone is removed.

Even at high concentrations, ozone may have no effect on biological contaminants embedded in porous material such as duct lining or ceiling tiles. In other words, ozone produced by ozone generators may inhibit the growth of some biological agents while it is present, but it is unlikely to fully decontaminate the air unless concentrations are high enough to be a health concern if people are present. Even with high levels of ozone, contaminants embedded in porous material may not be affected at all.

If I Follow Manufacturers' Directions, Can I Be Harmed?

Results of some controlled studies show that concentrations of ozone considerably higher than these standards are possible even when a user follows the manufacturer's operating instructions. There are many brands and models of ozone generators on the market. They vary in the amount of ozone they can produce. In many circumstances, the use of an ozone generator may not result in ozone concentrations that exceed public health standards. But many factors affect the indoor concentration of ozone so that under some conditions ozone concentrations may exceed public health standards.

In one study, a large ozone generator recommended by the manufacturer for spaces "up to 3,000 square feet," was placed in a 350 square foot room and run at a high setting. The ozone in the room quickly reached concentrations that were exceptionally high—0.50 to 0.80 ppm which is 5-10 times higher than public health limits.

In an EPA study, several different devices were placed in a home environment, in various rooms, with doors alternately opened and closed, and with the central ventilation system fan alternately turned on and off. The results showed that some ozone generators, when run at a high setting with interior doors closed, would frequently produce concentrations of 0.20-0.30 ppm. A powerful unit set on high with the interior doors opened achieved values of 0.12 to 0.20 ppm in adjacent rooms. When units were not run on high, and interior doors were open, concentrations generally did not exceed public health standards.

The concentrations reported above were adjusted to exclude that portion of the ozone concentration brought in from the outdoors. Indoor concentrations of ozone brought in from outside are typically 0.01-0.02 ppm, but could be as high as 0.03-0.05 ppm. If the outdoor portion of ozone were included in the indoor concentrations reported above, the concentrations inside would have been correspondingly higher, increasing the risk of excessive ozone exposure.

None of the studies reported above involved the simultaneous use of more than one device. The simultaneous use of multiple devices increases the total ozone output and therefore greatly increases the risk of excessive ozone exposure.

Why Is it Difficult to Control Ozone Exposure?

The actual concentration of ozone produced by an ozone generator depends on many factors. Concentrations will be higher if a more
powerful device or more than one device is used, if a device is placed
in a small space rather than a large space, if interior doors are closed
rather than open and, if the room has fewer rather than more materials and furnishings that adsorb or react with ozone and, provided
that outdoor concentrations of ozone are low, if there is less rather
than more outdoor air ventilation.

The proximity of a person to the ozone generating device can also
affect one's exposure. The concentration is highest at the point where
the ozone exits from the device, and generally decreases as one moves
further away.

Manufacturers and vendors advise users to size the device properly to the space or spaces in which it is used. Unfortunately, some
manufacturers' recommendations about appropriate sizes for particular
spaces have not been sufficiently precise to guarantee that ozone concentrations will not exceed public health limits. Further, some literature
distributed by vendors suggests that users err on the side of operating a
more powerful machine than would normally be appropriate for the intended space, the rationale being that the user may move in the future,
or may want to use the machine in a larger space later on. Using a more
powerful machine increases the risk of excessive ozone exposure.

Ozone generators typically provide a control setting by which the
ozone output can be adjusted. The ozone output of these devices is
usually not proportional to the control setting. That is, a setting at
medium does not necessarily generate an ozone level that is halfway
between the levels at low and high. The relationship between the control setting and the output varies considerably among devices, although most appear to elevate the ozone output much more than one
would expect as the control setting is increased from low to high. In experiments to date, the high setting in some devices generated 10 times
the level obtained at the medium setting. Manufacturer's instructions
on some devices link the control setting to room size and thus indicate
what setting is appropriate for different room sizes. However, room size
is only one factor affecting ozone levels in the room.

In addition to adjusting the control setting to the size of the room,
users have sometimes been advised to lower the ozone setting if they
can smell the ozone. Unfortunately, the ability to detect ozone by smell
varies considerably from person to person, and one's ability to smell
ozone rapidly deteriorates in the presence of ozone. While the smell

of ozone may indicate that the concentration is too high, lack of odor does not guarantee that levels are safe.

At least one manufacturer is offering units with an ozone sensor that turns the ozone generator on and off with the intent of maintaining ozone concentrations in the space below health standards. EPA is currently evaluating the effectiveness and reliability of these sensors, and plans to conduct further research to improve society's understanding of ozone chemistry indoors. EPA will report its findings as the results of this research become available.

Can Ozone Be Used in Unoccupied Spaces?

Ozone has been extensively used for water purification, but ozone chemistry in water is not the same as ozone chemistry in air. High concentrations of ozone in air, when people are not present, are sometimes used to help decontaminate an unoccupied space from certain chemical or biological contaminants or odors (e.g., fire restoration). However, little is known about the chemical by-products left behind by these processes. While high concentrations of ozone in air may sometimes be appropriate in these circumstances, conditions should be sufficiently controlled to insure that no person or pet becomes exposed. Ozone can adversely affect indoor plants, and damage materials such as rubber, electrical wire coatings, and fabrics and art work containing susceptible dyes and pigments.

What Other Methods Can Be Used?

The three most common approaches to reducing indoor air pollution, in order of effectiveness, are:

- *Source Control:* Eliminate or control the sources of pollution;

- *Ventilation:* Dilute and exhaust pollutants through outdoor air ventilation, and

- *Air Cleaning:* Remove pollutants through proven air cleaning methods.

Of the three, the first approach—source control— is the most effective. This involves minimizing the use of products and materials that cause indoor pollution, employing good hygiene practices to minimize biological contaminants (including the control of humidity and moisture, and occasional cleaning and disinfection of wet or moist surfaces), and using good housekeeping practices to control particles.

The second approach—outdoor air ventilation—is also effective and commonly employed. Ventilation methods include installing an exhaust fan close to the source of contaminants, increasing outdoor air flows in mechanical ventilation systems, and opening windows, especially when pollutant sources are in use.

The third approach—air cleaning—is not generally regarded as sufficient in itself, but is sometimes used to supplement source control and ventilation. Air filters, electronic particle air cleaners and ionizers are often used to remove airborne particles, and gas adsorbing material is sometimes used to remove gaseous contaminants when source control and ventilation are inadequate.

Conclusions

Whether in its pure form or mixed with other chemicals, ozone can be harmful to health. When inhaled, ozone can damage the lungs. Relatively low amounts of ozone can cause chest pain, coughing, shortness of breath and, throat irritation. It may also worsen chronic respiratory diseases such as asthma as well as compromise the ability of the body to fight respiratory infections. Some studies show that ozone concentrations produced by ozone generators can exceed health standards even when one follows manufacturer's instructions. Many factors affect ozone concentrations including the amount of ozone produced by the machine(s), the size of the indoor space, the amount of material in the room with which ozone reacts, the outdoor ozone concentration, and the amount of ventilation. These factors make it difficult to control the ozone concentration in all circumstances.

Available scientific evidence shows that, at concentrations that do not exceed public health standards, ozone is generally ineffective in controlling indoor air pollution. The concentration of ozone would have to greatly exceed health standards to be effective in removing most indoor air contaminants. In the process of reacting with chemicals indoors, ozone can produce other chemicals that themselves can be irritating and corrosive.

Recommendation

The public is advised to use proven methods of controlling indoor air pollution. These methods include eliminating or controlling pollutant sources, increasing outdoor air ventilation, and using proven methods of air cleaning.

Chapter 95

Lung Disorders and Nutrition

Nutrition can be a special issue for some patients with chronic lung disease. While we don't generally think of breathing as an energy-consuming activity, patients with difficulty breathing can devote a significant portion of their metabolism to this usually effortless activity. Coupled with nutritional problems that may accompany some conditions, this can become a major limitation.

Emphysema

Patients with moderate to severe emphysema have normal or larger than normal lung capacities. However, their lungs operate at reduced capacity. Emphysema destroys the alveoli, the tiny air chambers that fill normal lung tissue. With fewer functional alveoli, less oxygen is absorbed and less carbon dioxide is expelled with each breath. To compensate for this, the patient with emphysema must breathe more quickly than normally. You can better appreciate how difficult this becomes if you try breathing rapidly for even thirty seconds at a time.

Patients with severe emphysema typically become emaciated as their disease progresses. Their fat reserves are depleted to supply the energy to continue breathing. This can lead to striking changes in appearance, and frank malnutrition in some cases.

"Lung Disease and Nutrition," by David A. Cooke, M.D. © 2001 Omnigraphics, Inc.

Adequate calorie intake is essential to prevent these problems. Regular meals are important, and can be supplemented with the use of nutritional shakes between meals. In contrast to the recommendations for most healthy people, a high-fat diet is often necessary and desirable. Fat has more calories per gram than any other kind of food, and is therefore an important dietary component in these patients. Adequate protein intake is also necessary, since muscle breakdown can occur if dietary intake is insufficient.

Cystic Fibrosis

The most serious nutritional deficiencies tend to occur patients with cystic fibrosis. There are several reasons for this. First, the same problems that patients with emphysema face challenge cystic fibrosis patients. Making matters worse, nearly all patients with cystic fibrosis also have serious digestive problems. Cystic fibrosis destroys the pancreas, a gland in the abdomen that produces digestive enzymes. Without these enzymes, a person cannot properly digest food, especially fats. Further complicating matters, many cystic fibrosis patients also develop diabetes. Finally, cystic fibrosis patients tend to develop chronic lung infections. The metabolic stress of constantly fighting smoldering infection also takes a toll.

Good nutrition is key to survival for cystic fibrosis patients. Nutritionally-compromised victims of this disease have much higher death rates and worse lung infections. There are several strategies that can help prevent these serious outcomes.

Pancreatic enzyme supplements are a must for nearly all cystic fibrosis patients. These are pills containing digestive enzymes normally produced by the pancreas. They need to be taken with every meal to allow full absorption of the food eaten. Strict adherence to the regimen prescribed by the patient's physician is essential.

High fat diets are also important for most cystic fibrosis patients. Fat intake is generally the only way to provide adequate numbers of calories to meet their demands. Specially-formulated, high fat, high calorie nutritional shakes are also usually prescribed to help supplement food intake.

Other Nutritional Issues in Lung Disease

Healthy persons may also wonder about nutritional issues that may impact lung health. Outside of serious lung diseases discussed above, the importance of specific dietary measures is less clear.

Vitamin A and Beta Carotene

Diets high in vitamin A or beta carotene (a precursor of vitamin A) have been advocated in hopes of preventing lung cancer. These vitamins can act as anti-oxidants, which some experimental evidence suggests may help prevent DNA damage that leads to cancer. On this basis, a large study was performed looking at the effect of beta carotene supplements on heavy smokers, considered to be at high risk for developing lung cancer. Unfortunately, the trial did not show any benefit within a five year period. In fact, the rate of lung cancer was actually higher in the patients receiving extra beta carotene.

It's difficult to know what to conclude at this point regarding vitamin A and lung disease. It is still possible that it has benefits not seen in this trial. However, this dashes cold water on the high hopes many had for vitamin A supplementation.

It is worth knowing that vitamin A is stored in human fat tissues, and can accumulate over time. Doses higher than 20,000 units per day can result in vitamin A poisoning, which can be quite serious. Additionally, excess vitamin A in pregnancy can cause birth defects. It is worth discussing your plans with a physician if you choose to take supplemental vitamin A.

Vitamin C

Vitamin C is another vitamin with antioxidant properties. Based on theories similar to those for vitamin A use, it has been advocated as a potential cancer preventative. However, there is very little evidence at this point that it actually has an anticancer effect.

Vitamin C has been long recommended for prevention and treatment of the common cold. Scientific studies of this use have given mixed results. Taking supplemental vitamin C does not appear to reduce the likelihood of catching a cold. It is less clear whether it will lead to faster recovery once a cold develops. About half the studies done on the subject have found a benefit, while the other half have shown no effect.

Vitamin C appears to be relatively safe in doses of 100 to 2000 mg per day. "Megadoses" in excess of 2000 mg per day, may increase the risk for kidney stones.

Vitamin E

Yet another vitamin with antioxidant properties, with hopes that it might be a cancer preventative. Like vitamin A and C, there is little evidence that it actually works in this manner.

Like vitamin A, it is also possible to overdose on vitamin E. Doses in excess of 1000 units per day should be discussed with a doctor first.

B-Vitamins and Trace Minerals

B-complex vitamins such as thiamine, folic acid, and vitamin B12 are necessary for normal immune function. Similarly, trace elements such as copper, magnesium, and selenium also have roles in immune cell function. Deficiency of any of these can be problematic. However, there is no evidence that taking them in quantities beyond those found in a typical multivitamin give any additional benefit for immune function.

Chapter 96

Pneumonococcal Vaccine

Pneumonia Prevention: It's Worth a Shot

Pneumococcal (pronounced new-mo-KOK-al) disease is an infection caused by bacteria. These bacteria can attack different parts of the body. When they invade the lungs, they cause the most common kind of bacterial pneumonia. When the same bacteria enter the blood, they cause an infection called bacteremia (bak-ter-E-me-ah). In the brain, they cause meningitis. Pneumococcal pneumonia is a serious illness that kills thousands of older people in the United States each year.

Can Pneumonia Be Prevented?

For some causes of pneumonia, yes. The pneumococcal vaccine is safe, it works, and one shot lasts most people up to 10 years. People who get the vaccine are protected against almost all of the bacteria that cause pneumococcal pneumonia and other pneumococcal diseases as well. The shot, which is covered by Medicare, can be a lifesaver.

Some experts say it may be best to get the shot before age 65 — anytime after age 50 — since the younger you are, the better the results. They also say people should have this shot even if they have had pneumonia before. There are many different kinds of pneumonia, and having one kind does not protect against the others. The

"Pneumonia Prevention: It's Worth a Shot," *Age Page*, National Institute on Aging (NIA). 1996. Text available online at http://www.nih.gov/nia/health/pubpub/pneum.htm; cited April 2000.

vaccine, however, does protect against 88 percent of the pneumococcal bacteria that cause pneumonia. It does not guarantee that you will never get pneumonia. It does not protect against viral pneumonia. Most people need to get the shot only once. However some older people may need a booster; check with your doctor to find out if this is necessary.

Who Should Get the Vaccine?

According to the Centers for Disease Control and Prevention, everyone age 65 and older should get it the pneumonia vaccine. Some younger people should get it also.

Ask a doctor for the vaccine if you:

• Are age 65 or older.

• Have a chronic illness, such as heart or lung disease or diabetes.

• Have a weak immune system. (This can be caused by certain kidney diseases, some cancers, HIV infections organ transplant medicines, and other disease.)

Are There Side Effects?

Some people have mild side effects from the shot, but these usually are minor and last only a very short time. In studies, about half of the people getting the vaccine had mild side effects—swelling and soreness at the spot where the shot was given, usually on the arm.

A few people (less than 1 percent) had fever and muscle pain as well as more serious swelling and pain on the arm. The pneumonia shot cannot cause pneumonia because it is not made from the bacteria itself, but from a bacterial component that is not infectious. The same is true of the flu shot; it cannot cause flu. In fact, people can get the pneumonia vaccine and a flu shot at the same time.

About the Disease and the Vaccine

There are two main kinds of pneumonia—viral pneumonia and bacterial pneumonia. Bacterial pneumonia is more serious. One kind of bacteria causes pneumococcal pneumonia. In older people, this type of pneumonia is a common cause of hospitalization and death.

About 20 to 30 percent of people over age 65 who have pneumococcal pneumonia develop bacteremia. At least 20 percent of those with bacteremia die from it, even though they get antibiotics.

People age 65 and older are at high risk. They are two to three time more likely than people in general to get pneumococcal infections.

A recent, large study by the National Institutes of Health suggests that the vaccine prevents most cases of pneumococcal pneumonia.

The U.S. Public Health Service, the National Coalition for Adult Immunization, and the American Lung Association now recommend that all people age 65 and older get this vaccine.

Key Facts

- Everyone age 65 and older should get the pneumonia vaccine.
- Anyone with chronic disease or a weak immune system should also get the vaccine.
- Most people need to get it only once.
- Most people have mild or no side effects.
- It is covered by Medicare.

Part Six

Additional Help and Information

Chapter 97

Glossary of Related Terms

Acinus: The berrylike ending of a tiny airway in the lung, where the alveoli (air sacs) are located.

Acute: Severe or with sudden onset and short time span.

Airways: Tubes that carry air into and out of the lungs.

Alveoli: Tiny sac-like air spaces in the lung where carbon dioxide and oxygen are exchanged.

Amniotic fluid: The liquid that surrounds and cushions the fetus in its mother's womb.

Antibiotic: A drug that kills or inhibits the growth of bacteria.

Antibodies: Specific proteins produced by the body's immune system that bind with foreign proteins (antigens).

Artery: A blood vessel that carries blood from the heart to the rest of the body.

Asthma: Respiratory condition caused by narrowing of the airways; symptoms include recurrent attacks of wheezing, coughing, shortness of breath, and labored breathing.

Bronchiole: The smaller airways of the lungs.

From an undated fact sheet produced by the National Heart, Lung, and Blood Institute (NHLBI). Text available online at http://www.nhlbi.nih.gov/health/public/lung/other/bpd/glossary.htm; cited April 2000.

Bronchiolitis: Inflammation of the bronchioles, usually caused by a viral infection.

Bronchodilator: A drug that relaxes the smooth muscles of the airways and relieves constriction of the bronchi.

Bronchopulmonary: Pertaining to the lungs and air passages.

Capillaries: The tiniest blood vessels; capillary networks connect the arterioles (the smallest arteries) and the venules (the smallest veins).

Cell: Basic subunit of every living organism; the simplest unit that can exist as an independent living system.

Chronic: Of long duration; frequently recurring.

Cor pulmonale: Heart disease that results from resistance to the passage of blood through the lungs; it often leads to right heart failure.

Corticosteroids: Drugs that mimic the action of a group of hormones produced by adrenal glands; they are anti-inflammatory and act as bronchodilators.

Cyanosis: Bluish color of the skin due to insufficient oxygen in the blood.

Cystic fibrosis: A serious genetic disease of excretory glands, affecting lungs and other organs; it causes production of very thick mucus that interferes with normal digestion and breathing.

Diuretic: A drug that promotes the excretion of salt and water by the kidney.

Duct: A passage or tube with well-defined walls for the passage of air or liquids.

Dysplasia: Abnormal development or growth.

Edema: Abnormal accumulation of fluid in body tissues.

Emphysema: Chronic lung disease in which there is permanent destruction of alveoli.

Fetus: Unborn offspring from 7 or 8 weeks after conception until birth.

Gas exchange: Primary function of the lungs; transfer of oxygen from inhaled air into the blood and of carbon dioxide from the blood into the lungs.

Genetic: Inherited through genes passed on by one or both parents.

Gestation period: The period of development of the young from the time of conception until birth.

Hyaline membrane disease: A respiratory disease of newborns, especially premature infants, in which a membrane composed of proteins and dead cells forms and lines the alveoli making gas exchange difficult or impossible.

Hypertension: High blood pressure.

Immunization: Protection from disease by administering vaccines that induce the body to form antibodies against infectious agents.

Inflammation: Response of the body tissues to injury; typical signs are swelling, redness, and pain.

Mechanical ventilation: Use of a machine called a ventilator or respirator to improve the exchange of air between the lungs and the atmosphere.

Membrane: Thin, flexible film of proteins and lipids that encloses the contents of a cell; it controls the substances that go into and come out of the cell. Also, a thin layer of tissue that covers the surface or lines the cavity of an organ.

Mucus: A thick fluid produced by the lining of some organs of the body.

Neonatal period: The first 4 weeks after birth.

Neonatologist: Doctor who specializes in treating the diseases and disorders of newborn babies.

Oxygen: Colorless odorless gas that makes up about 20 percent of the air we breathe; it is essential to life because it is used for the chemical reactions that occur in the cells of the body.

Patent ductus arteriosus: Abnormal persistence of the opening in the arterial duct that connects the pulmonary artery to the descending aorta; this opening normally closes within 24 hours of birth.

Pathogenesis: The cellular events and reactions that occur in the development of disease.

Pathophysiology: Altered functions in an individual or an organ due to disease.

Placenta: The special tissue that joins the mother to her fetus; it provides the fetus with oxygen, water, and nutrients (food) from the mother's blood and secretes the hormones necessary for successful pregnancy.

611

Pneumonia: Inflammation of the lungs.

Pneumothorax: Accumulation of air or gas in the space between the lung and chest wall, resulting in partial or complete collapse of the lung.

Positive pressure ventilation: Provision of oxygen under pressure by a mechanical respirator.

Prenatal: Occurring before birth.

Progressive: Increasing in severity.

Pulmonary: Pertaining to the lungs.

Pulmonary hypertension: Abnormally high blood pressure in the arteries of the lungs.

Respiration: Process of exchanging oxygen from the air for carbon dioxide from the body; includes the mechanical process of breathing, gas exchange, and oxygen and carbon dioxide transport to and from the cells.

Respiratory distress syndrome: A lung disease that occurs primarily in premature infants; the newborn must struggle for each breath and blueing of its skin reflects the baby's inability to get enough oxygen.

Respiratory failure: Inability of the lungs to conduct gas exchange.

Retina: The inner layer of tissue at the back of the eye that is sensitive to light.

Risk factors: Habits, traits, or conditions in a person or in the environment that are associated with an increased chance (risk) of disease.

Surfactant: Fluid secreted by the cells of the alveoli that reduces the surface tension of pulmonary fluids; it contributes to the elastic properties of pulmonary tissue.

Symptom: Any indication of disease noticed or felt by a patient; in contrast, a sign of an illness is an objective observation.

Symptomatic treatment: Therapy that eases symptoms without addressing the cause of disease.

Ventilation: Exchange of air between the lungs and the atmosphere so that oxygen can be exchanged for carbon dioxide at the alveoli.

Ventilator: A breathing machine that is used to treat respiratory failure by promoting ventilation; also called a respirator.

Wheezing: Breathing with a rasp or whistling sound; a sign of airway constriction or obstruction.

Chapter 98

National Organizations that Offer Information to People with Lung Cancer

People with cancer and their families sometimes need assistance coping with the emotional as well as the practical aspects of their disease. This fact sheet includes some of the national organizations that provide this type of support. It is not intended to be a comprehensive listing of all organizations that offer these services in the United States, nor does inclusion of any particular organization imply endorsement by the National Cancer Institute, the National Institutes of Health, or the Department of Health and Human Services. The intent of this fact sheet is to provide information useful to individuals nationally. For that reason, it does not include the many local groups that offer valuable assistance to patients and their families in individual states or cities.

Alliance for Lung Cancer Advocacy, Support, and Education (ALCASE)
P.O. Box 849
Vancouver, WA 98666
Toll Free: 800-298-2436
Tel: 360-696-2436
Internet: http://www.alcase.org
E-Mail: info@alcase.org

The ALCASE offers programs designed to help improve the quality of life of people with lung cancer and their families. Programs include

National Cancer Institute (NCI), June 2001; all contact information verified and updated in November 2001.

613

education about the disease, psychosocial support, and advocacy about issues that concern lung cancer survivors.

American Cancer Society (ACS)

1599 Clifton Road, NE.
Atlanta, GA 30329-4251
Tel: 404-320-3333
Toll Free:800-ACS-2345 (1-800-227-2345)
Internet: http://www.cancer.org

The ACS is a voluntary organization that offers a variety of services to patients and their families. The ACS also supports research, provides printed materials, and conducts educational programs. Staff can accept calls and distribute publications in Spanish. A local ACS unit may be listed in the white pages of the telephone directory under "American Cancer Society."

American Cancer Society (ACS) Supported Programs:

Cancer Survivors Network

Toll Free: 800-ACS-2345 or 877-7333 (HOPE)
Internet: http://www.acscsn.org

This is both a telephone and Web-based service for cancer survivors, their families, caregivers, and friends. The telephone component (877-333-HOPE) provides survivors and families access to pre-recorded discussions. The Web-based component offers live online chat sessions, virtual support groups, pre-recorded talk shows, and personal stories.

I Can Cope

Tel: 734-647-8587 (registration and information)
Internet: http://www.med.umich.edu/1libr/cancer/cct04.htm

I Can Cope is a patient education program that is designed to help patients, families, and friends cope with the day-to-day issues of living with cancer.

International Association of Laryngectomees

8900 Thornton Road, Box 99311
Stockton, CA 95209
Toll Free: (866)IAL-FORU (425-3678)
Fax: 209-472-0516
Internet: http://larynxlink.com
E-Mail: IAL@larynxlink.com

This program assists people who have lost their voice as a result of cancer. It provides information on the skills needed by laryngectomees and works toward total rehabilitation of patients.

Look Good. . .Feel Better
Toll Free: 800-395-LOOK
Internet: http://www.lookgoodfeelbetter.org

This program was developed by the Cosmetic, Toiletry, and Fragrance Association Foundation in cooperation with ACS and the National Cosmetology Association. It focuses on techniques that can help people undergoing cancer treatment improve their appearance.

Reach to Recovery
1020 9th Avenue
Greeley, CO 80631
Tel: 970-356-9727

The Reach to Recovery Program is a rehabilitation program for women who have or have had breast cancer. The program helps breast cancer patients meet the physical, emotional, and cosmetic needs related to their disease and its treatment.

American Institute for Cancer Research (AICR)
1759 R Street, NW.
Washington, DC 20009
Toll Free: 800-843-8114
Tel: 202-328-7744
Internet: http://www.aicr.org
E-Mail: aicrweb@aicr.org

The AICR provides information about cancer prevention, particularly through diet and nutrition. They offer a toll-free nutrition hotline, pen pal support network, funding of research grants, and a wide array of consumer and health professional brochures and health aids about diet and nutrition and its link to cancer and cancer prevention. The AICR also offers the AICR Cancer Resource, an information and resource program for cancer patients. A limited selection of Spanish-language publications is available.

Cancer Care, Inc.
National Office
275 Seventh Avenue
New York, NY 10001

Tel: 212-302-2400 or 212 221-3300
Toll Free:800-813-HOPE (800-813-4673)
Fax: 212-719-0263
Internet: http://www.cancercare.org
E-Mail: info@cancercare.org

Cancer Care is a national nonprofit agency that offers free support, information, financial assistance, and practical help to people with cancer and their loved ones. Services are provided by oncology social workers and are available in person, over the telephone, and through the agency's Web site. Cancer Care's reach also extends to professionals-providing education, information, and assistance. A section of the Cancer Care Web site and some publications are available in Spanish, and staff can respond to calls and e-mails in Spanish.

Cancer Hope Network

Two North Road, Suite A
Chester, NJ 07930
Toll Free: 877-HOPENET (877-467-3638)
Internet: http://www.cancerhopenetwork.org
E-Mail: info@cancerhopenetwork.org

The Cancer Hope Network provides individual support to cancer patients and their families by matching them with trained volunteers who have undergone and recovered from a similar cancer experience. Such matches are based on the type and stage of cancer, treatments used, side effects experienced, and other factors.

Cancer Information and Counseling Line (CICL)
(a service of the AMC Cancer Research Center)

1600 Pierce Street
Denver, CO 80214
Toll Free: 800-525-3777
Fax: (303) 233-1863
Internet: http://www.amc.org/cicl.htm
E-Mail: cicl@amc.org

The CICL, part of the Psychosocial Program of the AMC Cancer Research Center, is a toll-free telephone service for cancer patients, their family members and friends, cancer survivors, and the general public. Professional counselors provide up-to-date medical information, emotional support through short-term counseling, and resource referrals to callers nationwide between the hours of 8:30 a.m. and 5:00

p.m. MST. Individuals may also submit questions about cancer and request resources via e-mail.

Cancer Research Foundation of America
1600 Duke Street, Suite 110
Alexandria, VA 22314
Toll Free: 800-227-CRFA (1-800-227-2732)
Tel: 703-836-4412
Internet: http://www.preventcancer.org
E-Mail: sweisel@crfa.org

The Cancer Research Foundation of America seeks to prevent cancer by funding research and providing educational materials on early detection and nutrition.

Candlelighters Childhood Cancer Foundation (CCCF)
3910 Warner Street
Kensington, MD 20895
Tel: 301-962-3520
Toll Free: 800-366-CCCF (800-366-2223)
Fax: 301-962-3521
Internet: http://www.candlelighters.org
E-Mail: info@candlelighters.org

The CCCF is a nonprofit organization that provides information, peer support, and advocacy through publications, an information clearing-house, and a network of local support groups. A financial aid list is available that lists organizations to which eligible families may apply for assistance.

Children's Hospice International
2202 Mount Vernon Avenue, Suite 3C
Alexandria, VA 22301
Tel: 703-684-0330
Toll Free: 800-2-4-CHILD (800-242-4453)
Fax: 703-684-0226
Internet: http://www.chionline.org
E-Mail: chiorg@aol.com

Children's Hospice International provides a network of support for dying children and their families. It serves as a clearinghouse for research programs and support groups, and offers educational materials and training programs on pain management and the care of seriously ill children.

617

Cure For Lymphoma Foundation (CFL)
215 Lexington Avenue
New York, NY 10016-6023
Tel: 212-213-9595
Toll Free: 800-CFL-6848 (800-235-6848)
Fax: 212-213-1987
Internet: http://www.cfl.org
E-Mail: infocfl@cfl.org

The CFL offers support and education programs and services to patients and caregivers. Materials and services include: "Understanding Lymphoma" booklets and fact sheets; lymphoma family forums; teleconferences; lymphoma Q & A's; a nationwide Patient-to-Patient Telephone Network; biweekly support groups; monthly lymphoma networking groups; patient aid; a quarterly newsletter, Together; and a toll-free information line. CFL also funds lymphoma research and collaborates with researchers, clinicians, social workers, and nurses. The CFL works to increase public awareness of lymphoma through grassroots public education campaigns.

Foundation for the Children's Oncology Group (FCOG)
[Formerly National Childhood Cancer Foundation (NCCF)]
440 East Huntington Drive
Suite 300
Post Office Box 60012
Arcadia, CA 91066-6012
Tel: 626-447-1674
Toll Free:800-458-6223
Fax: 626-447-6359 (the Foundation)
Fax: 626-445-4334 (Children's Oncology Group)
Internet: http://www.ConquerKidsCancer.org
E-Mail: info@ConquerKidsCancer.org

The NCCF supports research conducted by a network of institutions, each of which has a team of doctors, scientists, and other specialists with the special skills required for the diagnosis, treatment, supportive care, and research on the cancers of infants, children, and young adults. Advocating for children with cancer and the centers that treat them is also a focus of the NCCF. A limited selection of Spanish-language publications is available.

HOSPICELINK

Hospice Education Institute
190 Westbrook Road
Essex, CT 06426-1510
Tel: 860-767-1620
Toll Free: 800-331-1620
Fax: 203-767-2746
Internet: http://www.hospiceworld.org
E-Mail: HOSPICEALL@aol.com

Hospice Link helps patients and their families find support services in their communities. They offer information about hospice and palliative care and can refer cancer patients and their families to local hospice and palliative care programs.

National Asian Women's Health Organization (NAWHO)

250 Montgomery Street, Suite 900
San Francisco, CA 94104
Tel: 415-989-9747
Fax: 415-989-9758
Internet: http://www.nawho.org
E-Mail: nawho@nawho.org

NAWHO is working to improve the health status of Asian women and families through research, education, leadership, and public policy programs. They have resources for Asian women in English, Cantonese, Laotian, Vietnamese, and Korean. Publications on subjects such as reproductive rights, breast and cervical cancer, and tobacco control are available.

National Coalition for Cancer Survivorship (NCCS)

1010 Wayne Avenue, Suite 770
Silver Spring, MD 20910-5600
Toll Free: 877-NCCS-YES (877-622-7937)
Fax: 301-565-9670
Internet: http://www.cansearch.org
E-Mail: info@cansearch.org

NCCS is a network of groups and individuals that offer support to cancer survivors and their loved ones. It provides information and resources on cancer support, advocacy, and quality of life issues. A section of the NCCS Web site and a limited selection of publications are available in Spanish.

National Hospice and Palliative Care Organization (NHPCO)
1700 Diagonal Road, Suite 300
Alexandria, VA 22314
Tel: 703-837-1500
Toll Free: 800-658-8898 (Helpline)
Fax: 703-525-5762
Internet: http://www.nhpco.org
E-Mail: info@nhpco.org

The NHPCO is an association of programs that provide hospice and palliative care. It is designed to increase awareness about hospice services and to champion the rights and issues of terminally ill patients and their family members. They offer discussion groups, publications, information about how to find a hospice, and information about the financial aspects of hospice. Some Spanish-language publications are available, and staff are able to answer calls in Spanish.

Patient Advocate Foundation (PAF)
753 Thimble Shoals Boulevard, Suite B
Newport News, VA 23606
Tel: 757-873-6668
Toll Free: 800-532-5274
Fax: 757-873-8999
Internet: http://www.patientadvocate.org
E-Mail: help@patientadvocate.org

The PAF provides education, legal counseling, and referrals to cancer patients and survivors concerning managed care, insurance, financial issues, job discrimination, and debt crisis matters.

R. A. Bloch Cancer Foundation, Inc.
4435 Main Street, Suite 500
Kansas City, MO 64111
Tel: 816-WE-BUILD (816-932-8453)
Toll Free: 800-433-0464
Fax: 816-931-7486
Internet: http://www.blochcancer.org
E-Mail: hotline@hrblock.com

The R. A. Bloch Cancer Foundation matches newly diagnosed cancer patients with trained, home-based volunteers who have been treated for the same type of cancer. They also distribute informational materials, including a multidisciplinary list of institutions that offer second opinions. Information is available in Spanish.

STARBRIGHT Foundation
1990 South Bundy Drive, Suite 100
Los Angeles, CA 90025
Tel: 310-442-1560
Toll Free: 800-315-2580
Internet: http://www.starbright.org
E-Mail: ford@starbright.org

The STARBRIGHT Foundation creates projects that are designed to help seriously ill children and adolescents cope with the psychosocial and medical challenges they face. The STARBRIGHT Foundation produces materials such as interactive educational CD-ROMs and videos about medical conditions and procedures, advice on talking with a health professional, and other issues related to children and adolescents who have serious medical conditions. All materials are available to children, adolescents, and their families free of charge. Staff can respond to calls in Spanish.

The Wellness Community
35 East Seventh Street, Suite 412
Cincinnati, OH 45202
Tel: 513-421-7111
Toll Free: 888-793-WELL (888-793-9355)
Fax: 513-421-7119
Internet: http://www.wellness-community.org
E-Mail: help@wellness-community.org

The Wellness Community provides free psychological and emotional support to cancer patients and their families. They offer support groups facilitated by licensed therapists, stress reduction and cancer education workshops, nutrition guidance, exercise sessions, and social events.

Vital Options and "The Group Room" Cancer Radio Talk Show
P.O. Box 19233
Encino, CA 91416-9233
Tel: 818-508-5657
Toll Free: 800-GRP-ROOM (800-477-7666)
Internet: http://www.vitaloptions.org
E-Mail: geninfo@vitaloptions.org

The mission of Vital Options is to use communications technology to reach people dealing with cancer. This organization holds a weekly syndicated call-in cancer radio talk show called "The Group Room," which provides a forum for patients, long-term survivors, family members, physicians, and therapists to discuss cancer issues. Listeners can participate in the show during its broadcast every Sunday from 4 p.m.- 6 p.m., ET by calling either of the telephone numbers. A live Web simulcast of "The Group Room" can be heard by logging onto the Vital Options Web site.

Chapter 99

Asthma Resources

For More Information about Asthma

National Asthma Education and Prevention Program
NHLBI Information Center
P.O. Box 30105
Bethesda, MD 20824-0105
Tel: 301-251-1222
Internet: http://www.nhlbi.nih.gov/nhlbi/nhlbi.htm

Allergy and Asthma Network/Mothers of Asthmatics, Inc.
814 W. Diamond Avenue
Suite 150
Gaithersburg, MD 20878
Tel: 301-590-2770
Fax: 301-590-2776
Internet: http://www.podi.com

American Academy of Allergy, Asthma, and Immunology
611 East Wells Street
Milwaukee, WI 53202
Toll Free: 800-822-2762
Internet: http://www.aaaai.org

National Institutes of Health (NIH), NIH Publication No. 97-2339, 1997; contact information verified and updated in November 2001.

American College of Allergy, Asthma, and Immunology
85 West Algonquin Road
Suite 550
Arlington Heights, IL 60005
Toll Free: 800-842-7777
Internet: http://allergy.mcg.edu
E-Mail: mail@acaai.org

American Lung Association
1740 Broadway
New York, NY 10019
Toll Free: 800-586-4872
Tel: 212-315-8700
Internet: http://www.lungusa.org
E-Mail: info@lungusa.org

Asthma and Allergy Foundation of America
1233 20th Street
Suite 402
Washington, D.C. 20036
Toll Free: 800-727-8462
Tel: 202-466-7643
Fax: 202-466-8940
Internet: http://www.aafa.org

National Jewish Medical and Research Center (Lung Line)
1400 Jackson Street
Denver, CO 80206
Toll Free: 800-222-5864
Tel: 303-388-4461
Internet: http://www.njc.org

Chapter 100

Sleep Disorders Clinics

The major purposes of respiratory sleep disorders clinics are:

- Respiratory function assessment
- Investigation and management of disorders associated with sleep including snoring, sleep apnea, sleep hypoventilation, narcolepsy and related conditions.

Respiratory Sleep Disorders

There are two basic varieties of sleep apnea: obstructive and central. Obstructive sleep apnea is the most common, occurring in approximately 5% of adults. It is characterized by episodic collapse (partial or complete) of the upper airway during sleep and is usually associated with loud habitual snoring, daytime tiredness and lethargy and an excess morbidity and mortality, particularly from vascular disease. Central sleep apnea refers to inadequate ventilation during sleep due to diminished or absent respiratory effort, and is usually seen in the context of severe respiratory muscle weakness, chest wall deformity, or advanced lung disease.

A sleep disorders clinic arranges investigation and management of these disorders on referral. After referral the patient is assessed

From "Department of Pulmonary Physiology and Respiratory Sleep Disorders Clinic," at Sir Charles Gairdner Hospital, Verdun St., Nedlands, Western Australia 6009. © 2000 Sir Charles Gairdner Hospital; reprinted with permission. Text available online at http://www.scgh.health.wa.gov.au/csu/heart/rsdc2.html.

by one of the clinic's medical staff. If appropriate an overnight sleep study is arranged. In some cases this may involve simple assessment of breathing during sleep (oro-nasal airflow, chest wall motion, arterial O2 saturation).

More usually it involves assessment of these respiratory parameters together with sleep quality (using EEG, EOG, submental EMG), body position, sound, leg movements and, in some cases, transcutaneous CO2 and other measurements.

If significant sleep apnea is identified appropriate treatment is arranged and supervised by the Clinic. Other expertise is involved where necessary, in consultation with the referring doctor.

Management of Respiratory Failure

In individuals with pleural fibrosis, abnormalities of the chest wall such as kyphoscoliosis, respiratory muscle weakness, and some forms of severe chronic lung disease, respiratory failure is due to sleep hypoventilation. This can be controlled, respiratory and right heart failure reversed and life expectancy and quality substantially improved by non-invasive assisted ventilation delivered during sleep, via a face or nose mask, at home. Medical staff have particular expertise and long experience in this aspect of respiratory medicine.

Who Should Be Referred

- Patients with known or suspected respiratory disease requiring respiratory function testing as part of their initial or ongoing management
- Screening of patients exposed to drugs with potential pulmonary toxicity
- Screening of workforces potentially or actually exposed to noxious dusts or gases
- Fitness assessment for occupational or leisure pursuits with respiratory implications

Respiratory Function Assessment

Why Measure Respiratory Function?

- To identify the presence of respiratory disease and help define its cause

- To assess severity

- To monitor changes with time and/or treatment

The presence of respiratory disease may be known or suspected: measurement provides an objective assessment of the degree of functional impairment. This is indispensable in assessing respiratory symptoms, which are often an imprecise guide to severity. Measurement allows the effects of therapeutic interventions or changes with time to be accurately monitored. The pattern of functional impairment provides important information as to underlying causes. In cases where the symptoms are of multifactorial origin, the relative contribution of each component factor can be defined.

Measurement allows any clinician to make more precise and confident assessment of patients with respiratory disease and provides a rational basis for treatment and assessment of treatment outcomes.

Respiratory function testing is also used as a tool to screen for the presence of respiratory disease, for example in assessment for fitness for diving, screening patients exposed to agents with potential pulmonary toxic effects (e.g. cytotoxic drugs, amiodarone), and screening workforces with potential occupational exposure to noxious dusts and gases.

What Respiratory Function Services Are Available

Spirometry

This test measures the volume exhaled in the first second of forced expiration (FEV1), the forced vital capacity (FVC) and the maximum expiratory flow-volume relationship (flow-volume loop) before and after bronchodilator.

This basic assessment examines for the presence and severity of airflow obstruction and the response to bronchodilator. It is a useful but non-specific screening test for the presence of other respiratory disorders.

General Assessment of Lung Function

This group of tests includes measurement of lung volumes (including total lung capacity and residual volume), maximum expiratory flow rates, uniformity of gas distribution within the lung, transfer factor (diffusing capacity), and pulse oximetry.

627

These tests comprehensively assess resting lung function, including ventilatory capacity (the capacity to move air into and out of the lungs) and gas exchange (the capacity to transfer of gas across the alveolar-capillary interface). Characteristic patterns distinguish diseases primarily affecting airways from those affecting the lung parenchyma or vasculature and lung diseases from those of the pleura or chest wall.

Maximum Inspiratory and Expiratory Flow-Volume Curves

These tests diagnose the presence and assess the effect of large (central) airway obstruction. Characteristic patterns distinguish fixed from variable obstruction and extra- from intra-thoracic location.

Arterial Blood Gases

These tests define the presence and severity of respiratory failure and involve arterial blood gas sampling and analysis of the following:

- PO_2, PCO_2, pH, HCO_3-, base excess
- Arterial O_2 saturation (direct measurement by cooximeter)
- Hb and abnormal Hb forms (HbCO, metHb)
- Special calculations (eg shunt, O_2 content)

Bronchial Provocation Testing

These tests assess bronchial responsiveness by measuring the changes in maximum expiratory flow rates in response to increasing doses of inhaled agents:

- Histamine, Methacholine for the diagnosis of asthma
- Hypertonic Saline to assess the potential for asthma in scuba divers
- Occupational dusts/gases to assess effect of exposure to agents in the workplace

Exercise Testing (progressive cycle ergometry)

The cardio-respiratory responses to exercise are assessed to define the patient's maximum achievable workload, and the cause of any limitation. The test distinguishes between respiratory and cardiac causes of exercise limitation.

It allows the nature of the respiratory limitation to be determined (e.g. ventilatory abnormality, abnormality of gas exchange), as well as the magnitude of the abnormality and, with serial testing, the changes with time and treatment.

It is a very sensitive test with which to assess severity of interstitial lung disease or pulmonary vascular disease. It is useful in assessing fitness of patients with respiratory disability for non-sedentary occupations.

Simulated Altitude Testing

The ambient PO2 is reduced to simulate that found in commercial aircraft to assess air travel fitness in patients with severe respiratory disease who wish to fly. The effect of gentle exercise and requirement for oxygen supplementation are determined during this test.

Nasal Resistance

This test measures the resistance to airflow through each nasal airway to assess the significance of symptoms of nasal obstruction and/or anatomic abnormality in nasal cavity.

Control of Breathing

These tests assess ventilatory control by measuring the ventilatory responses to hypercapnic and/or hypoxic stimuli to breathing.

Lung Mechanics

These tests measure the lungs' elastic and flow resistive properties.

- Respiratory Muscle Function, Maximum Mouth pressures

  These are simple tests and are often performed in conjunction with the "Routine Assessment" where respiratory muscle weakness is known or suspected.

- Transdiaphragmatic pressure, phrenic n. conduction

  These tests are performed to investigate known or suspected weakness of the diaphragm or intercostal muscles and assess the clinical significance of any weakness.

Other Tests

Other tests of respiratory function are occasionally applied according to clinical presentation. These include specific tests of gas exchange.

Links to Sleep Disorders

The following website contains links to clinics and further information.

http://www.sleepnet.com/links.htm

Index

Index

633

C

P

R

Health Reference Series
COMPLETE CATALOG

Adolescent Health Sourcebook

Basic Consumer Health Information about Common Medical, Mental, and Emotional Concerns in Adolescents, Including Facts about Acne, Body Piercing, Mononucleosis, Nutrition, Eating Disorders, Stress, Depression, Behavior Problems, Peer Pressure, Violence, Gangs, Drug Use, Puberty, Sexuality, Pregnancy, Learning Disabilities, and More

Along with a Glossary of Terms and Other Resources for Further Help and Information

Edited by Chad T. Kimball. 700 pages. 2002. 0-7808-0248-9. $78.

AIDS Sourcebook, 1st Edition

Basic Information about AIDS and HIV Infection, Featuring Historical and Statistical Data, Current Research, Prevention, and Other Special Topics of Interest for Persons Living with AIDS

Along with Source Listings for Further Assistance

Edited by Karen Bellenir and Peter D. Dresser. 831 pages. 1995. 0-7808-0031-1. $78.

"One strength of this book is its practical emphasis. The intended audience is the lay reader . . . useful as an educational tool for health care providers who work with AIDS patients. Recommended for public libraries as well as hospital or academic libraries that collect consumer materials."
— *Bulletin of the Medical Library Association, Jan '96*

"This is the most comprehensive volume of its kind on an important medical topic. Highly recommended for all libraries."
— *Reference Book Review, '96*

"Very useful reference for all libraries."
— *Choice, Association of College and Research Libraries, Oct '95*

"There is a wealth of information here that can provide much educational assistance. It is a must book for all libraries and should be on the desk of each and every congressional leader. Highly recommended."
— *AIDS Book Review Journal, Aug '95*

"Recommended for most collections."
— *Library Journal, Jul '95*

AIDS Sourcebook, 2nd Edition

Basic Consumer Health Information about Acquired Immune Deficiency Syndrome (AIDS) and Human Immunodeficiency Virus (HIV) Infection, Featuring Updated Statistical Data, Reports on Recent Research and Prevention Initiatives, and Other Special Topics of Interest for Persons Living with AIDS, Including New Antiretroviral Treatment Options, Strategies for Combating Opportunistic Infections, Information about Clinical Trials, and More

Along with a Glossary of Important Terms and Resource Listings for Further Help and Information

Edited by Karen Bellenir. 751 pages. 1999. 0-7808-0225-X. $78.

"Highly recommended."
— *American Reference Books Annual, 2000*

"Excellent sourcebook. This continues to be a highly recommended book. There is no other book that provides as much information as this book provides."
— *AIDS Book Review Journal, Dec-Jan 2000*

"Recommended reference source."
— *Booklist, American Library Association, Dec '99*

"A solid text for college-level health libraries."
— *The Bookwatch, Aug '99*

Cited in *Reference Sources for Small and Medium-Sized Libraries, American Library Association, 1999*

Alcoholism Sourcebook

Basic Consumer Health Information about the Physical and Mental Consequences of Alcohol Abuse, Including Liver Disease, Pancreatitis, Wernicke-Korsakoff Syndrome (Alcoholic Dementia), Fetal Alcohol Syndrome, Heart Disease, Kidney Disorders, Gastrointestinal Problems, and Immune System Compromise and Featuring Facts about Addiction, Detoxification, Alcohol Withdrawal, Recovery, and the Maintenance of Sobriety

Along with a Glossary and Directories of Resources for Further Help and Information

Edited by Karen Bellenir. 613 pages. 2000. 0-7808-0325-6. $78.

"This title is one of the few reference works on alcoholism for general readers. For some readers this will be a welcome complement to the many self-help books on the market. Recommended for collections serving general readers and consumer health collections."
— *E-Streams, Mar '01*

"This book is an excellent choice for public and academic libraries."
— *American Reference Books Annual, 2001*

"Recommended reference source."
— *Booklist, American Library Association, Dec '00*

"Presents a wealth of information on alcohol use and abuse and its effects on the body and mind, treatment, and prevention."
— *SciTech Book News, Dec '00*

"Important new health guide which packs in the latest consumer information about the problems of alcoholism."
— *Reviewer's Bookwatch, Nov '00*

SEE ALSO *Drug Abuse Sourcebook, Substance Abuse Sourcebook*

Allergies Sourcebook, 1st Edition

Basic Information about Major Forms and Mechanisms of Common Allergic Reactions, Sensitivities, and Intolerances, Including Anaphylaxis, Asthma, Hives and Other Dermatologic Symptoms, Rhinitis, and Sinusitis Along with Their Usual Triggers Like Animal Fur, Chemicals, Drugs, Dust, Foods, Insects, Latex, Pollen, and Poison Ivy, Oak, and Sumac; Plus Information on Prevention, Identification, and Treatment

Edited by Allan R. Cook. 611 pages. 1997. 0-7808-0036-2. $78.

■

Allergies Sourcebook, 2nd Edition

Basic Consumer Health Information about Allergic Disorders, Triggers, Reactions, and Related Symptoms, Including Anaphylaxis, Rhinitis, Sinusitis, Asthma, Dermatitis, Conjunctivitis, and Multiple Chemical Sensitivity

Along with Tips on Diagnosis, Prevention, and Treatment, Statistical Data, a Glossary, and a Directory of Sources for Further Help and Information

Edited by Annemarie S. Muth. 598 pages. 2002. 0-7808-0376-0. $78.

■

Alternative Medicine Sourcebook

Basic Consumer Health Information about Alternatives to Conventional Medicine, Including Acupressure, Acupuncture, Aromatherapy, Ayurveda, Bioelectromagnetics, Environmental Medicine, Essence Therapy, Food and Nutrition Therapy, Herbal Therapy, Homeopathy, Imaging, Massage, Naturopathy, Reflexology, Relaxation and Meditation, Sound Therapy, Vitamin and Mineral Therapy, and Yoga, and More

Edited by Allan R. Cook. 737 pages. 1999. 0-7808-0200-4. $78.

"Recommended reference source."
—Booklist, American Library Association, Feb '00

"A great addition to the reference collection of every type of library." —American Reference Books Annual, 2000

■

Alzheimer's, Stroke & 29 Other Neurological Disorders Sourcebook, 1st Edition

Basic Information for the Layperson on 31 Diseases or Disorders Affecting the Brain and Nervous System, First Describing the Illness, Then Listing Symptoms, Diagnostic Methods, and Treatment Options, and Including Statistics on Incidences and Causes

Edited by Frank E. Bair. 579 pages. 1993. 1-55888-748-2. $78.

"Nontechnical reference book that provides reader-friendly information."
—Family Caregiver Alliance Update, Winter '96

"Should be included in any library's patient education section." —American Reference Books Annual, 1994

"Written in an approachable and accessible style. Recommended for patient education and consumer health collections in health science center and public libraries." —Academic Library Book Review, Dec '93

"It is very handy to have information on more than thirty neurological disorders under one cover, and there is no recent source like it." —Reference Quarterly, American Library Association, Fall '93

SEE ALSO Brain Disorders Sourcebook

■

Alzheimer's Disease Sourcebook, 2nd Edition

Basic Consumer Health Information about Alzheimer's Disease, Related Disorders, and Other Dementias, Including Multi-Infarct Dementia, AIDS-Related Dementia, Alcoholic Dementia, Huntington's Disease, Delirium, and Confusional States

Along with Reports Detailing Current Research Efforts in Prevention and Treatment, Long-Term Care Issues, and Listings of Sources for Additional Help and Information

Edited by Karen Bellenir. 524 pages. 1999. 0-7808-0223-3. $78.

"Provides a wealth of useful information not otherwise available in one place. This resource is recommended for all types of libraries."
—American Reference Books Annual, 2000

"Recommended reference source."
—Booklist, American Library Association, Oct '99

■

Arthritis Sourcebook

Basic Consumer Health Information about Specific Forms of Arthritis and Related Disorders, Including Rheumatoid Arthritis, Osteoarthritis, Gout, Polymyalgia Rheumatica, Psoriatic Arthritis, Spondyloarthropathies, Juvenile Rheumatoid Arthritis, and Juvenile Ankylosing Spondylitis

Along with Information about Medical, Surgical, and Alternative Treatment Options, and Including Strategies for Coping with Pain, Fatigue, and Stress

Edited by Allan R. Cook. 550 pages. 1998. 0-7808-0201-2. $78.

". . . accessible to the layperson."
—Reference and Research Book News, Feb '99

■

Asthma Sourcebook

Basic Consumer Health Information about Asthma, Including Symptoms, Traditional and Nontraditional Remedies, Treatment Advances, Quality-of-Life Aids, Medical Research Updates, and the Role of Allergies, Exercise, Age, the Environment, and Genetics in the Development of Asthma

Along with Statistical Data, a Glossary, and Directories of Support Groups, and Other Resources for Further Information

Edited by Annemarie S. Muth. 628 pages. 2000. 0-7808-0381-7. $78.

"A worthwhile reference acquisition for public libraries and academic medical libraries whose readers desire a quick introduction to the wide range of asthma information." — Choice, Association of College & esearch Libraries, Jun '01

"Recommended reference source."
— Booklist, American Library Association, Feb '01

"Highly recommended." — The Bookwatch, Jan '01

"There is much good information for patients and their families who deal with asthma daily."
— American Medical Writers Association Journal, Winter '01

"This informative text is recommended for consumer health collections in public, secondary school, and community college libraries and the libraries of universities with a large undergraduate population."
— American Reference Books Annual, 2001

Back & Neck Disorders Sourcebook

Basic Information about Disorders and Injuries of the Spinal Cord and Vertebrae, Including Facts on Chiropractic Treatment, Surgical Interventions, Paralysis, and Rehabilitation

Along with Advice for Preventing Back Trouble

Edited by Karen Bellenir. 548 pages. 1997. 0-7808-0202-0. $78.

"The strength of this work is its basic, easy-to-read format. Recommended."
— Reference and User Services Quarterly, American Library Association, Winter '97

Blood & Circulatory Disorders Sourcebook

Basic Information about Blood and Its Components, Anemias, Leukemias, Bleeding Disorders, and Circulatory Disorders, Including Aplastic Anemia, Thalassemia, Sickle-Cell Disease, Hemochromatosis, Hemophilia, Von Willebrand Disease, and Vascular Diseases

Along with a Special Section on Blood Transfusions and Blood Supply Safety, a Glossary, and Source Listings for Further Help and Information

Edited by Karen Bellenir and Linda M. Shin. 554 pages. 1998. 0-7808-0203-9. $78.

"Recommended reference source."
— Booklist, American Library Association, Feb '99

"An important reference sourcebook written in simple language for everyday, non-technical users. "
— Reviewer's Bookwatch, Jan '99

Brain Disorders Sourcebook

Basic Consumer Health Information about Strokes, Epilepsy, Amyotrophic Lateral Sclerosis (ALS/Lou Gehrig's Disease), Parkinson's Disease, Brain Tumors, Cerebral Palsy, Headache, Tourette Syndrome, and More

Along with Statistical Data, Treatment and Rehabilitation Options, Coping Strategies, Reports on Current Research Initiatives, a Glossary, and Resource Listings for Additional Help and Information

Edited by Karen Bellenir. 481 pages. 1999. 0-7808-0229-2. $78.

"Belongs on the shelves of any library with a consumer health collection." — E-Streams, Mar '00

"Recommended reference source."
— Booklist, American Library Association, Oct '99

SEE ALSO Alzheimer's, Stroke & 29 Other Neurological Disorders Sourcebook, 1st Edition

---

Breast Cancer Sourcebook

Basic Consumer Health Information about Breast Cancer, Including Diagnostic Methods, Treatment Options, Alternative Therapies, Self-Help Information, Related Health Concerns, Statistical and Demographic Data, and Facts for Men with Breast Cancer

Along with Reports on Current Research Initiatives, a Glossary of Related Medical Terms, and a Directory of Sources for Further Help and Information

Edited by Edward J. Prucha and Karen Bellenir. 580 pages. 2001. 0-7808-0244-6. $78.

"Recommended reference source."
— Booklist, American Library Association, Jan '02

"This reference source is highly recommended. It is quite informative, comprehensive and detailed in nature, and yet it offers practical advice in easy-to-read language. It could be thought of as the 'bible' of breast cancer for the consumer." — E-Streams, Jan '02

"From the pros and cons of different screening methods and results to treatment options, Breast Cancer Sourcebook provides the latest information on the subject."
— Library Bookwatch, Dec '01

"This thoroughgoing, very readable reference covers all aspects of breast health and cancer. . . . Readers will find much to consider here. Recommended for all public and patient health collections."
— Library Journal, Sep '01

SEE ALSO Cancer Sourcebook for Women, 1st and 2nd Editions, Women's Health Concerns Sourcebook

Breastfeeding Sourcebook

Basic Consumer Health Information about the Benefits of Breastmilk, Preparing to Breastfeed, Breastfeeding as a Baby Grows, Nutrition, and More, Including Information on Special Situations and Concerns Such as Mastitis, Illness, Medications, Allergies, Multiple Births, Prematurity, Special Needs, and Adoption

Along with a Glossary and Resources for Additional Help and Information

Edited by Jenni Lynn Colson. 350 pages. 2002. 0-7808-0332-9. $78.

SEE ALSO Pregnancy & Birth Sourcebook

■

Burns Sourcebook

Basic Consumer Health Information about Various Types of Burns and Scalds, Including Flame, Heat, Cold, Electrical, Chemical, and Sun Burns

Along with Information on Short-Term and Long-Term Treatments, Tissue Reconstruction, Plastic Surgery, Prevention Suggestions, and First Aid

Edited by Allan R. Cook. 604 pages. 1999. 0-7808-0204-7. $78.

"This is an exceptional addition to the series and is highly recommended for all consumer health collections, hospital libraries, and academic medical centers."
— *E-Streams, Mar '00*

"This key reference guide is an invaluable addition to all health care and public libraries in confronting this ongoing health issue."
— *American Reference Books Annual, 2000*

"Recommended reference source."
— *Booklist, American Library Association, Dec '99*

SEE ALSO Skin Disorders Sourcebook

■

Cancer Sourcebook, 1st Edition

Basic Information on Cancer Types, Symptoms, Diagnostic Methods, and Treatments, Including Statistics on Cancer Occurrences Worldwide and the Risks Associated with Known Carcinogens and Activities

Edited by Frank E. Bair. 932 pages. 1990. 1-55888-888-8. $78.

Cited in *Reference Sources for Small and Medium-Sized Libraries*, American Library Association, 1999

"Written in nontechnical language. Useful for patients, their families, medical professionals, and librarians."
— *Guide to Reference Books, 1996*

"Designed with the non-medical professional in mind. Libraries and medical facilities interested in patient education should certainly consider adding the *Cancer Sourcebook* to their holdings. This compact collection of reliable information . . . is an invaluable tool for helping patients and patients' families and friends to take the first steps in coping with the many difficulties of cancer."
— *Medical Reference Services Quarterly, Winter '91*

"Specifically created for the nontechnical reader . . . an important resource for the general reader trying to understand the complexities of cancer."
— *American Reference Books Annual, 1991*

"This publication's nontechnical nature and very comprehensive format make it useful for both the general public and undergraduate students."
— *Choice, Association of College and Research Libraries, Oct '90*

■

New Cancer Sourcebook, 2nd Edition

Basic Information about Major Forms and Stages of Cancer, Featuring Facts about Primary and Secondary Tumors of the Respiratory, Nervous, Lymphatic, Circulatory, Skeletal, and Gastrointestinal Systems, and Specific Organs; Statistical and Demographic Data; Treatment Options; and Strategies for Coping

Edited by Allan R. Cook. 1,313 pages. 1996. 0-7808-0041-9. $78.

"An excellent resource for patients with newly diagnosed cancer and their families. The dialogue is simple, direct, and comprehensive. Highly recommended for patients and families to aid in their understanding of cancer and its treatment."
— *Booklist Health Sciences Supplement, American Library Association, Oct '97*

"The amount of factual and useful information is extensive. The writing is very clear, geared to general readers. Recommended for all levels."
— *Choice, Association of College and Research Libraries, Jan '97*

■

Cancer Sourcebook, 3rd Edition

Basic Consumer Health Information about Major Forms and Stages of Cancer, Featuring Facts about Primary and Secondary Tumors of the Respiratory, Nervous, Lymphatic, Circulatory, Skeletal, and Gastrointestinal Systems, and Specific Organs

Along with Statistical and Demographic Data, Treatment Options, Strategies for Coping, a Glossary, and a Directory of Sources for Additional Help and Information

Edited by Edward J. Prucha. 1,069 pages. 2000. 0-7808-0227-6. $78.

"This title is recommended for health sciences and public libraries with consumer health collections."
— *E-Streams, Feb '01*

". . . can be effectively used by cancer patients and their families who are looking for answers in a language they can understand. Public and hospital libraries should have it on their shelves."
— *American Reference Books Annual, 2001*

"Recommended reference source."
— *Booklist, American Library Association, Dec '00*

Cancer Sourcebook for Women, 1st Edition

Basic Information about Specific Forms of Cancer That Affect Women, Featuring Facts about Breast Cancer, Cervical Cancer, Ovarian Cancer, Cancer of the Uterus and Uterine Sarcoma, Cancer of the Vagina, and Cancer of the Vulva; Statistical and Demographic Data; Treatments, Self-Help Management Suggestions, and Current Research Initiatives

Edited by Allan R. Cook and Peter D. Dresser. 524 pages. 1996. 0-7808-0076-1. $78.

"... written in easily understandable, non-technical language. Recommended for public libraries or hospital and academic libraries that collect patient education or consumer health materials."
— *Medical Reference Services Quarterly, Spring '97*

"Would be of value in a consumer health library. . . . written with the health care consumer in mind. Medical jargon is at a minimum, and medical terms are explained in clear, understandable sentences."
— *Bulletin of the Medical Library Association, Oct '96*

"The availability under one cover of all these pertinent publications, grouped under cohesive headings, makes this certainly a most useful sourcebook."
— *Choice, Association of College and Research Libraries, Jun '96*

"Presents a comprehensive knowledge base for general readers. Men and women both benefit from the gold mine of information nestled between the two covers of this book. Recommended."
— *Academic Library Book Review, Summer '96*

"This timely book is highly recommended for consumer health and patient education collections in all libraries."
— *Library Journal, Apr '96*

SEE ALSO *Breast Cancer Sourcebook, Women's Health Concerns Sourcebook*

■

Cancer Sourcebook for Women, 2nd Edition

Basic Consumer Health Information about Gynecologic Cancers and Related Concerns, Including Cervical Cancer, Endometrial Cancer, Gestational Trophoblastic Tumor, Ovarian Cancer, Uterine Cancer, Vaginal Cancer, Vulvar Cancer, Breast Cancer, and Common Non-Cancerous Uterine Conditions, with Facts about Cancer Risk Factors, Screening and Prevention, Treatment Options, and Reports on Current Research Initiatives

Along with a Glossary of Cancer Terms and a Directory of Resources for Additional Help and Information

Edited by Karen Bellenir. 604 pages. 2002. 0-7808-0226-8. $78.

SEE ALSO *Breast Cancer Sourcebook, Women's Health Concerns Sourcebook*

Cardiovascular Diseases & Disorders Sourcebook, 1st Edition

Basic Information about Cardiovascular Diseases and Disorders, Featuring Facts about the Cardiovascular System, Demographic and Statistical Data, Descriptions of Pharmacological and Surgical Interventions, Lifestyle Modifications, and a Special Section Focusing on Heart Disorders in Children

Edited by Karen Bellenir and Peter D. Dresser. 683 pages. 1995. 0-7808-0032-X. $78.

". . . comprehensive format provides an extensive overview on this subject." — *Choice, Association of College & Research Libraries, Jun '96*

". . . an easily understood, complete, up-to-date resource. This well executed public health tool will make valuable information available to those that need it most, patients and their families. The typeface, sturdy non-reflective paper, and library binding add a feel of quality found wanting in other publications. Highly recommended for academic and general libraries. "
— *Academic Library Book Review, Summer '96*

SEE ALSO *Healthy Heart Sourcebook for Women, Heart Diseases & Disorders Sourcebook, 2nd Edition*

■

Caregiving Sourcebook

Basic Consumer Health Information for Caregivers, Including a Profile of Caregivers, Caregiving Responsibilities and Concerns, Tips for Specific Conditions, Care Environments, and the Effects of Caregiving

Along with Facts about Legal Issues, Financial Information, and Future Planning, a Glossary, and a Listing of Additional Resources

Edited by Joyce Brennfleck Shannon. 600 pages. 2001. 0-7808-0331-0. $78.

"An ideal addition to the reference collection of any public library. Health sciences information professionals may also want to acquire the *Caregiving Sourcebook* for their hospital or academic library for use as a ready reference tool by health care workers interested in aging and caregiving." — *E-Streams, Jan '02*

"Recommended reference source."
— *Booklist, American Library Association, Oct '01*

■

Colds, Flu & Other Common Ailments Sourcebook

Basic Consumer Health Information about Common Ailments and Injuries, Including Colds, Coughs, the Flu, Sinus Problems, Headaches, Fever, Nausea and Vomiting, Menstrual Cramps, Diarrhea, Constipation, Hemorrhoids, Back Pain, Dandruff, Dry and Itchy Skin, Cuts, Scrapes, Sprains, Bruises, and More

Along with Information about Prevention, Self-Care, Choosing a Doctor, Over-the-Counter Medications, Folk Remedies, and Alternative Therapies, and Including a Glossary of Important Terms and a Directory of Resources for Further Help and Information

Edited by Chad T. Kimball. 638 pages. 2001. 0-7808-0435-X. $78.

"Will prove valuable to any library seeking to maintain a current, comprehensive reference collection of health resources. . . . Excellent reference."
— *The Bookwatch, Aug '01*

"Recommended reference source."
— *Booklist, American Library Association, July '01*

■

Communication Disorders Sourcebook

Basic Information about Deafness and Hearing Loss, Speech and Language Disorders, Voice Disorders, Balance and Vestibular Disorders, and Disorders of Smell, Taste, and Touch

Edited by Linda M. Ross. 533 pages. 1996. 0-7808-0077-X. $78.

"This is skillfully edited and is a welcome resource for the layperson. It should be found in every public and medical library."
— *Booklist Health Sciences Supplement, American Library Association, Oct '97*

■

Congenital Disorders Sourcebook

Basic Information about Disorders Acquired during Gestation, Including Spina Bifida, Hydrocephalus, Cerebral Palsy, Heart Defects, Craniofacial Abnormalities, Fetal Alcohol Syndrome, and More

Along with Current Treatment Options and Statistical Data

Edited by Karen Bellenir. 607 pages. 1997. 0-7808-0205-5. $78.

"Recommended reference source."
— *Booklist, American Library Association, Oct '97*

SEE ALSO Pregnancy & Birth Sourcebook

■

Consumer Issues in Health Care Sourcebook

Basic Information about Health Care Fundamentals and Related Consumer Issues, Including Exams and Screening Tests, Physician Specialties, Choosing a Doctor, Using Prescription and Over-the-Counter Medications Safely, Avoiding Health Scams, Managing Common Health Risks in the Home, Care Options for Chronically or Terminally Ill Patients, and a List of Resources for Obtaining Help and Further Information

Edited by Karen Bellenir. 618 pages. 1998. 0-7808-0221-7. $78.

"Both public and academic libraries will want to have a copy in their collection for readers who are interested in self-education on health issues."
— *American Reference Books Annual, 2000*

"The editor has researched the literature from government agencies and others, saving readers the time and effort of having to do the research themselves. Recommended for public libraries."
— *Reference and User Services Quarterly, American Library Association, Spring '99*

"Recommended reference source."
— *Booklist, American Library Association, Dec '98*

■

Contagious & Non-Contagious Infectious Diseases Sourcebook

Basic Information about Contagious Diseases like Measles, Polio, Hepatitis B, and Infectious Mononucleosis, and Non-Contagious Infectious Diseases like Tetanus and Toxic Shock Syndrome, and Diseases Occurring as Secondary Infections Such as Shingles and Reye Syndrome

Along with Vaccination, Prevention, and Treatment Information, and a Section Describing Emerging Infectious Disease Threats

Edited by Karen Bellenir and Peter D. Dresser. 566 pages. 1996. 0-7808-0075-3. $78.

■

Death & Dying Sourcebook

Basic Consumer Health Information for the Layperson about End-of-Life Care and Related Ethical and Legal Issues, Including Chief Causes of Death, Autopsies, Pain Management for the Terminally Ill, Life Support Systems, Insurance, Euthanasia, Assisted Suicide, Hospice Programs, Living Wills, Funeral Planning, Counseling, Mourning, Organ Donation, and Physician Training

Along with Statistical Data, a Glossary, and Listings of Sources for Further Help and Information

Edited by Annemarie S. Muth. 641 pages. 1999. 0-7808-0230-6. $78.

"Public libraries, medical libraries, and academic libraries will all find this sourcebook a useful addition to their collections."
— *American Reference Books Annual, 2001*

"An extremely useful resource for those concerned with death and dying in the United States."
— *Respiratory Care, Nov '00*

"Recommended reference source."
— *Booklist, American Library Association, Aug '00*

"This book is a definite must for all those involved in end-of-life care." — *Doody's Review Service, 2000*

■

Diabetes Sourcebook, 1st Edition

Basic Information about Insulin-Dependent and Non-insulin-Dependent Diabetes Mellitus, Gestational Diabetes, and Diabetic Complications, Symptoms, Treatment, and Research Results, Including Statistics on Prevalence, Morbidity, and Mortality

Along with Source Listings for Further Help and Information

Edited by Karen Bellenir and Peter D. Dresser. 827 pages. 1994. 1-55888-751-2. $78.

". . . very informative and understandable for the layperson without being simplistic. It provides a comprehensive overview for laypersons who want a general understanding of the disease or who want to focus on various aspects of the disease."
— *Bulletin of the Medical Library Association, Jan '96*

■

Diabetes Sourcebook, 2nd Edition

Basic Consumer Health Information about Type 1 Diabetes (Insulin-Dependent or Juvenile-Onset Diabetes), Type 2 (Noninsulin-Dependent or Adult-Onset Diabetes), Gestational Diabetes, and Related Disorders, Including Diabetes Prevalence Data, Management Issues, the Role of Diet and Exercise in Controlling Diabetes, Insulin and Other Diabetes Medicines, and Complications of Diabetes Such as Eye Diseases, Periodontal Disease, Amputation, and End-Stage Renal Disease

Along with Reports on Current Research Initiatives, a Glossary, and Resource Listings for Further Help and Information

Edited by Karen Bellenir. 688 pages. 1998. 0-7808-0224-1. $78.

"An invaluable reference." — *Library Journal, May '00*

Selected as one of the 250 "Best Health Sciences Books of 1999." — *Doody's Rating Service, Mar-Apr 2000*

"This comprehensive book is an excellent addition for high school, academic, medical, and public libraries. This volume is highly recommended."
—*American Reference Books Annual, 2000*

"Provides useful information for the general public."
— *Healthlines, University of Michigan Health Management Research Center, Sep/Oct '99*

". . . provides reliable mainstream medical information . . . belongs on the shelves of any library with a consumer health collection." — *E-Streams, Sep '99*

"Recommended reference source."
— *Booklist, American Library Association, Feb '99*

■

Diet & Nutrition Sourcebook, 1st Edition

Basic Information about Nutrition, Including the Dietary Guidelines for Americans, the Food Guide Pyramid, and Their Applications in Daily Diet, Nutritional Advice for Specific Age Groups, Current Nutritional Issues and Controversies, the New Food Label and How to Use It to Promote Healthy Eating, and Recent Developments in Nutritional Research

Edited by Dan R. Harris. 662 pages. 1996. 0-7808-0084-2. $78.

"Useful reference as a food and nutrition sourcebook for the general consumer." — *Booklist Health Sciences Supplement, American Library Association, Oct '97*

"Recommended for public libraries and medical libraries that receive general information requests on nutrition. It is readable and will appeal to those interested in learning more about healthy dietary practices."
— *Medical Reference Services Quarterly, Fall '97*

"An abundance of medical and social statistics is translated into readable information geared toward the general reader." — *Bookwatch, Mar '97*

"With dozens of questionable diet books on the market, it is so refreshing to find a reliable and factual reference book. Recommended to aspiring professionals, librarians, and others seeking and giving reliable dietary advice. An excellent compilation." — *Choice, Association of College and Research Libraries, Feb '97*

SEE ALSO Digestive Diseases & Disorders Sourcebook, Gastrointestinal Diseases & Disorders Sourcebook

■

Diet & Nutrition Sourcebook, 2nd Edition

Basic Consumer Health Information about Dietary Guidelines, Recommended Daily Intake Values, Vitamins, Minerals, Fiber, Fat, Weight Control, Dietary Supplements, and Food Additives

Along with Special Sections on Nutrition Needs throughout Life and Nutrition for People with Such Specific Medical Concerns as Allergies, High Blood Cholesterol, Hypertension, Diabetes, Celiac Disease, Seizure Disorders, Phenylketonuria (PKU), Cancer, and Eating Disorders, and Including Reports on Current Nutrition Research and Source Listings for Additional Help and Information

Edited by Karen Bellenir. 650 pages. 1999. 0-7808-0228-4. $78.

"This book is an excellent source of basic diet and nutrition information." — *Booklist Health Sciences Supplement, American Library Association, Dec '00*

"This reference document should be in any public library, but it would be a very good guide for beginning students in the health sciences. If the other books in this publisher's series are as good as this, they should all be in the health sciences collections."
—*American Reference Books Annual, 2000*

"This book is an excellent general nutrition reference for consumers who desire to take an active role in their health care for prevention. Consumers of all ages who select this book can feel confident they are receiving current and accurate information." — *Journal of Nutrition for the Elderly, Vol. 19, No. 4, '00*

"Recommended reference source."
—*Booklist, American Library Association, Dec '99*

SEE ALSO Digestive Diseases & Disorders Sourcebook, Gastrointestinal Diseases & Disorders Sourcebook

Digestive Diseases & Disorders Sourcebook

Basic Consumer Health Information about Diseases and Disorders that Impact the Upper and Lower Digestive System, Including Celiac Disease, Constipation, Crohn's Disease, Cyclic Vomiting Syndrome, Diarrhea, Diverticulosis and Diverticulitis, Gallstones, Heartburn, Hemorrhoids, Hernias, Indigestion (Dyspepsia), Irritable Bowel Syndrome, Lactose Intolerance, Ulcers, and More

Along with Information about Medications and Other Treatments, Tips for Maintaining a Healthy Digestive Tract, a Glossary, and Directory of Digestive Diseases Organizations

Edited by Karen Bellenir. 335 pages. 2000. 0-7808-0327-2. $78.

"This title would be an excellent addition to all public or patient-research libraries."
— *American Reference Books Annual, 2001*

"This title is recommended for public, hospital, and health sciences libraries with consumer health collections."
— *E-Streams, Jul-Aug '00*

"Recommended reference source."
— *Booklist, American Library Association, May '00*

SEE ALSO *Diet & Nutrition Sourcebook, 1st and 2nd Editions, Gastrointestinal Diseases & Disorders Sourcebook*

∎

Disabilities Sourcebook

Basic Consumer Health Information about Physical and Psychiatric Disabilities, Including Descriptions of Major Causes of Disability, Assistive and Adaptive Aids, Workplace Issues, and Accessibility Concerns

Along with Information about the Americans with Disabilities Act, a Glossary, and Resources for Additional Help and Information

Edited by Dawn D. Matthews. 616 pages. 2000. 0-7808-0389-2. $78.

"A much needed addition to the Omnigraphics *Health Reference Series*. A current reference work to provide people with disabilities, their families, caregivers or those who work with them, a broad range of information in one volume, has not been available until now. . . . It is recommended for all public and academic library reference collections."
— *E-Streams, May '01*

"An excellent source book in easy-to-read format covering many current topics; highly recommended for all libraries."
— *Choice, Association of College and Research Libraries, Jan '01*

"Recommended reference source."
— *Booklist, American Library Association, Jul '00*

"An involving, invaluable handbook."
— *The Bookwatch, May '00*

Domestic Violence & Child Abuse Sourcebook

Basic Consumer Health Information about Spousal/ Partner, Child, Sibling, Parent, and Elder Abuse, Covering Physical, Emotional, and Sexual Abuse, Teen Dating Violence, and Stalking; Includes Information about Hotlines, Safe Houses, Safety Plans, and Other Resources for Support and Assistance, Community Initiatives, and Reports on Current Directions in Research and Treatment

Along with a Glossary, Sources for Further Reading, and Governmental and Non-Governmental Organizations Contact Information

Edited by Helene Henderson. 1,064 pages. 2001. 0-7808-0235-7. $78.

"This is important information. The Web has many resources but this sourcebook fills an important societal need. I am not aware of any other resources of this type."
— *Doody's Review Service, Sep '01*

"Recommended for all libraries, scholars, and practitioners."
— *Choice, Association of College & Research Libraries, Jul '01*

"Recommended reference source."
— *Booklist, American Library Association, Apr '01*

"Important pick for college-level health reference libraries."
— *The Bookwatch, Mar '01*

"Because this problem is so widespread and because this book includes a lot of issues within one volume, this work is recommended for all public libraries."
— *American Reference Books Annual, 2001*

∎

Drug Abuse Sourcebook

Basic Consumer Health Information about Illicit Substances of Abuse and the Diversion of Prescription Medications, Including Depressants, Hallucinogens, Inhalants, Marijuana, Narcotics, Stimulants, and Anabolic Steroids

Along with Facts about Related Health Risks, Treatment Issues, and Substance Abuse Prevention Programs, a Glossary of Terms, Statistical Data, and Directories of Hotline Services, Self-Help Groups, and Organizations Able to Provide Further Information

Edited by Karen Bellenir. 629 pages. 2000. 0-7808-0242-X. $78.

"Containing a wealth of information, this book will be useful to the college student just beginning to explore the topic of substance abuse. This resource belongs in libraries that serve a lower-division undergraduate or community college clientele as well as the general public."
— *Choice, Association of College and Research Libraries, Jun '01*

"Recommended reference source."
— *Booklist, American Library Association, Feb '01*

"Highly recommended." — *The Bookwatch, Jan '01*

"Even though there is a plethora of books on drug abuse, this volume is recommended for school, public, and college libraries."
— *American Reference Books Annual, 2001*

SEE ALSO *Alcoholism Sourcebook, Substance Abuse Sourcebook*

Ear, Nose & Throat Disorders Sourcebook

Basic Information about Disorders of the Ears, Nose, Sinus Cavities, Pharynx, and Larynx, Including Ear Infections, Tinnitus, Vestibular Disorders, Allergic and Non-Allergic Rhinitis, Sore Throats, Tonsillitis, and Cancers That Affect the Ears, Nose, Sinuses, and Throat

Along with Reports on Current Research Initiatives, a Glossary of Related Medical Terms, and a Directory of Sources for Further Help and Information

Edited by Karen Bellenir and Linda M. Shin. 576 pages. 1998. 0-7808-0206-3. $78.

"Overall, this sourcebook is helpful for the consumer seeking information on ENT issues. It is recommended for public libraries."
—*American Reference Books Annual, 1999*

"Recommended reference source."
—*Booklist, American Library Association, Dec '98*

Eating Disorders Sourcebook

Basic Consumer Health Information about Eating Disorders, Including Information about Anorexia Nervosa, Bulimia Nervosa, Binge Eating, Body Dysmorphic Disorder, Pica, Laxative Abuse, and Night Eating Syndrome

Along with Information about Causes, Adverse Effects, and Treatment and Prevention Issues, and Featuring a Section on Concerns Specific to Children and Adolescents, a Glossary, and Resources for Further Help and Information

Edited by Dawn D. Matthews. 322 pages. 2001. 0-7808-0335-3. $78.

"This volume is another convenient collection of excerpted articles. Recommended for school and public library patrons; lower-division undergraduates; and two-year technical program students."
—*Choice, Association of College & Research Libraries, Jan '02*

"Recommended reference source." —*Booklist, American Library Association, Oct '01*

Endocrine & Metabolic Disorders Sourcebook

Basic Information for the Layperson about Pancreatic and Insulin-Related Disorders Such as Pancreatitis, Diabetes, and Hypoglycemia; Adrenal Gland Disorders Such as Cushing's Syndrome, Addison's Disease, and Congenital Adrenal Hyperplasia; Pituitary Gland Disorders Such as Growth Hormone Deficiency, Acromegaly, and Pituitary Tumors; Thyroid Disorders Such as Hypothyroidism, Graves' Disease, Hashimoto's Disease, and Goiter; Hyperparathyroidism; and Other Diseases and Syndromes of Hormone Imbalance or Metabolic Dysfunction

Along with Reports on Current Research Initiatives

Edited by Linda M. Shin. 574 pages. 1998. 0-7808-0207-1. $78.

"Omnigraphics has produced another needed resource for health information consumers."
—*American Reference Books Annual, 2000*

"Recommended reference source."
—*Booklist, American Library Association, Dec '98*

Environmentally Induced Disorders Sourcebook

Basic Information about Diseases and Syndromes Linked to Exposure to Pollutants and Other Substances in Outdoor and Indoor Environments Such as Lead, Asbestos, Formaldehyde, Mercury, Emissions, Noise, and More

Edited by Allan R. Cook. 620 pages. 1997. 0-7808-0083-4. $78.

"Recommended reference source."
—*Booklist, American Library Association, Sep '98*

"This book will be a useful addition to anyone's library." —*Choice Health Sciences Supplement, Association of College and Research Libraries, May '98*

". . . a good survey of numerous environmentally induced physical disorders . . . a useful addition to anyone's library."
—*Doody's Health Sciences Book Reviews, Jan '98*

". . . provide[s] introductory information from the best authorities around. Since this volume covers topics that potentially affect everyone, it will surely be one of the most frequently consulted volumes in the *Health Reference Series*." —*Rettig on Reference, Nov '97*

Ethnic Diseases Sourcebook

Basic Consumer Health Information for Ethnic and Racial Minority Groups in the United States, Including General Health Indicators and Behaviors, Ethnic Diseases, Genetic Testing, the Impact of Chronic Diseases, Women's Health, Mental Health Issues, and Preventive Health Care Services

Along with a Glossary and a Listing of Additional Resources

Edited by Joyce Brennfleck Shannon. 664 pages. 2001. 0-7808-0336-1. $78.

"Recommended for health sciences libraries where public health programs are a priority."
—*E-Streams, Jan '02*

"Recommended reference source."
—*Booklist, American Library Association, Oct '01*

"Will prove valuable to any library seeking to maintain

a current, comprehensive reference collection of health resources. . . . An excellent source of health information about genetic disorders which affect particular ethnic and racial minorities in the U.S."

—The Bookwatch, Aug '01

■

Family Planning Sourcebook

Basic Consumer Health Information about Planning for Pregnancy and Contraception, Including Traditional Methods, Barrier Methods, Hormonal Methods, Permanent Methods, Future Methods, Emergency Contraception, and Birth Control Choices for Women at Each Stage of Life

Along with Statistics, a Glossary, and Sources of Additional Information

Edited by Amy Marcaccio Keyzer. 520 pages. 2001. 0-7808-0379-5. $78.

"Recommended reference source."

— Booklist, American Library Association, Oct '01

"Will prove valuable to any library seeking to maintain a current, comprehensive reference collection of health resources. . . . Excellent reference."

— The Bookwatch, Aug '01

SEE ALSO Pregnancy & Birth Sourcebook

■

Fitness & Exercise Sourcebook, 1st Edition

Basic Information on Fitness and Exercise, Including Fitness Activities for Specific Age Groups, Exercise for People with Specific Medical Conditions, How to Begin a Fitness Program in Running, Walking, Swimming, Cycling, and Other Athletic Activities, and Recent Research in Fitness and Exercise

Edited by Dan R. Harris. 663 pages. 1996. 0-7808-0186-5. $78.

"A good resource for general readers." *— Choice, Association of College and Research Libraries, Nov '97*

"The perennial popularity of the topic . . . make this an appealing selection for public libraries."

— Rettig on Reference, Jun/Jul '97

■

Fitness & Exercise Sourcebook, 2nd Edition

Basic Consumer Health Information about the Fundamentals of Fitness and Exercise, Including How to Begin and Maintain a Fitness Program, Fitness as a Lifestyle, the Link between Fitness and Diet, Advice for Specific Groups of People, Exercise as It Relates to Specific Medical Conditions, and Recent Research in Fitness and Exercise

Along with a Glossary of Important Terms and Resources for Additional Help and Information

Edited by Kristen M. Gledhill. 646 pages. 2001. 0-7808-0334-5. $78.

"Highly recommended for public, consumer, and school grades fourth through college."

—E-Streams, Nov '01

"Recommended reference source." *— Booklist, American Library Association, Oct '01*

"The information appears quite comprehensive and is considered reliable. . . . This second edition is a welcomed addition to the series."

—Doody's Review Service, Sep '01

"This reference is a valuable choice for those who desire a broad source of information on exercise, fitness, and chronic-disease prevention through a healthy lifestyle." *—American Medical Writers Association Journal, Fall '01*

"Will prove valuable to any library seeking to maintain a current, comprehensive reference collection of health resources. . . . Excellent reference."

— The Bookwatch, Aug '01

■

Food & Animal Borne Diseases Sourcebook

Basic Information about Diseases That Can Be Spread to Humans through the Ingestion of Contaminated Food or Water or by Contact with Infected Animals and Insects, Such as Botulism, E. Coli, Hepatitis A, Trichinosis, Lyme Disease, and Rabies

Along with Information Regarding Prevention and Treatment Methods, and Including a Special Section for International Travelers Describing Diseases Such as Cholera, Malaria, Travelers' Diarrhea, and Yellow Fever, and Offering Recommendations for Avoiding Illness

Edited by Karen Bellenir and Peter D. Dresser. 535 pages. 1995. 0-7808-0033-8. $78.

"Targeting general readers and providing them with a single, comprehensive source of information on selected topics, this book continues, with the excellent caliber of its predecessors, to catalog topical information on health matters of general interest. Readable and thorough, this valuable resource is highly recommended for all libraries."

— Academic Library Book Review, Summer '96

"A comprehensive collection of authoritative information." *— Emergency Medical Services, Oct '95*

■

Food Safety Sourcebook

Basic Consumer Health Information about the Safe Handling of Meat, Poultry, Seafood, Eggs, Fruit Juices, and Other Food Items, and Facts about Pesticides, Drinking Water, Food Safety Overseas, and the Onset, Duration, and Symptoms of Foodborne Illnesses, Including Types of Pathogenic Bacteria, Parasitic Protozoa, Worms, Viruses, and Natural Toxins

Along with the Role of the Consumer, the Food Handler, and the Government in Food Safety; a Glossary, and Resources for Additional Help and Information

Edited by Dawn D. Matthews. 339 pages. 1999. 0-7808-0326-4. $78.

"This book is recommended for public libraries and universities with home economic and food science programs." —*E-Streams, Nov '00*

"Recommended reference source." —*Booklist, American Library Association, May '00*

"This book takes the complex issues of food safety and foodborne pathogens and presents them in an easily understood manner. [It does] an excellent job of covering a large and often confusing topic." —*American Reference Books Annual, 2000*

Forensic Medicine Sourcebook

Basic Consumer Information for the Layperson about Forensic Medicine, Including Crime Scene Investigation, Evidence Collection and Analysis, Expert Testimony, Computer-Aided Criminal Identification, Digital Imaging in the Courtroom, DNA Profiling, Accident Reconstruction, Autopsies, Ballistics, Drugs and Explosives Detection, Latent Fingerprints, Product Tampering, and Questioned Document Examination

Along with Statistical Data, a Glossary of Forensics Terminology, and Listings of Sources for Further Help and Information

Edited by Annemarie S. Muth. 574 pages. 1999. 0-7808-0232-2. $78.

"Given the expected widespread interest in its content and its easy to read style, this book is recommended for most public and all college and university libraries." —*E-Streams, Feb '01*

"Recommended for public libraries." —*Reference & User Services Quarterly, American Library Association, Spring 2000*

"Recommended reference source." —*Booklist, American Library Association, Feb '00*

"A wealth of information, useful statistics, references are up-to-date and extremely complete. This wonderful collection of data will help students who are interested in a career in any type of forensic field. It is a great resource for attorneys who need information about types of expert witnesses needed in a particular case. It also offers useful information for fiction and nonfiction writers whose work involves a crime. A fascinating compilation. All levels." —*Choice, Association of College and Research Libraries, Jan 2000*

"There are several items that make this book attractive to consumers who are seeking certain forensic data. . . . This is a useful current source for those seeking general forensic medical answers." —*American Reference Books Annual, 2000*

Gastrointestinal Diseases & Disorders Sourcebook

Basic Information about Gastroesophageal Reflux Disease (Heartburn), Ulcers, Diverticulosis, Irritable Bowel Syndrome, Crohn's Disease, Ulcerative Colitis, Diarrhea, Constipation, Lactose Intolerance, Hemorrhoids, Hepatitis, Cirrhosis, and Other Digestive Problems, Featuring Statistics, Descriptions of Symptoms,

and Current Treatment Methods of Interest for Persons Living with Upper and Lower Gastrointestinal Maladies

Edited by Linda M. Ross. 413 pages. 1996. 0-7808-0078-8. $78.

". . . very readable form. The successful editorial work that brought this material together into a useful and understandable reference makes accessible to all readers information that can help them more effectively understand and obtain help for digestive tract problems." —*Choice, Association of College and Research Libraries, Feb '97*

SEE ALSO Diet & Nutrition Sourcebook, 1st and 2nd Editions, Digestive Diseases & Disorders

Genetic Disorders Sourcebook, 1st Edition

Basic Information about Heritable Diseases and Disorders Such as Down Syndrome, PKU, Hemophilia, Von Willebrand Disease, Gaucher Disease, Tay-Sachs Disease, and Sickle-Cell Disease, Along with Information about Genetic Screening, Gene Therapy, Home Care, and Including Source Listings for Further Help and Information on More Than 300 Disorders

Edited by Karen Bellenir. 642 pages. 1996. 0-7808-0034-6. $78.

"Recommended for undergraduate libraries or libraries that serve the public." —*Science & Technology Libraries, Vol. 18, No. 1, '99*

"Provides essential medical information to both the general public and those diagnosed with a serious or fatal genetic disease or disorder." —*Choice, Association of College and Research Libraries, Jan '97*

"Geared toward the lay public. It would be well placed in all public libraries and in those hospital and medical libraries in which access to genetic references is limited." —*Doody's Health Sciences Book Review, Oct '96*

Genetic Disorders Sourcebook, 2nd Edition

Basic Consumer Health Information about Hereditary Diseases and Disorders, Including Cystic Fibrosis, Down Syndrome, Hemophilia, Huntington's Disease, Sickle Cell Anemia, and More; Facts about Genes, Gene Research and Therapy, Genetic Screening, Ethics of Gene Testing, Genetic Counseling, and Advice on Coping and Caring

Along with a Glossary of Genetic Terminology and a Resource List for Help, Support, and Further Information

Edited by Kathy Massimini. 768 pages. 2001. 0-7808-0241-1. $78.

"Recommended for public libraries and medical and hospital libraries with consumer health collections." —*E-Streams, May '01*

"Recommended reference source." —*Booklist, American Library Association, Apr '01*

Head Trauma Sourcebook

Basic Information for the Layperson about Open-Head and Closed-Head Injuries, Treatment Advances, Recovery, and Rehabilitation

Along with Reports on Current Research Initiatives

Edited by Karen Bellenir. 414 pages. 1997. 0-7808-0208-X. $78.

Headache Sourcebook

Basic Consumer Health Information about Migraine, Tension, Cluster, Rebound and Other Types of Headaches, with Facts about the Cause and Prevention of Headaches, the Effects of Stress and the Environment, Headaches during Pregnancy and Menopause, and Childhood Headaches

Along with a Glossary and Other Resources for Additional Help and Information

Edited by Dawn D. Matthews. 350 pages. 2002. 0-7808-0337-X. $78.

Health Insurance Sourcebook

Basic Information about Managed Care Organizations, Traditional Fee-for-Service Insurance, Insurance Portability and Pre-Existing Conditions Clauses, Medicare, Medicaid, Social Security, and Military Health Care

Along with Information about Insurance Fraud

Edited by Wendy Wilcox. 530 pages. 1997. 0-7808-0222-5. $78.

Health Reference Series Cumulative Index 1999

A Comprehensive Index to the Individual Volumes of the Health Reference Series, Including a Subject Index, Name Index, Organization Index, and Publication Index

Along with a Master List of Acronyms and Abbreviations

Edited by Edward J. Prucha, Anne Holmes, and Robert Rudnick. 990 pages. 2000. 0-7808-0382-5. $78.

Healthy Aging Sourcebook

Basic Consumer Health Information about Maintaining Health through the Aging Process, Including Advice on Nutrition, Exercise, and Sleep, Help in Making Decisions about Midlife Issues and Retirement, and Guidance Concerning Practical and Informed Choices in Health Consumerism

Along with Data Concerning the Theories of Aging, Different Experiences in Aging by Minority Groups, and Facts about Aging Now and Aging in the Future; and Featuring a Glossary, a Guide to Consumer Help, Additional Suggested Reading, and Practical Resource Directory

Edited by Jenifer Swanson. 536 pages. 1999. 0-7808-0390-6. $78.

SEE ALSO Physical & Mental Issues in Aging Sourcebook

Healthy Heart Sourcebook for Women

Basic Consumer Health Information about Cardiac Issues Specific to Women, Including Facts about Major Risk Factors and Prevention, Treatment and Control Strategies, and Important Dietary Issues

Along with a Special Section Regarding the Pros and Cons of Hormone Replacement Therapy and Its Impact on Heart Health, and Additional Help, Including Recipes, a Glossary, and a Directory of Resources

Edited by Dawn D. Matthews. 336 pages. 2000. 0-7808-0329-9. $78.

SEE ALSO *Cardiovascular Diseases & Disorders Sourcebook, 1st Edition, Heart Diseases & Disorders Sourcebook, 2nd Edition, Women's Health Concerns Sourcebook*

Heart Diseases & Disorders Sourcebook, 2nd Edition

Basic Consumer Health Information about Heart Attacks, Angina, Rhythm Disorders, Heart Failure, Valve Disease, Congenital Heart Disorders, and More, Including Descriptions of Surgical Procedures and Other Interventions, Medications, Cardiac Rehabilitation, Risk Identification, and Prevention Tips

Along with Statistical Data, Reports on Current Research Initiatives, a Glossary of Cardiovascular Terms, and Resource Directory

Edited by Karen Bellenir. 612 pages. 2000. 0-7808-0238-1. $78.

SEE ALSO *Cardiovascular Diseases & Disorders Sourcebook, 1st Edition; Healthy Heart Sourcebook for Women*

Household Safety Sourcebook

Basic Consumer Health Information about Household Safety, Including Information about Poisons, Chemicals, Fire, and Water Hazards in the Home

Along with Advice about the Safe Use of Home Maintenance Equipment, Choosing Toys and Nursery Furniture, Holiday and Recreation Safety, a Glossary, and Resources for Further Help and Information

Edited by Dawn D. Matthews. 606 pages. 2002. 0-7808-0338-8. $78.

Immune System Disorders Sourcebook

Basic Information about Lupus, Multiple Sclerosis, Guillain-Barré Syndrome, Chronic Granulomatous Disease, and More

Along with Statistical and Demographic Data and Reports on Current Research Initiatives

Edited by Allan R. Cook. 608 pages. 1997. 0-7808-0209-8. $78.

Infant & Toddler Health Sourcebook

Basic Consumer Health Information about the Physical and Mental Development of Newborns, Infants, and Toddlers, Including Neonatal Concerns, Nutrition Recommendations, Immunization Schedules, Common Pediatric Disorders, Assessments and Milestones, Safety Tips, and Advice for Parents and Other Caregivers

Along with a Glossary of Terms and Resource Listings for Additional Help

Edited by Jenifer Swanson. 585 pages. 2000. 0-7808-0246-2. $78.

Injury & Trauma Sourcebook

Basic Consumer Health Information about the Impact of Injury, the Diagnosis and Treatment of Common and Traumatic Injuries, Emergency Care, and Specific Injuries Related to Home, Community, Workplace, Transportation, and Recreation

Along with Guidelines for Injury Prevention, a Glossary, and a Directory of Additional Resources

Edited by Joyce Brennfleck Shannon. 700 pages. 2002. 0-7808-0421-X. $78.

Kidney & Urinary Tract Diseases & Disorders Sourcebook

Basic Information about Kidney Stones, Urinary Incontinence, Bladder Disease, End Stage Renal Disease, Dialysis, and More

Along with Statistical and Demographic Data and Reports on Current Research Initiatives

Edited by Linda M. Ross. 602 pages. 1997. 0-7808-0079-6. $78.

Learning Disabilities Sourcebook

Basic Information about Disorders Such as Dyslexia, Visual and Auditory Processing Deficits, Attention Deficit/Hyperactivity Disorder, and Autism

Along with Statistical and Demographic Data, Reports on Current Research Initiatives, an Explanation of the Assessment Process, and a Special Section for Adults with Learning Disabilities

Edited by Linda M. Shin. 579 pages. 1998. 0-7808-0210-1. $78.

"An excellent candidate for inclusion in a public library reference section. It's a great source of information. Teachers will also find the book useful. Definitely worth reading."
—*Journal of Adolescent & Adult Literacy, Feb 2000*

"Readable . . . provides a solid base of information regarding successful techniques used with individuals who have learning disabilities, as well as practical suggestions for educators and family members. Clear language, concise descriptions, and pertinent information for contacting multiple resources add to the strength of this book as a useful tool." —*Choice, Association of College and Research Libraries, Feb '99*

"Recommended reference source."
—*Booklist, American Library Association, Sep '98*

"A useful resource for libraries and for those who don't have the time to identify and locate the individual publications." —*Disability Resources Monthly, Sep '98*

Liver Disorders Sourcebook

Basic Consumer Health Information about the Liver and How It Works; Liver Diseases, Including Cancer, Cirrhosis, Hepatitis, and Toxic and Drug Related Diseases; Tips for Maintaining a Healthy Liver; Laboratory Tests, Radiology Tests, and Facts about Liver Transplantation

Along with a Section on Support Groups, a Glossary, and Resource Listings

Edited by Joyce Brennfleck Shannon. 591 pages. 2000. 0-7808-0383-3. $78.

"A valuable resource."
—*American Reference Books Annual, 2001*

"This title is recommended for health sciences and public libraries with consumer health collections."
—*E-Streams, Oct '00*

"Recommended reference source."
—*Booklist, American Library Association, Jun '00*

Lung Disorders Sourcebook

Basic Consumer Health Information about Emphysema, Pneumonia, Tuberculosis, Asthma, Cystic Fibrosis, and Other Lung Disorders, Including Facts about Diagnostic Procedures, Treatment Strategies, Disease Prevention Efforts, and Such Risk Factors as Smoking, Air Pollution, and Exposure to Asbestos, Radon, and Other Agents

Along with a Glossary and Resources for Additional Help and Information

Edited by Dawn D. Matthews. 678 pages. 2002. 0-7808-0339-6. $78.

Medical Tests Sourcebook

Basic Consumer Health Information about Medical Tests, Including Periodic Health Exams, General Screening Tests, Tests You Can Do at Home, Findings of the U.S. Preventive Services Task Force, X-ray and Radiology Tests, Electrical Tests, Tests of Blood and Other Body Fluids and Tissues, Scope Tests, Lung Tests, Genetic Tests, Pregnancy Tests, Newborn Screening Tests, Sexually Transmitted Disease Tests, and Computer Aided Diagnoses

Along with a Section on Paying for Medical Tests, a Glossary, and Resource Listings

Edited by Joyce Brennfleck Shannon. 691 pages. 1999. 0-7808-0243-8. $78.

"Recommended for hospital and health sciences libraries with consumer health collections."
—*E-Streams, Mar '00*

"This is an overall excellent reference with a wealth of general knowledge that may aid those who are reluctant to get vital tests performed."
—*Today's Librarian, Jan 2000*

"A valuable reference guide."
—*American Reference Books Annual, 2000*

Men's Health Concerns Sourcebook

Basic Information about Health Issues That Affect Men, Featuring Facts about the Top Causes of Death in Men, Including Heart Disease, Stroke, Cancers, Prostate Disorders, Chronic Obstructive Pulmonary Disease, Pneumonia and Influenza, Human Immunodeficiency Virus and Acquired Immune Deficiency Syndrome, Diabetes Mellitus, Stress, Suicide, Accidents and Homicides; and Facts about Common Concerns for Men, Including Impotence, Contraception, Circumcision, Sleep Disorders, Snoring, Hair Loss, Diet, Nutrition, Exercise, Kidney and Urological Disorders, and Backaches

Edited by Allan R. Cook. 738 pages. 1998. 0-7808-0212-8. $78.

"This comprehensive resource and the series are highly recommended."
—*American Reference Books Annual, 2000*

"Recommended reference source."
—*Booklist, American Library Association, Dec '98*

Mental Health Disorders Sourcebook, 1st Edition

Basic Information about Schizophrenia, Depression, Bipolar Disorder, Panic Disorder, Obsessive-Compulsive Disorder, Phobias and Other Anxiety Disorders, Paranoia and Other Personality Disorders, Eating Disorders, and Sleep Disorders

Along with Information about Treatment and Therapies

Edited by Karen Bellenir. 548 pages. 1995. 0-7808-0040-0. $78.

"This is an excellent new book . . . written in easy-to-understand language."
— *Booklist Health Sciences Supplement, American Library Association, Oct '97*

". . . useful for public and academic libraries and consumer health collections."
— *Medical Reference Services Quarterly, Spring '97*

"The great strengths of the book are its readability and its inclusion of places to find more information. Especially recommended."
— *Reference Quarterly, American Library Association, Winter '96*

". . . a good resource for a consumer health library."
— *Bulletin of the Medical Library Association, Oct '96*

"The information is data-based and couched in brief, concise language that avoids jargon. . . . a useful reference source."
— *Readings, Sep '96*

"The text is well organized and adequately written for its target audience."
— *Choice, Association of College and Research Libraries, Jun '96*

". . . provides information on a wide range of mental disorders, presented in nontechnical language."
— *Exceptional Child Education Resources, Spring '96*

"Recommended for public and academic libraries."
— *Reference Book Review, 1996*

Mental Health Disorders Sourcebook, 2nd Edition

Basic Consumer Health Information about Anxiety Disorders, Depression and Other Mood Disorders, Eating Disorders, Personality Disorders, Schizophrenia, and More, Including Disease Descriptions, Treatment Options, and Reports on Current Research Initiatives

Along with Statistical Data, Tips for Maintaining Mental Health, a Glossary, and Directory of Sources for Additional Help and Information

Edited by Karen Bellenir. 605 pages. 2000. 0-7808-0240-3. $78.

"Well organized and well written."
— *American Reference Books Annual, 2001*

"Recommended reference source."
— *Booklist, American Library Association, Jun '00*

Mental Retardation Sourcebook

Basic Consumer Health Information about Mental Retardation and Its Causes, Including Down Syndrome, Fetal Alcohol Syndrome, Fragile X Syndrome, Genetic Conditions, Injury, and Environmental Sources

Along with Preventive Strategies, Parenting Issues, Educational Implications, Health Care Needs, Employment and Economic Matters, Legal Issues, a Glossary, and a Resource Listing for Additional Help and Information

Edited by Joyce Brennfleck Shannon. 642 pages. 2000. 0-7808-0377-9. $78.

"Public libraries will find the book useful for reference and as a beginning research point for students, parents, and caregivers."
— *American Reference Books Annual, 2001*

"The strength of this work is that it compiles many basic fact sheets and addresses for further information in one volume. It is intended and suitable for the general public. This sourcebook is relevant to any collection providing health information to the general public."
— *E-Streams, Nov '00*

"From preventing retardation to parenting and family challenges, this covers health, social and legal issues and will prove an invaluable overview."
— *Reviewer's Bookwatch, Jul '00*

Obesity Sourcebook

Basic Consumer Health Information about Diseases and Other Problems Associated with Obesity, and Including Facts about Risk Factors, Prevention Issues, and Management Approaches

Along with Statistical and Demographic Data, Information about Special Populations, Research Updates, a Glossary, and Source Listings for Further Help and Information

Edited by Wilma Caldwell and Chad T. Kimball. 376 pages. 2001. 0-7808-0333-7. $78.

"This is a very useful resource book for the lay public."
— *Doody's Review Service, Nov '01*

"Well suited for the health reference collection of a public library or an academic health science library that serves the general population."
— *E-Streams, Sep '01*

"Recommended reference source."
— *Booklist, American Library Association, Apr '01*

" Recommended pick both for specialty health library collections and any general consumer health reference collection."
— *The Bookwatch, Apr '01*

Ophthalmic Disorders Sourcebook

Basic Information about Glaucoma, Cataracts, Macular Degeneration, Strabismus, Refractive Disorders, and More

Along with Statistical and Demographic Data and Reports on Current Research Initiatives

Edited by Linda M. Ross. 631 pages. 1996. 0-7808-0081-8. $78.

Oral Health Sourcebook

Basic Information about Diseases and Conditions Affecting Oral Health, Including Cavities, Gum Disease, Dry Mouth, Oral Cancers, Fever Blisters, Canker Sores, Oral Thrush, Bad Breath, Temporomandibular Disorders, and other Craniofacial Syndromes

Along with Statistical Data on the Oral Health of Americans, Oral Hygiene, Emergency First Aid, In-

formation on Treatment Procedures and Methods of
Replacing Lost Teeth

Edited by Allan R. Cook. 558 pages. 1997. 0-7808-0082-
6. $78.

"Unique source which will fill a gap in dental sources
for patients and the lay public. A valuable reference tool
even in a library with thousands of books on dentistry.
Comprehensive, clear, inexpensive, and easy to read
and use. It fills an enormous gap in the health care literature." — Reference and User Services Quarterly,
American Library Association, Summer '98

"Recommended reference source."
—Booklist, American Library Association, Dec '97

∎

Osteoporosis Sourcebook

Basic Consumer Health Information about Primary
and Secondary Osteoporosis and Juvenile Osteoporosis
and Related Conditions, Including Fibrous Dysplasia,
Gaucher Disease, Hyperthyroidism, Hypophosphata-
sia, Myeloma, Osteopetrosis, Osteogenesis Imperfecta,
and Paget's Disease

Along with Information about Risk Factors, Treatments, Traditional and Non-Traditional Pain Management, a Glossary of Related Terms, and a Directory of
Resources

Edited by Allan R. Cook. 584 pages. 2001. 0-7808-
0239-X. $78.

"This would be a book to be kept in a staff or patient
library. The targeted audience is the layperson, but the
therapist who needs a quick bit of information on a particular topic will also find the book useful."
—Physical Therapy, Jan '02

"Recommended for all public libraries and general
health collections, especially those supporting patient
education or consumer health programs."
—E-Streams, Nov '01

"Will prove valuable to any library seeking to maintain
a current, comprehensive reference collection of health
resources. . . . From prevention to treatment and associated conditions, this provides an excellent survey."
—The Bookwatch, Aug '01

"Recommended reference source."
—Booklist, American Library Association, July '01

SEE ALSO Women's Health Concerns Sourcebook

∎

Pain Sourcebook

Basic Information about Specific Forms of Acute and
Chronic Pain, Including Headaches, Back Pain, Muscular Pain, Neuralgia, Surgical Pain, and Cancer Pain

Along with Pain Relief Options Such as Analgesics,
Narcotics, Nerve Blocks, Transcutaneous Nerve Stimulation, and Alternative Forms of Pain Control, Including Biofeedback, Imaging, Behavior Modification, and
Relaxation Techniques

Edited by Allan R. Cook. 667 pages. 1997. 0-7808-0213-
6. $78.

"The text is readable, easily understood, and well
indexed. This excellent volume belongs in all patient
education libraries, consumer health sections of public
libraries, and many personal collections."
—American Reference Books Annual, 1999

"A beneficial reference." — Booklist Health Sciences
Supplement, American Library Association, Oct '98

"The information is basic in terms of scholarship and is
appropriate for general readers. Written in journalistic
style . . . intended for non-professionals. Quite thorough
in its coverage of different pain conditions and summa-
rizes the latest clinical information regarding pain
treatment." — Choice, Association of College
and Research Libraries, Jun '98

"Recommended reference source."
—Booklist, American Library Association, Mar '98

∎

Pediatric Cancer Sourcebook

Basic Consumer Health Information about Leuke-
mias, Brain Tumors, Sarcomas, Lymphomas, and
Other Cancers in Infants, Children, and Adolescents,
Including Descriptions of Cancers, Treatments, and
Coping Strategies

Along with Suggestions for Parents, Caregivers, and
Concerned Relatives, a Glossary of Cancer Terms, and
Resource Listings

Edited by Edward J. Prucha. 587 pages. 1999. 0-7808-
0245-4. $78.

"An excellent source of information. Recommended for
public, hospital, and health science libraries with consumer health collections." — E-Streams, Jun '00

"Recommended reference source."
—Booklist, American Library Association, Feb '00

"A valuable addition to all libraries specializing in
health services and many public libraries."
—American Reference Books Annual, 2000

∎

Physical & Mental Issues in Aging Sourcebook

Basic Consumer Health Information on Physical and
Mental Disorders Associated with the Aging Process,
Including Concerns about Cardiovascular Disease,
Pulmonary Disease, Oral Health, Digestive Disorders,
Musculoskeletal and Skin Disorders, Metabolic
Changes, Sexual and Reproductive Issues, and
Changes in Vision, Hearing, and Other Senses

Along with Data about Longevity and Causes of
Death, Information on Acute and Chronic Pain,
Descriptions of Mental Concerns, a Glossary of Terms,
and Resource Listings for Additional Help

Edited by Jenifer Swanson. 660 pages. 1999. 0-7808-
0233-0. $78.

"This is a treasure of health information for the layperson." — Choice Health Sciences Supplement,
Association of College & Research Libraries, May 2000

SEE ALSO *Healthy Aging Sourcebook*

Podiatry Sourcebook

Basic Consumer Health Information about Foot Conditions, Diseases, and Injuries, Including Bunions, Corns, Calluses, Athlete's Foot, Plantar Warts, Hammertoes and Clawtoes, Clubfoot, Heel Pain, Gout, and More

Along with Facts about Foot Care, Disease Prevention, Foot Safety, Choosing a Foot Care Specialist, a Glossary of Terms, and Resource Listings for Additional Information

Edited by M. Lisa Weatherford. 380 pages. 2001. 0-7808-0215-2. $78.

Pregnancy & Birth Sourcebook

Basic Information about Planning for Pregnancy, Maternal Health, Fetal Growth and Development, Labor and Delivery, Postpartum and Perinatal Care, Pregnancy in Mothers with Special Concerns, and Disorders of Pregnancy, Including Genetic Counseling, Nutrition and Exercise, Obstetrical Tests, Pregnancy Discomfort, Multiple Births, Cesarean Sections, Medical Testing of Newborns, Breastfeeding, Gestational Diabetes, and Ectopic Pregnancy

Edited by Heather E. Aldred. 737 pages. 1997. 0-7808-0216-0. $78.

SEE ALSO *Congenital Disorders Sourcebook, Family Planning Sourcebook*

Prostate Cancer Sourcebook

Basic Consumer Health Information about Prostate Cancer, Including Information about the Associated Risk Factors, Detection, Diagnosis, and Treatment of Prostate Cancer

Along with Information on Non-Malignant Prostate Conditions, and Featuring a Section Listing Support and Treatment Centers and a Glossary of Related Terms

Edited by Dawn D. Matthews. 358 pages. 2001. 0-7808-0324-8. $78.

Public Health Sourcebook

Basic Information about Government Health Agencies, Including National Health Statistics and Trends, Healthy People 2000 Program Goals and Objectives, the Centers for Disease Control and Prevention, the Food and Drug Administration, and the National Institutes of Health

Along with Full Contact Information for Each Agency

Edited by Wendy Wilcox. 698 pages. 1998. 0-7808-0220-9. $78.

Reconstructive & Cosmetic Surgery Sourcebook

Basic Consumer Health Information on Cosmetic and Reconstructive Plastic Surgery, Including Statistical Information about Different Surgical Procedures, Things to Consider Prior to Surgery, Plastic Surgery Techniques and Tools, Emotional and Psychological Considerations, and Procedure-Specific Information

Along with a Glossary of Terms and a Listing of Resources for Additional Help and Information

Edited by M. Lisa Weatherford. 374 pages. 2001. 0-7808-0214-4. $78.

Rehabilitation Sourcebook

Basic Consumer Health Information about Rehabilitation for People Recovering from Heart Surgery, Spinal Cord Injury, Stroke, Orthopedic Impairments, Amputation, Pulmonary Impairments, Traumatic Injury, and More, Including Physical Therapy, Occupational Therapy, Speech/ Language Therapy, Massage Therapy, Dance Therapy, Art Therapy, and Recreational Therapy

Along with Information on Assistive and Adaptive Devices, a Glossary, and Resources for Additional Help and Information

Edited by Dawn D. Matthews. 531 pages. 1999. 0-7808-0236-5. $78.

Respiratory Diseases & Disorders Sourcebook

Basic Information about Respiratory Diseases and Disorders, Including Asthma, Cystic Fibrosis, Pneumonia, the Common Cold, Influenza, and Others, Featuring Facts about the Respiratory System, Statistical and Demographic Data, Treatments, Self-Help Management Suggestions, and Current Research Initiatives

Edited by Allan R. Cook and Peter D. Dresser. 771 pages. 1995. 0-7808-0037-0. $78.

"Designed for the layperson and for patients and their families coping with respiratory illness. . . . an extensive array of information on diagnosis, treatment, management, and prevention of respiratory illnesses for the general reader." — *Choice, Association of College and Research Libraries, Jun '96*

"A highly recommended text for all collections. It is a comforting reminder of the power of knowledge that good books carry between their covers." — *Academic Library Book Review, Spring '96*

"A comprehensive collection of authoritative information presented in a nontechnical, humanitarian style for patients, families, and caregivers." — *Association of Operating Room Nurses, Sep/Oct '95*

Sexually Transmitted Diseases Sourcebook, 1st Edition

Basic Information about Herpes, Chlamydia, Gonorrhea, Hepatitis, Nongonoccocal Urethritis, Pelvic Inflammatory Disease, Syphilis, AIDS, and More

Along with Current Data on Treatments and Preventions

Edited by Linda M. Ross. 550 pages. 1997. 0-7808-0217-9. $78.

Sexually Transmitted Diseases Sourcebook, 2nd Edition

Basic Consumer Health Information about Sexually Transmitted Diseases, Including Information on the Diagnosis and Treatment of Chlamydia, Gonorrhea, Hepatitis, Herpes, HIV, Mononucleosis, Syphilis, and Others

Along with Information on Prevention, Such as Condom Use, Vaccines, and STD Education; And Featuring a Section on Issues Related to Youth and Adolescents, a Glossary, and Resources for Additional Help and Information

Edited by Dawn D. Matthews. 538 pages. 2001. 0-7808-0249-7. $78.

"Every school and public library should have a copy of this comprehensive and user-friendly reference book." — *Choice, Association of College & Research Libraries, Sep '01*

"This is a highly recommended book. This is an especially important book for all school and public libraries." — *AIDS Book Review Journal, Jul-Aug '01*

"Recommended reference source." — *Booklist, American Library Association, Apr '01*

"Recommended pick both for specialty health library collections and any general consumer health reference collection." — *The Bookwatch, Apr '01*

Skin Disorders Sourcebook

Basic Information about Common Skin and Scalp Conditions Caused by Aging, Allergies, Immune Reactions, Sun Exposure, Infectious Organisms, Parasites, Cosmetics, and Skin Traumas, Including Abrasions, Cuts, and Pressure Sores

Along with Information on Prevention and Treatment

Edited by Allan R. Cook. 647 pages. 1997. 0-7808-0080-X. $78.

". . . comprehensive, easily read reference book." — *Doody's Health Sciences Book Reviews, Oct '97*

SEE ALSO *Burns Sourcebook*

Sleep Disorders Sourcebook

Basic Consumer Health Information about Sleep and Its Disorders, Including Insomnia, Sleepwalking, Sleep Apnea, Restless Leg Syndrome, and Narcolepsy

Along with Data about Shiftwork and Its Effects, Information on the Societal Costs of Sleep Deprivation, Descriptions of Treatment Options, a Glossary of Terms, and Resource Listings for Additional Help

Edited by Jenifer Swanson. 439 pages. 1998. 0-7808-0234-9. $78.

"This text will complement any home or medical library. It is user-friendly and ideal for the adult reader." — *American Reference Books Annual, 2000*

"A useful resource that provides accurate, relevant, and accessible information on sleep to the general public. Health care providers who deal with sleep disorders patients may also find it helpful in being prepared to answer some of the questions patients ask." — *Respiratory Care, Jul '99*

"Recommended reference source." — *Booklist, American Library Association, Feb '99*

Sports Injuries Sourcebook

Basic Consumer Health Information about Common Sports Injuries, Prevention of Injury in Specific Sports, Tips for Training, and Rehabilitation from Injury

Along with Information about Special Concerns for Children, Young Girls in Athletic Training Programs, Senior Athletes, and Women Athletes, and a Directory of Resources for Further Help and Information

Edited by Heather E. Aldred. 624 pages. 1999. 0-7808-0218-7. $78.

"While this easy-to-read book is recommended for all libraries, it should prove to be especially useful for public, high school, and academic libraries; certainly it should be on the bookshelf of every school gymnasium." —*E-Streams, Mar '00*

"Public libraries and undergraduate academic libraries will find this book useful for its nontechnical language." —*American Reference Books Annual, 2000*

■

Substance Abuse Sourcebook

Basic Health-Related Information about the Abuse of Legal and Illegal Substances Such as Alcohol, Tobacco, Prescription Drugs, Marijuana, Cocaine, and Heroin; and Including Facts about Substance Abuse Prevention Strategies, Intervention Methods, Treatment and Recovery Programs, and a Section Addressing the Special Problems Related to Substance Abuse during Pregnancy

Edited by Karen Bellenir. 573 pages. 1996. 0-7808-0038-9. $78.

"A valuable addition to any health reference section. Highly recommended." —*The Book Report, Mar/Apr '97*

". . . a comprehensive collection of substance abuse information that's both highly readable and compact. Families and caregivers of substance abusers will find the information enlightening and helpful, while teachers, social workers and journalists should benefit from the concise format. Recommended." —*Drug Abuse Update, Winter '96/'97*

SEE ALSO *Alcoholism Sourcebook, Drug Abuse Sourcebook*

■

Transplantation Sourcebook

Basic Consumer Health Information about Organ and Tissue Transplantation, Including Physical and Financial Preparations, Procedures and Issues Relating to Specific Solid Organ and Tissue Transplants, Rehabilitation, Pediatric Transplant Information, the Future of Transplantation, and Organ and Tissue Donation

Along with a Glossary and Listings of Additional Resources

Edited by Joyce Brennfleck Shannon. 628 pages. 2002. 0-7808-0322-1. $78.

■

Traveler's Health Sourcebook

Basic Consumer Health Information for Travelers, Including Physical and Medical Preparations, Transportation Health and Safety, Essential Information about Food and Water, Sun Exposure, Insect and Snake Bites, Camping and Wilderness Medicine, and Travel with Physical or Medical Disabilities

Along with International Travel Tips, Vaccination Recommendations, Geographical Health Issues, Disease Risks, a Glossary, and a Listing of Additional Resources

Edited by Joyce Brennfleck Shannon. 613 pages. 2000. 0-7808-0384-1. $78.

"Recommended reference source." —*Booklist, American Library Association, Feb '01*

"This book is recommended for any public library, any travel collection, and especially any collection for the physically disabled." —*American Reference Books Annual, 2001*

■

Women's Health Concerns Sourcebook

Basic Information about Health Issues That Affect Women, Featuring Facts about Menstruation and Other Gynecological Concerns, Including Endometriosis, Fibroids, Menopause, and Vaginitis; Reproductive Concerns, Including Birth Control, Infertility, and Abortion; and Facts about Additional Physical, Emotional, and Mental Health Concerns Prevalent among Women Such as Osteoporosis, Urinary Tract Disorders, Eating Disorders, and Depression

Along with Tips for Maintaining a Healthy Lifestyle

Edited by Heather E. Aldred. 567 pages. 1997. 0-7808-0219-5. $78.

"Handy compilation. There is an impressive range of diseases, devices, disorders, procedures, and other physical and emotional issues covered . . . well organized, illustrated, and indexed." —*Choice, Association of College and Research Libraries, Jan '98*

SEE ALSO *Breast Cancer Sourcebook, Cancer Sourcebook for Women, 1st and 2nd Editions, Healthy Heart Sourcebook for Women, Osteoporosis Sourcebook*

■

Workplace Health & Safety Sourcebook

Basic Consumer Health Information about Workplace Health and Safety, Including the Effect of Workplace Hazards on the Lungs, Skin, Heart, Ears, Eyes, Brain, Reproductive Organs, Musculoskeletal System, and Other Organs and Body Parts

Along with Information about Occupational Cancer, Personal Protective Equipment, Toxic and Hazardous Chemicals, Child Labor, Stress, and Workplace Violence

Edited by Chad T. Kimball. 626 pages. 2000. 0-7808-0231-4. $78.

"As a reference for the general public, this would be useful in any library." —*E-Streams, Jun '01*

"Provides helpful information for primary care physicians and other caregivers interested in occupational medicine. . . . General readers; professionals." —*Choice, Association of College & Research Libraries, May '01*

"Recommended reference source."
—Booklist, American Library Association, Feb '01

"Highly recommended."   *— The Bookwatch, Jan '01*

Worldwide Health Sourcebook

Basic Information about Global Health Issues, Including Malnutrition, Reproductive Health, Disease Dispersion and Prevention, Emerging Diseases, Risky Health Behaviors, and the Leading Causes of Death

Along with Global Health Concerns for Children, Women, and the Elderly, Mental Health Issues, Research and Technology Advancements, and Economic, Environmental, and Political Health Implications, a Glossary, and a Resource Listing for Additional Help and Information

Edited by Joyce Brennfleck Shannon. 614 pages. 2001. 0-7808-0330-2. $78.

"Named an Outstanding Academic Title."
—Choice, Association of College & Research Libraries, Jan '02

"Yet another handy but also unique compilation in the extensive Health Reference Series, this is a useful work because many of the international publications reprinted or excerpted are not readily available. Highly recommended."
—Choice, Association of College & Research Libraries, Nov '01

"Recommended reference source."
—Booklist, American Library Association, Oct '01

Health Reference Series